ADVANCES IN
MEDICAL ONCOLOGY, RESEARCH
AND EDUCATION

Volume IX

DIGESTIVE CANCER

ADVANCES IN MEDICAL ONCOLOGY, RESEARCH AND EDUCATION

Proceedings of the 12th International Cancer Congress,
Buenos Aires, 1978

General Editors: A. CANONICO, O. ESTEVEZ, R. CHACON and S. BARG, Buenos Aires

---

Volumes and Editors:

   I - CARCINOGENESIS. *Editor:* G. P. Margison

  II - CANCER CONTROL. *Editors:* A. Smith and C. Alvarez

 III - EPIDEMIOLOGY. *Editor:* Jillian M. Birch

  IV - BIOLOGICAL BASIS FOR CANCER DIAGNOSIS. *Editor:* Margaret Fox

   V - BASIS FOR CANCER THERAPY 1. *Editor:* B. W. Fox

  VI - BASIS FOR CANCER THERAPY 2. *Editor:* M. Moore

 VII - LEUKEMIA AND NON-HODGKIN LYMPHOMA. *Editor:* D. G. Crowther

VIII - GYNECOLOGICAL CANCER. *Editor:* N. Thatcher

  IX - DIGESTIVE CANCER. *Editor:* N. Thatcher

   X - CLINICAL CANCER - PRINCIPAL SITES 1. *Editor:* S. Kumar

  XI - CLINICAL CANCER - PRINCIPAL SITES 2. *Editor:* P. M. Wilkinson

 XII - ABSTRACTS

(Each volume is available separately.)

Pergamon Journals of Related Interest

ADVANCES IN ENZYME REGULATION
COMPUTERIZED TOMOGRAPHY
EUROPEAN JOURNAL OF CANCER
INTERNATIONAL JOURNAL OF RADIATION ONCOLOGY, BIOLOGY, PHYSICS
LEUKEMIA RESEARCH

ADVANCES IN MEDICAL ONCOLOGY, RESEARCH AND EDUCATION

Proceedings of the 12th International Cancer Congress,
Buenos Aires, 1978

Volume IX

DIGESTIVE CANCER

Editor:

N. THATCHER

Cancer Research Campaign Department of Medical Oncology
Christie Hospital and Holt Radium Institute, Manchester

PERGAMON PRESS

OXFORD · NEW YORK · TORONTO · SYDNEY · PARIS · FRANKFURT

U.K.	Pergamon Press Ltd., Headington Hill Hall, Oxford OX3 0BW, England
U.S.A.	Pergamon Press Inc., Maxwell House, Fairview Park, Elmsford, New York 10523, U.S.A.
CANADA	Pergamon of Canada, Suite 104, 150 Consumers Road, Willowdale, Ontario M2J 1P9, Canada
AUSTRALIA	Pergamon Press (Aust.) Pty. Ltd., P.O. Box 544, Potts Point, N.S.W. 2011, Australia
FRANCE	Pergamon Press SARL, 24 rue des Ecoles, 75240 Paris, Cedex 05, France
FEDERAL REPUBLIC OF GERMANY	Pergamon Press GmbH, 6242 Kronberg-Taunus, Pferdstrasse 1, Federal Republic of Germany

First edition 1979

British Library Cataloguing in Publication Data

International Cancer Congress, 12th, Buenos Aires, 1978
Advances in medical oncology, research and education.
Vol. 9: Digestive cancer
1. Cancer - Congresses
I. Title   II. Thatcher, N
616.9'94   RC261.A1   79-40103

ISBN 0 08 024392 4
ISBN 0-08-023777-0 Set of 12 vols.

In order to make this volume available as economically and as rapidly as possible the authors' typescripts have been reproduced in their original forms. This method unfortunately has its typographical limitations but it is hoped that they in no way distract the reader.

*Printed and bound at William Clowes & Sons Limited
Beccles and London*

Contents

Contents

OESOPHAGEAL CANCER

Foreword

This book contains papers from the main meetings of the Scientific Programme presented during the 12th International Cancer Congress, which took place in Buenos Aires, Argentina, from 5 to 11 October 1978, and was sponsored by the International Union against Cancer (UICC).

This organisation, with headquarters in Geneva, gathers together from more than a hundred countries 250 medical associations which fight against Cancer and organizes every four years an International Congress which gives maximum coverage to oncological activity throughout the world.

The 11th Congress was held in Florence in 1974, where the General Assembly unanimously decided that Argentina would be the site of the 12th Congress. Argentina was chosen not only because of the beauty of its landscapes and the cordiality of its inhabitants, but also because of the high scientific level of its researchers and practitioners in the field of oncology.

From this Assembly a distinguished International Committee was appointed which undertook the preparation and execution of the Scientific Programme of the Congress.

The Programme was designed to be profitable for those professionals who wished to have a general view of the problem of Cancer, as well as those who were specifically orientated to an oncological subspeciality. It was also conceived as trying to cover the different subjects related to this discipline, emphasizing those with an actual and future gravitation on cancerology.

The scientific activity began every morning with a Special Lecture (5 in all), summarizing some of the subjects of prevailing interest in Oncology, such as Environmental Cancer, Immunology, Sub-clinical Cancer, Modern Cancer Therapy Concepts and Viral Oncogenesis. Within the 26 Symposia, new acquisitions in the technological area were incorporated; such acquisitions had not been exposed in previous Congresses.

15 Multidisciplinary Panels were held studying the more frequent sites in Cancer, with an approach to the problem that included biological and clinical aspects, and concentrating on the following areas: aetiology, epidemiology, pathology, prevention, early detection, education, treatment and results. Proferred Papers were presented as Workshops instead of the classical reading, as in this way they could be discussed fully by the participants. 66 Workshops were held, this being the first time that free communications were presented in this way in a UICC Congress.

The Programme also included 22 "Meet the Experts", 7 Informal Meetings and more than a hundred films.

METHODOLOGY

The methodology used for the development of the Meeting and to make the scientific works profitable, had some original features that we would like to mention.

The methodology used in Lectures, Panels and Symposia was the usual one utilized in previous Congresses and functions satisfactorily. Lectures lasted one hour each. Panels were seven hours long divided into two sessions, one in the morning and one in the afternoon. They had a Chairman and two Vice-chairmen (one for each session). Symposia were three hours long. They had a Chairman, a Vice-chairman and a Secretary

Of the 8164 registered members, many sent proferred papers of which over 2000 were presented. They were grouped in numbers of 20 or 25, according to the subject, and discussed in Workshops. The International Scientific Committee studied the abstracts of all the papers, and those which were finally approved were sent to the Chairman of the corresponding Workshop who, during the Workshop gave an introduction and commented on the more outstanding works. This was the first time such a method had been used in an UICC Cancer Congress.

"Meet the Experts" were two hours long, and facilitated the approach of young professionals to the most outstanding specialists. The congress was also the ideal place for an exchange of information between the specialists of different countries during the Informal Meetings. Also more than a hundred scientific films were shown.

The size of the task carried out in organising this Congress is reflected in some statistical data: More than 18,000 letters were sent to participants throughout the world; more than 2000 abstracts were published in the Proceedings of the Congress; more than 800 scientists were active participants of the various meetings.

There were 2246 papers presented at the Congress by 4620 authors from 80 countries.

The Programme lasted a total of 450 hours, and was divided into 170 scientific meetings where nearly all the subjects related to Oncology were discussed.

All the material gathered for the publication of these Proceedings has been taken from the original papers submitted by each author. The material has been arranged in 12 volumes, in various homogenous sections, which facilitates the reading of the most interesting individual chapters. Volume XII deals only with the abstracts of proffered papers submitted for Workshops and Special Meetings. The titles of each volume offer a clear view of the extended and multidisciplinary contents of this collection which we are sure will be frequently consulted in the scientific libraries.

We are grateful to the individual authors for their valuable collaboration as they have enabled the publication of these Proceedings, and we are sure Pergamon Press was a perfect choice as the Publisher due to its responsibility and efficiency.

Argentina   Dr Abel Canónico
March 1979   Dr Roberto Estevez
                                   Dr Reinaldo Chacon
                                   Dr Solomon Barg

                                   General Editors

Introduction

This volume is concerned with gastro-intestinal malignancy and features colo-rectal, hepatocellular, pancreatic, gastric and oesophageal carcinomata. Aetiological considerations, epidemiological factors and different methods for early diagnosis, radiological, biochemical etc. are included. The treatment options, surgery, radiotherapy, chemotherapy, the use of irradiation to the primary site and combination modality therapy are discussed.

N. THATCHER
March 1979

Colorectal Cancer

Colorectal Cancer: Early Diagnosis

F. P. Rossini

Division of Gastroenterology, Dept. of Oncology
Ospedale Maggiore di S. Giovanni Battista e della
Città di Torino, Turin - Italy

ABSTRACT

The Author summarizes the results of surgery of colorectal carcinoma, which are linked with an early diagnosis.
A review is then done of the available diagnostic procedures, which can lead to an early diagnosis (Clinic, Radiology, Endoscopy and its subsidiary techniques).
The conclusions may be of use in achieving a diagnosis early enough for effective therapy.

Key words: Colorectal cancer. Early diagnosis. Radiology. Endoscopy. Histology. Brush cytology. Endoscopic polypectomy. Perendoscopic CEA test. Endoscopic dye spraying method.

COLORECTAL CANCER : EARLY DIAGNOSIS

This Panel, as well as all the meetings about colorectal cancer that take place all over the world, is motivated by several factors:
- the high incidence of colorectal cancer, which is, moreover, on the increase,
- the lack of adequate therapeutic results which have not come up to expectation,
- the strong conviction that only an early diagnosis can assure a much better prognosis.

ANNUAL INCIDENCE OF COLORECTAL CANCER PER 100.000 INHABITANTS

USA   38-46

URSS   20

ITALY   20.7 (Mortality data - ISTAT, 1971)

In Piedmont (Italy) the annual incidence of colorectal cancer per 100.000 inhabitants is 35.18 cases.

COLORECTAL CANCER (RECTUM INCLUDED) 1965-1971

CANCER OF THE LARGE BOWEL (RECTUM INCLUDED 1965 - 1971						
TOTAL NUMBER OF CASES			INCIDENCE PER 100.000 INHABITANTS			
SEX \ AGE	M	F	MF	M	F	MF
0-19	7	46	53	0.18	1.16	0.65
20-39	129	130	259	2.85	2.95	2.90
40-59	1.140	1.137	2.277	29.97	28.42	29.18
60-79	3.586	3.173	6.759	150.35	103.80	124.20
80-99	667	903	1.570	256.27	201.13	221.37
TOTAL	5.529	5.389	10.918	36.48	33.95	35.18

(FROM THE CANCER REGISTRY OF PIEDMONT - TORINO, ITALY)

In recent years, remarkable advances in colorectal cancer therapy have resulted from improved surgical techniques, adequate preparation of patients before surgery and anaesthesiological and resuscitational assistence. The results of surgery, however, are disappointing in that they have not shown constant improvement.

This statement is confirmed by a survey of over 100 American Hospitals done in 1972 (End Results in Cancer - Report n. 4): the five-year survival of 22.910 cases of rectal cancer was 29% in the years 1940-49, raised to 40% in the next ten years, but did not change significantly afterwards. To date, the only way to improve the results of therapy is an early diagnosis: reports and clinical casuistries all over the world are in agreement on this point.

The five and ten year survival rates have been (End Results in Cancer) 70% and 63% respectively in cases of localized carcinoma, 34% and 23% in cases in which lymphnodes and/or neighbouring tissues and organs were also affected. The results of therapy, therefore, are linked with the degree of invasion of the lesion (Dukes A, B, C) and hence with the promptness of the diagnosis. With reference to the degree of invasion (Dukes), the five-year survival rates are: Dukes A 61-81%, B 25-64%, C 6-28% (from the Technical Report UICC Colorectal Cancer, 1975).

The large bowel can be easily reached with the diagnostic tools that are now available; it is therefore surprising that colorectal cancer which can be so easily diagnosed, often undergoes the operation in an advanced stage. The average period elapsing between the first symptoms and the diagnosis - called "fatal pause" by Bokelmann - is about seven monts.

Nowadays, by means of the available diagnostic and therapeutic tools, a survival of over 5 years can be achieved in 75% of patients, if the diagnosis is prompt, that is early enough for effective therapy.

The diagnosis of early cancer can be made only on the surgically resected bowel and is obviously rare; the goal must be the detection of cancer before metastatic spread occurs.

At present the diagnostic procedures at our disposal can lead to a timely diagnosis, if employed as early as possible.

Diagnostic procedures

History
Digital rectal examination
Occult blood in the stools
Proctosigmoidoscopy with fiberscope
Double contrast barium enema
Coloscopy + subsidiary techniques

HISTORY - A carefully detailed history should always be taken, especially in the patient who has been previously labelled as "colitic".

Inquiries concerning the presence of gross or occult blood in the stools (never ascribe rectal bleeding to hemorrhoids without searching for additional lesions), the change in bowel habits, increased use of laxatives, irregular or alternating bowel habits, mucoid discharge, tenesmus, sense of incomplete or unsatisfactory evacuation, two-step defecation, decrease in the caliber of stools, anaemia of unknown aetiology, episodes of unexplained "colic" pain, "cramps" or gas distension pain, increasing constipation, episodes of incomplete obstruction, are mandatory.

Patients presenting one or more direct "warning" symptoms must be thoroughly examined in order to confirm or rule out a colorectal tumour. Obviously a careful examination will be the more justified if the warning symptoms mentioned are accompanied by indirect signs, such as familiarity for large bowel cancer or polyps or malignancy elsewhere, surface tumours, or previous diagnosis of high risk lesions.

According to personal experience, a period of time from six to fifteen months approximatively elapses between the first changes in bowel habits and the definitive diagnosis. After the diagnosis has been made, in many cases, a careful history will prove that one or more warning symptoms have been in existence for more than a year.

In our experience, such delay seems to be caused in about 40-45% of cases by the negligence of patients who underestimated their symptoms; an additional 10-15% of such patients had been treated for hemorrhoids; the other cases had not undergone diagnostic examinations at all, or

only a conventional Barium Enema, or the diagnostic work up had not
been completed by Endoscopy.

DIGITAL RECTAL EXAMINATION - Digital rectal examination in exceedingly
important. A high percentage of rectal cancers are within reach of
the examining finger and may be detected by this technique, which
must always be performed for all Patients with colorectal symptoms.

TESTS FOR OCCULT BLOOD IN THE STOOLS - The guaiac test seems to be
the most reliable and simple method of testing the faeces for blood.

This test decreases the false-positive results, it is practical and
hence acceptable to the patients, can be performed quickly and easily,
and proved very useful also as a routine office procedure.

PROCTOSIGMOIDOSCOPY WITH FIBERSCOPE - Conventional rigid
proctosigmoidoscopy, which has been for years the main procedure for
the early diagnosis of colorectal tumours, is now being replaced by
flexible fiberoptic sigmoidoscopy, which gives remarkable technical
and diagnostic advantages.

By means of the flexible sigmoidoscope a quick, careful, comfortable
exploration of the rectum, sigmoid colon and beyond, can be accomplished
at the same time, with the same preparation of the patient and with
better results - as compared to the rigid scope.

The availability of more effective fiberoptic instruments allows us
to plan the endoscopic examination of the large bowel according to
new criteria, particularly for the early diagnosis of tumours.

After an accurate Double contrast Barium Enema, the 'long'
fibercoloscope (160-185 cm) is indicated when lesions are suspected
between the splenic flexure and the caecum. 'Short' or 'medium'
fibercoloscopes (60-110 cm) are more effective for the routine
endoscopic examination of the rectum, sigmoid and discending colon,
as well as in screening and follow up procedures of patients affected
by high risk lesions, follow up of patients operated for colonic
cancer or polyps, first examination of patients showing direct or
indirect warning sign and symptoms.

The flexibility and easy manoeuvering of the fiberoptic instrument
allows a quick exploration up to the splenic flexure in 5-10 minutes,
that is at the same time as that of conventional rigid proctosigmoidoscopy.
Besides these advantages, the flexible sigmoidoscope is more
comfortable for the patient, allows a better view and magnification
of lesions, abolishes blind spots by means of the polydirectional
flexibility of the tip, permits a proper dosage of insufflated air
and an easy performance of all the endoscopic subsidiary techniques.

Thus, the effectiveness of the medium or short fibercoloscope in the
detection of cancer must be emphasized. It is well known, in fact,
that the majority of large bowel tumours are located in the left
colon, especially in the rectum and sigmoid.

FROM THE CANCER REGISTRY OF PIEDMONT

COLORECTAL   CARCINOMA

1965 - 1971

```
ASCENDING COLON .......................    775 ( 7.1%)
TRANSVERSE COLON ......................    561 ( 5.1%)
DESCENDING COLON ......................    409 ( 3.8%)
SIGMOID COLON .........................   2548 (23.3%)
RECTUM ................................   6625 (60.7%)
                                         ──────────────
                            TOTAL 10918 ( 100% )
```

(FROM THE CANCER REGISTRY OF PIEDMONT - TORINO, ITALY)

It appears from the personal series that out of 741 colonic polyps endoscopically resected between 1973 and 1978, about 87% were located in the left colon.

Similarly, out of 167 cancers diagnosed in the last 18 months, about 93% were found in the rectum, sigmoid and left colon. When only a conventional rigid proctosigmoidoscopy is performed up to 18-20 cm from the anal verge, a certain number of polyps and cancers will remain undetected a few centimetres beyond.

In a group of 200 patients, who underwent conventional proctosigmoidoscopy first and flexible sigmoidoscopy immediately after, cancer or polyps were detected beyond 20 cm in 25 cases(12.5%).

Flexible fiberoptic sigmoidoscopy, therefore,should be regarded as a routine examination, not a sophisticated supplement to conventional proctoscopy. Only in this way will a reliable early diagnosis of colorectal cancer become feasible.

DOUBLE CONTRAST BARIUM ENEMA - In the diagnosis of large bowel tumours a radiological study is the first examination to be performed: it is irreplaceable, easy and often more acceptable for the patient than endoscopy procedures.

The recent air contrast techniques represent real progress in radiology for they allow a careful study of the colonic walls and put into evidence any slight change in the mucosal surface. This method can assure a surprisingly high diagnostic accuracy.

Like all instrumental methods, however, radiological techniques have some limitations: organizational problems, failures caused by inadequate preparation of patients, difficulties in interpreting the films because of technical troubles (colonic areas left out from the films) or, more often, because of changes in the normal anatomic conformation and morphology of the bowel (diverticulosis, incomplete stenoses, shrinking of the ileo-pelvic segment, narrowed tracts, doubtful filling defects, superposition of the transverse upon the descending colon, etc.). For all these reasons (technical, organizational, interpretative factors), even the most careful radiological study may leave some diagnostic doubts. Endoscopy and its subsidiary techniques can clarify these doubts in a high percentage of cases.

As Miller and Winawer (1976) reported, the conventional Barium enema may overlook about 40% of precancerous lesions and 20% of carcinomas, in comparison with the Double contrast Barium enema.

As far as large bowel and precancerous lesions are concerned, endoscopy has proved one of the most effective diagnostic tools.

In reviewing the personal series only with reference to those patients in whom endoscopy was used as the conclusive and resolutive diagnostic procedure, and omitting, therefore, the cases in which cancer had been made evident by Barium enema, we have noted the following: out of 179 cases in whom Radiology roused the suspicion of carcinoma, Endoscopy confirmed the diagnosis of cancer in 115 (64.2%).

In 108 symptomatic patients the Barium enema suggested polyps: the endoscopic examination substantiated the diagnosis in 60% of cases, found a malignant lesion in 3.7%, no abnormality in about 35%. In 144 individuals affected by diverticulosis, the radiological study could not rule out a coexisting cancer. The difficult and incomplete bowel preparation, together with inflammation, perivisceritis and adhesions due to the diverticular disease itself, are an obvious obstacle to a technically correct radiological examination.

In cases od diverticular diesease even endoscopy is problematic : there are technical difficulties in performing the examination, difficulties in completely cleansing the bowel lumen, risk of perforation - problems and risks which usually increase when one or more complications of diverticulosis are present. Out of those 144 patients with diverticulosis and a radiological suspicion of cancer, endoscopy found a carcinoma in 12% of cases, polyps in 22%, diverticular disease alone in 50%.

Endoscopy is often indicated in diverticular disease and proves very useful to rule out an associated tumoral lesion: polyps frequently coexist with diverticula (20-27%), cancer and diverticula are associated in 8-15% of cases.

Out of 122 patients with warning symptoms, whose conventional barium enemas were within normal limits, endoscopy found neoplastic lesions in 22%.

The radiological techniques failed in 44 symptomatic patients because of complete incontinence on barium enema; diagnostic investigation was completed by endoscopy, and a malignant tumour was discovered in about 70% of cases.

The reported figures, drawn from the personal experience, emphasize the role of coloscopy as the second step examination, i.e. the complement and completion of the radiological investigations.

Endoscopy and its subsidiary techniques play a fundamental role in the evaluation of precancerous conditions.

Besides familial polyposis, which certainly evolves in cancer, the major causes which predispose to colorectal carcinoma are: Idiopathic Ulcerative Proctocolitis, Crohn's diesease of the colon and colorectal polyps.

When any of these three conditions exist an immediate endoscopic screening is indispensable.

In Ulcerative Proctocolitis proctoscopy will suffice to evaluate the acute stages of the disease. But in cases where there is inflammation of the whole colon and, especially if this condition has existed for many years (these are the main two factors which predispose to cancer), a careful exploration of the entire colon is mandatory, to evaluate: the degree of inflammation, the stage of evolution of the disease, the occurrence of villous or papillary changes on the mucosal surface, the pseudopolyps, the possible presence of true polyps and/ or areas of suspected infiltration.

Multiple directed biopsies taken with standard forceps provide enough material for a thorough histological examination.

Endoscopic brush cytology assures the twofold advantage of obtaining smears both directed by the endoscopic view and coming from wider mucosal areas than those explored by bioptic samples.

With both cytologic and histologic examinations it is possible to follow the inflammatory process at different stages, starting from inflammatory dysplasia, through precancer and intra-epithelial anaplasia, leading to cancer.

The dye spraying method with indigo-carmine is a useful technique to identify and underline suspicious mucosal areas with surface irregularities which must be exactly sampled histologically and cytologically, but may escape detection by conventional endoscopy.

The endoscopic dye spraying method is exceedingly useful in the diagnosis of 'micropolyps' which may be barely detected with the normal endoscopic view, but which become quite evident after the staining procedure.

In 1.3% of our series of Ulceratuve Colitis patients, coloscopy its subsidiary techniques revealed association with adenomatous polyps, demonstrating the coexistence of two precancerous lesions.

In 2.3% of case of Ulcerative Colitis a carcinoma was found by endoscopy.

A careful follow up is necessary in all the patients affected by Crohn's disease: the risk of malignancy is much greater in this illness than in the normal population, and increases according to the duration of the disease (1.6% reported in world literature).

In the personal series and a multicentric investigation done in Italy in 1975, no proven association between Crohn's disease and colorectal cancer was demonstrated.

In Crohn's disease the endoscopic examination has the same advantages as in Ulcerative Colitis, as well as biopsies, brush cytology and particularly the big particle biopsy technique with diathermic snare.

This method is very useful in cases of Crohn's disease, since it allows to obtain abundant bioptic material for a correct pathological diagnosis, without risk of hemorrhage. In a personal series of over 150 patients affected by Crohn's disease, cytological atypias were detected in only two cases, thus advising more frequent and repeated controls.

The perendoscopic CEA test is a subsidiary technique based on the association of endoscopic and radioimmunological methods. CEA determinations have been carried out on fluid collected in the different segments of the large bowel by means of colonic lavage during coloscopy. CEA levels in the lavage fluid of normal subjects have been less than 20 ng/ml in all cases. In the Patients affected by carcinoma high concentrations of CEA have been observed.

Normal CEA levels have been found in the coloscopic lavage fluid of benign colonic polyposis, high levels in cases of familial polyposis progressed to cancer. In Patients affected by Ulcerative Colitis for more than 5 years, above normal CEA concentrations have been detected, while normal values have been found in Ulcerative Colitis patients suggering from the disease for less than 5 years.

In 15 out of 18 cases of Crohn's disease of the colon CEA levels were found to be within normal limits; only in three Patients high concentrations were observed, together with cytologic finding of cellular atypias.

The reported data are the results of a preliminary study, which obviously need confirmation and further investigations. If such preliminary results are confirmed, bearing in mind that the risk of carcinoma increases according to the duration of Inflammatory Bowel Disease, the CEA test on endoscopic lavage fluid might be useful for a more specific selection of high risk patients.

Colorectal polyposis is undoubtedly the most important precancerous condition.

Literature data show that cancerization of polyps occurs in different but never negligible percentages, according to histological type, size and, perhaps, location. In all certain or suspected cases, therefore, a precise diagnosis is necessary.

Even if the radiological diagnosis is certain for polyps, coloscopy is still required to ascertain or exclude the presence of other polyps. During surgical operation for multiple discrete polyposis coloscopy is also indicated. The Surgeon, in fact, can not always feel and detect small new growths with only external palpation of the bowel.

Peroperative coloscopy - that is coloscopy performed during operation, on the open abdomen - allows a careful inspection of the whole colon, based on the strict co-operation of Surgeon and Endoscopist. The Surgeon examines the bowel wall from outside, by means of transillumination, the Endoscopist, watching the bowel lumen, gives the Surgeon exact information about site and size of polyps and the adequate bounds of resection.

In evaluating colorectal polyposis, coloscopy is also indicated to exclude a coexisting carcinoma. The importance of inspecting the whole colon when one or more polyps are discovered, is semonstrated by personal experience: out of 495 patients affected by colonic carcinoma, 119 (24%) had a 'sentry' polyp distal to the cancer.

In all cases of colorectal polyposis fibercoloscopy is indispensable to perform endoscopic polypectomies. Endoscopic polypectomy should always be done, when technically feasible, since it is the only complete and reliable diagnostic tool. On bioptic samples alone no definitive diagnosis can be made as far as a correct evaluation of histological type or cancerous transformation is concerned.

The endoscopic removal of one or more polypoid growths can solve many problems of diagnosis (correct histopathological classification) and therapy (disappearance of clinical symptoms, removal of a precancerous lesion, interruption of the adenoma-carcinoma sequence).

Taking into account the experience of reliable Authors, based on numerous series and a satisfactory follow up of many cases, the following therapeutic protocol is being applied at present.

- Endoscopic polypectomy whnever technically feasible, and nothing more than this procedure when the histological examination reasonably excludes invasion beyond the muscolaris mucosae.

- Surgery when endoscopic polypectomy is not technically feasible, or invasion of non-pedunculated polyps is clearly demonstrated beyond the muscolaris mucosae or beyond the muscolaris mucosae with the involvement of the stalk of pedunculated polyps.

- In doubtful cases, the procedure has to be decided for each individual patient by consultation of Endoscopist, Surgeon and Pathologist, taking into account the features of the polyp (size,

histological type, degree of dysplasia, depth of invasion, etc.)
and the condition of the patient.

Obviously, the validity of this therapeutic protocol must be further
investigated and confirmed. In any case, coloscopy and endoscopic
polypectomy, wisely employed in a screening and follow up program of
colorectal polyposis, can lead to an effective prophylaxis of
colorectal carcinoma.

The large bowel can be satisfactorily examined and easily studied by
the available diagnostic tools, which should all be employed in
symptomatic patients, who show with one or more warning signs and
in whom the occurrence of a tumour is already suspected on clinical
grounds.

The main diagnostic problem - which is obviously linked with the
problem of early diagnosis - concerns asymptomatic patients.

A mass screening, consisting in periodic examinations of the whole
population of a country, is very difficult and too expensive, since
the public costs are exceedingly high. Mass surveys, on the other
hand, being often uncontrolled observations of a large number of
persons, without a precise system, have little value.

At present, therefore, a mass screening with the aim of achieving
early diagnosis of colorectal cancer is practically impossible; a
planned examination of the population at risk, on the contrary, is
more feasible, and certainly should be done.

Testing stools of asymptomatic individuals for occult blood will pick
out a higher percentage of high risk patients, besides the ones
already identified.

In addition to the patients affected by precancerous conditions,
which may be regarded as high risk lesions (familial polyposis,
polyps, Ulcerative Colitis, Crohn's disease), and hence need the best
attention and a careful screening, other patients bearing 'risk
factors' must be further identified by a methodical and accurate
search.

RISK FACTORS

Age > 40 years

Familial History

As far as age is concerned, the threshold is conventionally indicated
at 40 years, since both reported series and the data drawn from the
Cancer Registry of Piedmont (Italy) underline the sharp increase of
colorectal cancer incidence after 40 years. The risk of cancer further
increases, if an age of over 40 years is associated with precancerous

conditions or with the second main risk factor, that is familiarity.

A deep careful family history must be taken from as many relatives as possible of patients affected by inheritable precancerous of cancerous syndromes, such as diffuse familial polyposis, Gardner's syndrome, Turcot's syndrome. Peutz-Jeghers' syndrome, and similarly from all the relatives of patients operated for colorectal carcinoma.

The occurrence of a colorectal cancer in relatives of patients operated for large bowel carcinoma is not uncommon: this observation, noticed time after time in the hospital and office practice,justifies systematic diagnostic investigations in all the relatives of patients affected by colorectal carcinoma, with the establishment of 'family--form' and the organization of Centres or Associations of patients operated for large bowel cancer. So, a twofold advantage may be obtained in following-up the operated patients and carrying out a familial screening. The knowledge of cancer risk for each member of the family, moreover, may be helpful in detecting an initial lesion at the earliest possible time.

In conclusion, what can we do for the early diagnosis of colorectal cancer at present?:

1. Careful screning of patients with warning symptoms. No examination is useless, if it allows the ruling out of lesions.

2. Identification, diagnostic investigation and following up high risk patients.

3. Information about the families and the family risk of patients affected by carcinoma and/or precancerous lesions.

4. Up to date education of the General Practitioner.
   The General Practitioner must always be supplied with informative and operative instruments, which can help him is actively working in this field. He should identify high risk individuals and/or patients with warning symptoms and send them to Specialized Centres, where cancer can be detected before metastases or irreparable injuries occur, so that a timely diagnosis can be achieved for an effective therapy.

REFERENCES

Appel, M.F. (1976). Preoperative and postoperative colonoscopy for colorectal carcinoma. Colon et Rectum 19, 664-666.

Banche, M., F.P. Rossini, and. A. Ferrari (1976). The role of coloscopy in the differential diagnosis between Idiopathic Ulcerative Colitis and Crohn's disease of the colon. Amer. J. Gastroent., 65, 539,1976.

Bohlman, T.W., et al. (1977). Fiberoptic pansigmoidoscopy. An evaluation and comparison with rigid sigmoidoscopy. Gastroenterology,72, 644-649.

Bokelmann D., H.U. Druner and U. Schulz (1972). Klinik und Prognose der Kolon-und Rectum-Karzinome. Dtsch. med. Wschr., 97, 1590.

Brooke, B.W. (1969). Ulcerative colitis and carcinoma of the colon. J.R. Coll. Surg. Edin., 14, 274-278.

Chevrel, B. (1974). Maladie de Crohn et transformation maligne. Méd. Chir. Dig.,3,431.

Colombo, C., S. Lombardo and A. Ramella (1973). Risultati a distanza della cura chirurgica del cancro del colon e del retto. Chir. Gastroenter.,7, 449.

Darke, S.D., A.G. Parks and J.J. Grongono (1973). Adenocarcinoma and Crohn's disease. A report of two cases and analysis of the literature. Brit. J. Surg., 60, 169.

Edwards, F.C. and S.C. Truelove (1964). Course and prognosis of Ulcerative Colitis. IV Carcinoma of the colon. Gut, 5, 1.

End results in cancer (1972). Report n.4 U.S. Department of Health, Education and Welfare.

Ferrari, A. and F.P. Rossini (1976). Indagine policentrica in tema di Rettocolite Ulcerosa Idiopatica e Malattia di Crohn del colon. Min. Med., 67, 505.

Fielding, J.F., P. Prior, J.A. Waterhouse and W.T. Cooke (1972). Malignancy in Crohn's disease. Scand. J. Gastroent., 7, 3.

Frotz, H., R. Philippen, H. Hockemeyen and Th. Gheorghin (1976). Partielle Koloskopie, eine etablierte untersuchung in der gastroenterologie? Acta Endoscopica et Radiocinematographica, tome VI, n. 2, 173-175.

Gabriellsson,N., S. Granqvist and H. Ohlsen (1976). Recurrent carcinoma of the colon in the anastomosis diagnosed by roentegen examination and colonoscopy. Endoscopy, 8, 47-52.

Gilbertsen, V.A. (1974). Proctosigmoidoscopy and polypectmy in reducing the incidence of rectal cancer. Cancer, 34, 936-939.

Gold, P. and S.O. Freedman (1965). Specific carcinoembryonic antigens of the human digestive system. J. Exp. Med., 122, 467-481.

Greegor, D.H. (1971). Occult blood testing for detection of asymptomatic colon cancer. Cancer, 28, 131.

Greegor, D.H. (1971). Occult blood testing for detection of asymptomatic colon cancer. Cancer, 28, 131-134.

Greenstein, A.J., A.E. Papatestas, S. Celler, I. Kreel and A.H.Aufses (1976). Cancer inflammatory bowel disease. III Int. Symp. on detection and prevention of cancer, New York.

Hutten, L., J. Kewenter and C. Ahren (1972). Precancer and carcinoma in chronic Ulcerative Colitis, Scand. J. Gastroent., 7, 663.

Kreel, L., H. Herlinger and J. Glanville (1973). Technique of the double contrast barium meal with examples of correlation with endoscopy. Clinical Radiology, 24, 307.

Laufer, J., N.C.W. Smith and J.E. Mullens (1976). The radiological demonstration of colorectal polyp undetected by endoscopy. Gastroenterology, 70, 167-170.

Lightdale, C.J., S.S. Sternberg, G. Posner and P. Sherlock (1975). Carcinoma complicating Crohn's disease. Report of seven cases and review of the literature. Amer. J. Med., 59, 262.

Miller, R.E. (1974). Detection of colon carcinoma and the barium enema. J.A.M.A., 230, 1195.

Morson, B.C. (1966). Cancer in Ulcerative Colitis. Gut. 7, 425.

Morson, B.C. and L.S.C. Pang (1967). Rectal biopsy as an aid to cancer control in Ulcerative Colitis. Gut, 8, 423.

Morson, B.C. (1971). Precancerous conditions of the large bowel. Proc. R. Soc. Med., 64, 959-962.

Morson, B.C. (1976). Pathology of the gastrointestinal tract. Current topics in Pathology, 63. Springer-Verlag. Berlin, Heidelberg, New York.

Ottenjann, R. (1972). Colonic polyps and coloscopic polypectomy. Endoscopy, 4, 212-216.

Otto, P. H. Huchzemeyer and D. Helmstaedt (1977). The new short flexible sigmoidoscopes of ACMI and Wolf in the endoscopic examination of the rectum and sigmoid colon (abstr.). Endoscopy,9, 193.

Overholt, B.F. (1973). Endoscopic diagnosis in gastrointestinal cancer. In: Proceedings Seventh National Cancer Conference. Philadelphia, J.B. Lippincott Co., pp. 475-480.

Overholt, B.F. (1971). Flexible fiberoptic sigmoidoscopy. Cancer, 28, 123-126.

Overholt, B.F.,and II M Pallard (1967). Cancer of the colon and rectum. Current procedures for detection and diagnosis. Cancer,20, 445-450.

Penfold J.C.B. et al. (1977). Early detection of colonic cancer by colonoscopy. Colon et Rectum, 20, 86-88.

Rider, J.A., J.B. Kirsner, H.C. Moeller and W.L. Palmer (1959). Polyps of the colon and rectum. A 4-Years to 9-years follow-up study of 537 patients. J.A.M.A., 170, 638.

Rossini, F.P. (1975). Atlas of coloscopy. Piccin Medical Books, Padova (Italy).

Rossini, F.P., A. Ferrari and G. Droetto (1976). Caratterizzazione
    coloscopica delle poliposi del grosso intestino. Aspetti macrosco
    pici e correlazioni istologiche. Min. Med., 67, 502.

Rossini, F.P. and A. Ferrari (1976). Use and limitation of coloscopy
    in the diagnosis and treatment of colonic polyps. Acta Endoscopica
    ed Radiocinematographica, 6, 133.

Rossini,F.P. and A. Ferrari (1976). Tecniche collaterali in coloscopia:
    reale ausilio diagnostico? Simp. Naz. su "Attualità diagnostica e
    terapeutica dell'Endoscopia Digestiva". Roma.

Rossini, F.P. and A. Ferrari (in press). Usefulness of the dye
    spraying method in coloscopy.

Rossini, F.P. and A. Ferrari (1978). Vantaggi diagnostici, Tecnici,
    economici della coloscopia parziale con fibroscopio medio.
    Giorn-Gastroent. End., 1 (n.2) (in press).

Sherlock, P., M. Lipkin and S.J. Winawez (1975). Predisposing factors
    in colon carcinoma, in Advances International Medicine. Edited by
    G.H. Stollerman, Chicago, Year Book Medical Publishers, 20, 121.

Theodore, W., M.D. Bohlman, M. Ronald, MD. Katon, R. Gilbert,
    M.D. Lipshutz, F. Michael, M.D. McCool, W. Frederick, MD. Smith
    and S. Clifford,MD. Melnyk (1977). Fiberoptic Pansigmoidoscopy -
    An evaluation and comparison with rigid sigmoidoscopy.
    Gastroenterology, 72, 644-649.

Welch, C.E. and S.E. Hedberg (1975). Polypoid lesions of the
    gastrointestinal tract. (pag. 46). 2nd edition Major Problems in
    clinical Surgery. W.B. Saunders Company, Philadelphia, London,
    Toronto.

Williams C.B., R.H. Hunt, H. Loose, R.H. Riddel, Y. Sakai and E.T.
    Swarbrick (1974). Colonoscopy in the management of colon polyps.
    Br. J. Surg., 61, 673.

Williams, C.B. and R.H. Riddel (1976). Coloscopic polypectomy in
    Topics in Gastrointestinal endoscopy. Ed.Salomon P.R. and Schiller,
    K.F.R., publ. Heinemann Medical, London.

Winawer, S.J., P. Sherlock, D. Schottenfeld and D.G. Miller (1976).
    Screening for colon cancer. Gastroenterology, 70, 783.

Winawer, S.J., P. Sherlock and D. Schottenfeld (1976.
    Screening for colon cancer. Gastroenterology,70, 783.

Wolff, W.I. and H. Shinya (1974). Earlier diagnosis of cancer the
    colon througt colonic endoscopy (colonoscopy). Cancer, 34, 913-
    -931.

Wolff, W.I. and H. Shinya (1973b).Plypectomy via the fiberoptic
    colonoscope. N. Engl. J. Med., 288, 329-332.

Second Look Operation for Colon Cancer

John Peter Minton

The Ohio State University Hosp., Department of Surgery,
410 W. 10th Ave., Columbus, Ohio 43210, USA

Since 1972 we have been carefully studying the carcinoembryonic antigen (CEA) values in patients with carcinoma of the colon and rectum (1). From these studies we have found that it is necessary to obtain a preoperation CEA value to determine if the patient's malignancy is making CEA. Cancers of the sigmoid colon usually have the highest CEA values and produce significantly elevated CEA values (2). In contrast, some cancers of the right colon and rectum do not produce significant CEA elevations even before surgery so the CEA may be unreliable as a marker in the postoperative period (3). A careful physical examination at each follow-up visit is the most reliable way to discover the presence of recurrent cancers which do not produce elevated levels of CEA. Serial CEA determinations have been shown to give the surgeon the earliest warning of recurrent colon cancer in patients who are known to make CEA by the presence of an elevated preoperation CEA value that falls to 2.5 ng/ml or less within the first month after colon or rectum resection. In this type of patient, by determining the serum CEA values at monthly intervals, or at least every two months, a new baseline level for each patient is established. Once the new baseline is known any significant increase from this lowest normal CEA value for a specific patient means there is a new source of CEA production which must be discovered. In our experience from a retrospective study which started in 1972 and a prospective study which started in 1976, there is no question that CEA alone is the single most reliable and informative indicator of recurrent cancer for these patients (4). Even though a careful physical re-evaluation is performed on each of these patients as well as bone and liver scans and G.I., chest and urologic x-ray studies plus blood studies, echography and a hepatic artery angiogram in many patients, the vast majority of these tests and examinations have demonstrated absolutely nothing abnormal. Only when the exploratory operation is performed is the recurrent disease found. Since two thirds of recurrences occur within the first 18 months after the primary resection, patients must have close CEA surveillance during this period of time. The ideal CEA follow-up to date is every month for the first two years and every two months for the next three years; after five years every six

months for two years, then once a year. This regression in frequency of sampling takes into account the likelihood of early recurrence from rapidly growing tumors and continues long enough to
detect slow-growing recurrent tumors.

Experience with the carcinoembryonic antigen radioimmunoassay
has enabled us to interpret values obtained in our laboratory and
to place reliable clinical significance on numerical value changes.
We (1) proposed a carcinoembryonic antigen nomogram as a simple
scale for evaluation of the significance of the carcinoembryonic
antigen value. If a follow-up determination exceeds two standard
deviations from the new low base line value established longer than
one month after resection, the rise is considered to signal a significant regrowth of the tumor. In the absence of other explanations
for the carcinoembryonic antigen elevation, reoperation is indicated.
If a new low, 2.5 milligrams per milliliter $\pm$ 2, base line value
does not occur, the surgeon must assume that there was a significant
amount of cancer left after operation.

Even though the two studies we initiated are small, the principle of second-look surgery that Dr. Wangensteen (5) demonstrated
has a new opportunity for very accurate application to today's
colorectal cancer patients using the CEA as an indicator for his
second-look surgery.

Operation

After the physical, laboratory and x-ray evaluations, patients
with no detectable evidence of unresectable metastatic disease are
taken to the operating room where a xyphoid to pubis midline incision is made. The entire intra-abdominal viscera are carefully
examined. The right and left lobes of the liver are examined.
Frequently, the right lobe must be detached from the diaphragm at
the bare area for a thorough bimanual examination of that lobe.
Two True Cut[R] needle biopsies are made randomly in each liver lobe
if it appears clinically free of tumor. If tumor is present in one
lobe or the other a lobectomy is done. If both lobes have a lesion
or two, wedge resections are done. If diffuse metastases are present biopsy both lobes then insert a Broviac[R] catheter into the
hepatic artery through a branch of the gastroduodenal artery and/or
a second catheter is placed into the portal vein via a mesenteric
vein for infusion of 5-FU. The retrobiliary nodes are biopsied,
the right colon is taken down from its gutter attachments and the
vena cava and periaortic nodes are biopsied. Any suspicious nodes
along the aorta or base of the small bowel mesentery are removed
for frozen section. The gastrohepatic ligament is divided and the
caudate lobe of the liver is inspected. The ureters are followed
into the pelvis and any remaining iliac and obturator lymph nodes
are examined and removed for frozen section. Any areas which suggest metastases to the peritoneum, mesentery, omentum, or bowel
wall are biopsied. At each place where recurrent cancer is confirmed by frozen section metal clips are placed to guide future
radiotherapy. When exploration in the hollow of the pelvis is clinically negative, multiple True Cut[R] needle biopsies of the soft
tissues on both sides of the pelvis are sent for frozen section.
This type of surgical exploration has been very effective in detecting and removing small amounts of recurrent malignant tumor.
Wherever recurrent tumor is present every attempt at total

resection is made. To facilitate bowel resections, a stapling device has been used. Each site of resected or unresectable tumor is marked with metal clips. Post operation management may include hyperalimentation and always includes chemotherapy, radiation therapy and immunotherapy. If the patient has not had an intestinal anastomosis, liver resection or ureteral anastomosis, chemotherapy is started a week or less after the operation. When anastomoses are present the treatments may start two to three weeks after operation. Chemotherapy is given at a total of 15 mg/kg/24 hrs for five consecutive days. The 5-FU is given in six equally divided doses every four hours. This is followed by radiation therapy to 4500 rads to the areas marked by the metal clips. During and after the course of radiation therapy, 50 mg of levamisole is taken by mouth three times per day on Saturday and Sunday, or the days when radiotherapy is not given. After the patient recovers from the acute radiation effects, he receives 15 mg/kg of 5-FU, IV push, each week plus levamisole at the same dosage (50 mg by mouth) indefinitely. Follow-up with CEA continues in the usual manner unless the patient was found to have incurable metastatic disease at the second-look procedure. If all detectable metastatic disease is not removed the patient is treated the same way as described above until there is evidence of progression. Then, other chemotherapeutic agents are used as indicated.

Results

In the retrospective study from 1972 through 1975, 22 patients underwent a CEA dictated second-look operation. Recurrent tumor was found in 19 (86%). Among these 19 patients, only 6 (26%) had a resectable tumor, the remaining 13 had distant disease and only confirmation of recurrent tumor was able to be done at reoperation. Of the three additional patients who underwent second-look with no tumor found, two have subsequently proved to have positive bone scans and one had a positive brain scan. All patients with unresectable disease were dead within 14 months. Of the patients with resectable tumor, four remain alive and free of disease, one longer than five years and three longer than three years.

In the retrospective study, the average CEA value of patients with unresectable recurrent cancer was greater than 20 nanograms per ml of serum. Whereas the six patients wit h resectable diseases had an average CEA value of 7.2 ng/ml. The average time delay in the 13 patients with unresectable disease was seven months compared to 3.5 months in the six patients with resectable disease.

In the prospective study started in 1976, 22 patients have had second-look procedures, 15 had localized disease and six had distant disease, one had no tumor discovered. In the prospective study the 15 with resectable disease had an average CEA of 8.2 ng/ml, the six with distant metastases had 18.8 ng/ml. The time delay after detection of an elevated CEA in patients with localized resectable tumor at second-look was 1.2 months and in patients with unresectable disease it was 4.8 months. The usual reason for time delay is the patient's unwillingness to have a second operation when the patient "feels so good" and all the tests are negative, except for the rising CEA. This delay needless to say has led to unresectable disease and death in every patient.

Comment

In summary, our patients had demonstrated that serial CEA determinations contributed to detection of recurrent tumor, and that
shortening of the delay between detection of CEA elevation and reoperation resulted in an increase from 6 of 22 patients to 15 of 22
patients with resectable recurrent tumor. If these results continue
to be substantiated, the CEA assay has made a significant contribution to control of this disease.

Serial CEA assays should be performed at least every two months,
preferably every month for the first 18 months. All benign inflammatory conditions that cause CEA elevations must be searched for and
ruled out before reoperation is decided upon. The physician must be
cognizant not only of the significance of the assay but also its
limitations. We find a rising CEA the earliest indication of many
recurrent colon cancers.

References

1. Martin EW Jr, James KK, Hurtubise PE, Catalano P and Minton JP.
    The use of CEA as an early indicator for gastrointestinal tumor
    recurrence and second-look procedures.   Cancer 39:440-446, 1977.

2. Martin EW Jr, Kibbey WE, Samson R, Stewart W, Hardy T and
    Minton JP.   Carcinoembryonic antigen in colorectal practice:
    Report of three cases.   Dis Colon Rectum 19:99-106, 1976.

3. Martin EW Jr, Kibbey WE, DiVecchia L, Anderson G, Catalano P
    and Minton JP.   Carcinoembryonic antigen: Clinical and histor-
    ical aspects.   Cancer 37:62-81, 1976.

4. Minton JP, James KK, Hurtubise PE, Rinker L, Joyce S and
    Martin EW Jr.   The use of serial carcinoembryonic antigen deter-
    minations to predict recurrence of carcinoma of the colon and the
    time for a second-look operation.   Surg Gynec Obstet 147:208-
    210, 1978.

5. Wangensteen OH, Lewis FJ, Arhelger SW, Muller JJ and MacLean LD.
    An interim report upon the "second-look" procedure for cancer of
    the stomach, colon and rectum for "limited intraperitoneal car-
    cinosis".   Surg Gynec Obstet 99:257, 1954.

Surgery of Colo-rectal Cancer

D. Bokelmann

Department of Surgery, University of Heidelberg, F.R.G.

ABSTRACT

More than 2000 patients treated in a period of 30 years in the Surgical Department of the Universität Heidelberg were analyzed. Surgery only does cure about 50 per cent of all colo-rectal cancers. Local, regional, and disseminated cancers unremoved or untreated by surgery and other modalities account for this unrelenting mortality for the past 20 years. In incurable cancers the tumour resection is the best palliative course of treatment. In lower rectal lesions for the majority of the patients radicality still has to be given priority over maintenance of continence, if we want to speak in terms of radical surgery. Local excision as a curative procedure is reserved only for a small number of selected patients.

After diagnosis of a colo-rectal cancer surgery alone is still the most frequent and effective therapy. The goal is to remove the involved part of the organ together with the regional lymphvessels and nodes. The principle of oncologic radical surgery can be reached, because of the especially favourable anatomical conditions in carcinomas of the colon and rectum. The so-called classical resections, introduced by MAYO (1908) and particularly by KOERTE (1913), still today are performed. According to the drainage of the lymphatics along with the great blood vessels the standard resections are: right hemicolectomy, resection of the transverse colon, left hemicolectomy and resection of the sigmoid colon. The extention of resection varies individually and depends upon the location and the stage of the tumour. The reconstruction is performed by an end-to-end-anastomosis with a single - or double-layered row of sutures. We use a synthetic, absorbable, atraumatic suture material from polyglycol-acid (DEXON) and in general carry out a single-layer sero-muscular suture. In general, resections of the colon are performed without establishing a colostomy. Only in emergency cases with bowel obstruction a defunctioning colostomy for decompression is necessary before the resection. The reconstruction of the normal bowel passage is possible in a third step after the recovery of the patient. Preoperative bowel antisepsis with nonabsorbable antibi-

otics leads to disturbances of the normal culture of bowel bacte-
rias. So this method is prefered by less surgeons. We prepare our
patients by an oral orthograde intestinal lavage in connection with
oral laxatives and by this we obtain an excellent bowel cleaning.
Careful medical treatment before operation is necessary, because
more than 80 per cent of our patients are above 60 years of age.

Therapeutic results essentially depend upon three factors:
1.) the possibility of either radical or only symptomatic surgery.
2.) the patients age and
3.) the tumour stage.

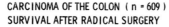
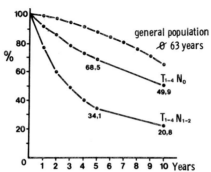

Fig. 1

Patients after radical surgery can have in comparison with the
general population a good prognosis (Fig. 1).
We found in tumours without metastases a 5-year-survival-rate of
68,5 per cent, while the 10-year-survival-rate was 49,9 per cent.
The prognosis is reduced even if radical surgery is performed in
all cases with positive lymph nodes to 20,8 per cent after 10 years.
This group showed a large number of these patients were not able to
undergo curative surgery. The deciding influence in the course of
the tumour disease occur in the first five years. After that one
can expect the patient to remain tumour-free.
Especially in the first two years after primary treatment we must
expect the appearance of a local tumour recurrence. In our patients
we observed this in 11,7 per cent of 609 radical tumour resections.
The cause for a local recurrence on one hand could be an incomplete
resection, so that parts of the intramural growing tumour or positive lymph nodes are not removed (Tab. 1).
On the other hand a seeding of tumour cells into the lumen of the
bowel, into the vessels or into the peritoneal cavity could occur
through manipulation of the tumour during surgery. Tumour cells can
finally implanted into the bowel wall by sutures. The very infrequent late recurrences in the area of the anastomosis are probably
not caused through manipulation of the tumour during the operation.
These are rather new primary tumours arising at the anastomosis
with possibly the same aetiologic factors as other primary tumours

of the colon. The development of these tumours requires a very long time interval (approximately 10-years). The incidence of local recurrences can be reduced by improved surgical technique (TURNBULL et al, 1967).
The principle is to eliminate the dissemination of tumour cells and to make the primary resection line at a distance sufficiently remote from the tumour. It is very important that the removal of all the lymph nodes of the drainage area in a mono-bloc-resection is accomplished (Tab. 2).

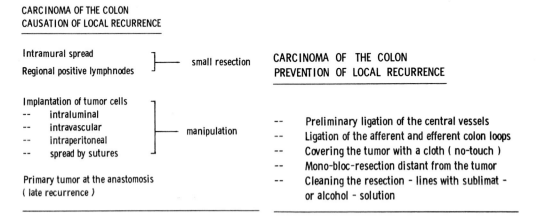

CARCINOMA OF THE COLON
CAUSATION OF LOCAL RECURRENCE

Intramural spread
Regional positive lymphnodes ⎱ small resection

Implantation of tumor cells
-- intraluminal
-- intravascular ⎱ manipulation
-- intraperitoneal
-- spread by sutures

Primary tumor at the anastomosis
(late recurrence)

CARCINOMA OF THE COLON
PREVENTION OF LOCAL RECURRENCE

-- Preliminary ligation of the central vessels
-- Ligation of the afferent and efferent colon loops
-- Covering the tumor with a cloth (no-touch)
-- Mono-bloc-resection distant from the tumor
-- Cleaning the resection - lines with sublimat - or alcohol - solution

Tab. 1   Tab. 2

However, in practice this maneuver is not always successful especially in cases concerning large tumours with adhesions to the surrounding tissues. With regular follow-ups including X-ray and endoscopy the capability for early detection of local recurrences is increased. Also the determination of the carcino-embryonic antigen (CEA) may indicate a recurrence.
With early diagnosis even local recurrences can have a favourable prognosis (Fig. 2).
We have found that those patients treated with another radical resection have a 5-year-survival-rate of 32 per cent, whereas the patient given only palliative operations - with or without resection - die within 3 years. All patients with inoperable recurrences die within the first year following diagnosis.
In the handling of patients with advanced tumours or distant metastases but in fairly good condition the best palliative course of treatment is still tumour resection.
The 5-year-survival-rate in patients treated with resection compared to those who were not resected are approximately the same - under 10 per cent (Fig. 3).
However, the patients with resections experienced a small improvement of the median survival time. The deciding argument in favour of palliative tumour resection is an improvement in quality of life. These patients can be freed from pain, bleeding and from other sequelae of the necrotizising tumour in the remaining life-span.

In addition, many patients will not require a colostomy. In cases
with obstruction and non-resectable primary tumours, the surgeon
should try to perform an internal anastomosis when ever possible
(for instance ileo-transversostomie).

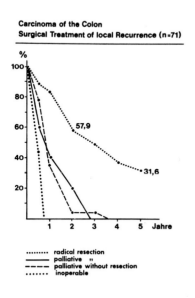

Fig. 2

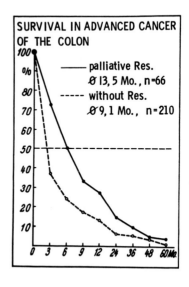

Fig. 3

The surgery of rectal cancer is governed by other principles.
Because of the position of the rectum in the pelvis and because
of the importance of attempting to preserve anal continence, the
spectrum of rectal tumour surgery is greater than in the colon
(Tab. 3).
We must differentiate between methods which result in loss of the
anus and a permanent sigmoid colostomy from those in which the
tumour can be surgically removed with preservation of anal function
These sphincter-preserving operations can generally be performed if
the lower tumour margin is localized 10 to 12 cm above the anus.
But also in lower situated tumours some surgeons try to perform
such operations, for example PARKS with a transanal anastomosis or
others using the pull-through-operation. These operations involving
supraanal anastomosis are burdened with a high postoperative compli
cation rate (Tab. 4). Frequently one observes a complete or partial
anal incontinence. Besides, these methods, especially in advanced
tumour-stages, are associated with a higher rate of recurrences.
The other complications, too, show that such operations should only
be performed in selected cases.
Due to the fact that in Heidelberg not only elective, but very many
emergency patients are treated, a curative surgical intervention
was no more possible in 27 per cent of our cases, because the patients were in poor condition or had extensive metastases. In the
other 73 per cent anterior resection or radical rectum exstirpation
was performed. In more than 80 per cent of these cases radicality

was given priority over the maintenance of continence. According to
KRASKE and BAUER the sacral-abdominal-amputation was performed more
often than the abdominal-perineal-resection.
The overall postoperative mortality was 13,8 per cent in male and
9,1 per cent in female patients.

CARCINOMA OF THE RECTUM
SURGICAL METHODS

A. With permanent colostomy:

   abdomino - perineal resection
   synchron. abdom. -perineal resection
   sacro - abdominal resection

B. Spincter - preserving - procedures:

   anterior resection   ——   abdominal anastomosis
                          ——   transanal anastomosis
   pull - through operation
   rectotomia posterior
   transanal local excision / coagulation

Tab. 3

COMPLICATIONS OF THE " LOWER " ANASTOMOSIS
(less than 7 cm)

High incontinence rate (sensory)
High recurrence rate
Nekrosis of the colon
Retraction
Prolaps of the mucosa
Disturbed wound healing (stenosis)

Tab. 4

The prognosis depends directly upon the tumour stage. We have classified the tumours of our patients in accordance with the "Heidelberg TNM-proposal", which is nearly identical with the new proposal
of the UICC (1978). We found in colon tumours without regional metastases a 30 per cent difference in 5-year-survival rate between
the stage T_1 and T_4. The difference in rectal tumours was 49 per
cent (Tab. 5).
With the occurrence of regional metastases the prognosis decreases
sharply. In patients where distant metastases are present the 5-
year-survival-rate in colon as well as in rectal cancer is less
than 5 per cent. Tumour recurrences in the pelvis occur after radical surgical handling almost exclusively in advanced tumour stages
(T_3, T_4). The incidence is approximately 10 - 12 per cent.
The diagnosis is very difficult, because sacral or perineal pains
could present themselves also without recurrence. The determination
of carcino-embryonic antigen (CEA) is an important diagnostic aid
also in this cases. In many patients the use of computertomography
is successful in providing evidence of local recurrence.
In inoperable patients, local tumour excision or reduction by electrocoagulation, frequently in repeated applications, can sometimes
help to avoid a colostomy and to extend the life-span of the patient (Fig. 4). The average age of our patients with this procedure
was 1 decade higher than those with other palliative procedures
(74 years). Wether or not the electrocoagulation simply reduces the
size of the tumour, or also activates immunological carcinoma re-
jection, is still an unproven speculation. Due to the questionable
radicality of electrocoagulation, it should not be used in operable
cases.

GROUPING OF TUMOUR - STAGES IN COLO - RECTAL CANCER
5 - YEAR - SURVIVAL - RATES (Surg. Departm., HEIDELBERG)

STAGE	n	COLON 5-year - survival	n	RECTUM 5 - year - survival
$T_1N_0M_0$	26	19 (73,1 %)	124	82 (66,1 %)
$T_2N_0M_0$	51	33 (65,8 %)	204	120 (58,8 %)
$T_3N_0M_0$	138	72 (52,8 %)	293	135 (46,7 %)
$T_4N_0M_0$	94	41 (43,6 %)	23	4 (17,4 %)
$T_{1-4}N_1M_0$	34	11 (32,3 %)	88	31 (36,3 %)
$T_{1-4}N_2M_0$	135	26 (19,3 %)	399	95 (23,8 %)
$T_{1-4}N_xM_1$	194	6 (3,1 %)	215	10 (4,6 %)

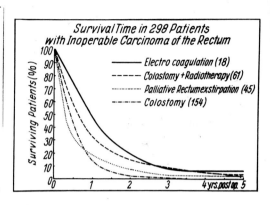

Survival Time in 298 Patients
with Inoperable Carcinoma of the Rectum

—— Electro coagulation (18)
----- Colostomy + Radiotherapy (61)
······· Palliative Rectumexstirpation (45)
—·—· Colostomy (154)

Tab. 5   Fig. 4

After a proctectomy, the colostomy patients are confronted with a
series of well known problems (Tab. 6).
Astonishingly, 92 per cent of our patients had scarcely any change
in their bowel habits postoperatively.
The majority of patients consider a daily enema to be just as unnecessary as before the operation. With modern colostomy bags the
hygienic care and use is relatively unproblematic. The inconve-
nient and often embarassing release of gas from the colostomy can
be prevented through the implantation of the Erlangen magnetic
ring closure device.
But unfortunately not all patients are suitable for this operation

---

COMPLICATIONS AND MORBIDITY
AFTER EXSTIRPATION
OF THE RECTUM

I. Colostomy : Control of Bowel Action
Hernia
Prolaps
Retraction
Stenosis

II. Perineal Hernia
Coccygodynia

III. Disorder of Bladder Function

IV. Sexual Dysfunction (♂ 25-80%)

V. Individual and Professional
Rehabilitation

GROUPING OF THE TUMOUR - STAGES IN
1346 PATIENTS WITH RECTAL CARCINOMA

T_1 = 147 (11 %) (Surg. Departm., HEIDELBERG)

	N_0	N_1	N_2	N_3	M_1
T_1	124	5	13	0	5
T_2	204	11	16	0	33
T_3	293	64	316	0	101
T_4	23	8	54	27	49

Tab. 6   Tab. 7

According to the literature postoperative micturition is altered in 20 per cent of the patients. Besides chronic infection mechanical factors such as posterior caudal kinking of the bladder or prostatic hypertrophic could be responsible for this change.
Furthermore intraoperative lesions of the sympathetic and parasympathetic nerves may play a role.
An exact differentiation between mechanical and neurological factors is essential to choose a specific therapy.
For this purpose it is important to measure simultaneous uroflow, micturition volume, bladder-pressure as well as the so called differential pressure as a parameter for the detrusor muscle activity. The differential pressure becomes negative as a sign of neurogenic damage.
Unfortunately disturbances of sexual function are another consequence of these operations. This again shows the requirement of a thoughtful psychological care. The many complications and also the fact that the postoperative mortality continously increases with increasing age, has recently become a subject of scientific discussion to change the strategy of treatment.

Is it allowed to perform local excision of lower rectal malignant lesions with sphincter preservation?

In our patients we see early carcinoma (stage T_1) in 11 per cent of all rectal carcinoma (Tab. 7).
In 15,7 per cent of these tumours histological examination by the pathologist determined metastatic involvement was already present. GREANEY and IRVING (1977) reported that in ulcerated T_1-tumours metastases were present in 50 per cent. In addition NIVATVONGS and GOLDBERG (1978) found that in polypoid adenomas with malignant invasion of the stalk (stage T_1) in 10 to 15 per cent metastases were present. Certainly in patients with distant metastases the local excision is acceptable. But preoperatively the lymphnode involvement or its absence is in practice impossible to ascertain. The local tumour excision either transanal or after rectotomia posterior has a low postoperative mortality, but includes in regional limited cancer a high risk factor.

TREATMENT OF MALIGNANT ADENOMA VERSUS RECURRENCE
(JAHADI, BALDWIN, 1975)

TREATMENT	NUMBER OF PATIENTS	NUMBER OF RECURRENCES
Local excision	48	14 (29,2 %)
Anterior or segmental resection	52	3 (5,7 %)
Abdominoperineal resection	18	0
Colotomy and excision	13	5 (38,4 %)
Pull-through	2	0
(Colectomy)	1	0
TOTAL	145	22 (15,2 %)

Tab. 8

SELECTIONSCRITERIA FOR LOCAL TUMOREXCISION IN LOWER RECTAL LESIONS

Adenomas with severe cellular dysplasia
Small polypoid carcinomas (border - line - lesions)
Highly differentiated carcinomas (T_1 = <2 cm)
Advanced patient age (> 75 years)
High operation risk
Refusal of colostomy
Palliation in advanced carcinomas

Tab. 9

In a group of unselected patients JAHADI and BALDWIN (1975) found
that after local excision almost 30 per cent displayed recurrence.
However, after anterier or segmental resection only 5,7 and after
colotomy with excision 38,4 per cent of the cases developed local
recurrences (Tab. 8).
Usually rectal tumours have a relatively low tendency towards infiltration into the rectal wall. Very early they dissiminate
tumour cells into the submucosa which form colonies proximal and
distal from the tumour (WESTHUES, 1934, GOLIGHER et al, 1951).
BLACK and WAUGH (1948) found that the tumour spread is greatest
to the submucosa and can exceed the palpable tumour margin by a
distance up to 2 cm. In anaplastic carcinomas they observed a
lateral spreading up to 7,5 cm.
The indication for local excision should only be decided according
to strict selective criteria (Tab. 9).
An exact histological diagnosis by the pathologist is the first
condition. In highly differentiated carcinomas, in my opinion, we
must consider advanced patient age or high operation risk.
Especially in sessile tumours and ulcerative growth there is no
indication in younger patients, if we want to speak in terms of
radical surgery. In patients with advanced age local excision is
acceptable. In this age group the tumour doubling time is so long
that the patient will die from natural causes more likely before
the cancer reaches an advanced stage.
Of course, in advanced cancer palliative handling is also indicated.
Finally I would like to emphasize that in lower rectal cancer for
the majority of the patients radicality still has to be given priority over maintenance of continence.
Local tumour excision as a curative surgical treatment is reserved
only for a small number of selected patients.

References

Black, W.A., J.M. Waugh (1948). Intramural extension of carcinoma
    of descending colon, sigmoid and rectosigmoid: a pathologic
    study. Surg. Gynecol. Obstet., 87, 457.
Bokelmann, D. (1977). Möglichkeiten der operativen Krebshehandlung:
    Dickdarmcarcinome. Münch.med.Wschr., 119, 623.
Bokelmann, D. (1978). Kolon- und Rektum-Tumoren. Diagnostik, 11, 3.
Goligher, J.H., L.E. Dukes, H.J.R. Bussey (1951). Local recurrence
    after sphinctersaving excissions for carcinoma of the rectum
    and rectosigmoid. Brit. J. Surg., 39, 199.
Greaney, M.G., T.T. Irving (1977). Criteria for selection of rectal
    cancer for local treatment. Dis. Colon Rectum, 20, 463.
Jahadi, M.R., A. Baldwin (1975). Villous adenomas of colon and
    rectum. Amer. J. Surg., 130, 729.
Nivatvongs, S., S.M. Goldberg (1978). Management of patients who
    have polyps containing invasive carcinoma removed via colonos
    copy. Dis. Colon Rectum, 21, 8.
Turnbull, R.B., K. Kyle, F.R. Watson, J. Spratt (1967). Cancer of
    the colon: the influence of no-touch isolation technic on sur-
    vival rates. Ann. Surg., 166, 420.
UICC (1978). TNM-Klassifizierung der malignen Tumoren. Springer
    Berlin-Heidelberg-New-York.
Westhues, H. (1934). Die pathologisch-anatomischen Grundlagen der
    Chirurgie des Rectumcarcinoms. Thieme, Leipzig.

Radiation Therapy of Colo-rectal Carcinoma

Leonard L. Gunderson

*Department of Radiation Medicine, Massachusetts General
Hospital and Harvard Medical School, Boston, MA 02114, USA*

ABSTRACT

Recent developments have led to marked interest in a combined modality approach for
colo-rectal carcinoma: 1) Increasing data that "radical" operations do not necessarily prevent tumor regrowth in the tumor bed and regional lymph nodes; 2) Acceptance of the "subclinical disease" radiation dose concept and 3) Preliminary data of
various pre- and post-operative radiation series which suggest that the incidence
of local recurrence can be markedly reduced by moderate to high radiation doses although distant metastases continue to be a problem. The therapeutic "gains" with
radiation might be offset by an increase in complications unless wisdom is used in
treatment planning. Use of techniques to improve both tumor and normal tissue localization is dove-tailed with a discussion of optimization of radiation portals
with shaped multiple fields, "shrinking field" techniques, etc. Future possibilities of radiation for colorectal carcinomas are discussed.

KEYWORDS

Ca colo-rectum, operative failures, radiation pre- and post-op, radiation treatment planning, therapeutic ratio.

INTRODUCTION

Survival rates for colorectal carcinoma have improved slightly over the past 25 to
30 years. Such improvements, however, have been the result of an increase in operability, with little improvement by stage of disease in those patients who have
survived a "curative resection". (Polk and others, 1973).

Until recently, radiation has played a very minor role in the initial treatment of
colorectal lesions. Its major role has been its marked palliative (75-80%) and
occasional curative value (5-30%) for residual, inoperable and/or recurrent lesions.
(Gunderson, 1976) As a single modality of treatment, however, irradiation with
conventional supervoltage equipment is not a competitive alternative to surgery in
many patients since the limited tolerance of the surrounding organs and initial
tumor bulk can prevent a suitable therapeutic ratio between cure and complications.
Radiation, however, has considerable potential when combined with surgery for lesions which are resectable but at high risk for recurrence.

The purpose of this discussion is to develop a logical approach to the use of rad-

29

iation therapy in colo-rectal malignancies by discussing areas of treatment failure
in re-operative and clinical series with subsequent implications for adjuvant therapy. A comparison of common staging systems utilized in these malignancies is
shown in Table I. A modification of the Astler-Coller rectal system (Astler and
Coller, 1954; Gunderson and Sosin, 1974) applicable to all carcinomas of the alimentary tract is preferred in analyzing data because it reflects more accurately
the influence that initial extent of disease has on later patterns and incidence of
failure as well as on survival rates. The modified system differentiates by degree
of extra rectal or extra colonic involvement in the B_2 or C_2 group be it microscopic only (m), gross extension confirmed by microscopy (m&g) or adherence to or
invasion of surrounding organs or structures (B_3 or C_3).

TABLE 1   Comparison of Dukes' Staging Scheme (3) with a Modification of the Astler-
Coller System (1) by Gunderson and Sosin (8)

Staging System

Dukes'	Modified Astler-Coller	Description
A	A	Nodes negative; lesion limited to mucosa
	B_1	Nodes negative; extension of lesion through mucosa but still within bowel wall
B	B_2*	Nodes negative; extension through the entire bowel wall (including serosa if present)
C	C_1	Nodes positive; lesion limited to bowel wall
	C_2*	Nodes positive; extension of lesion through the entire bowel wall (including serosa)

* Separate notation is made regarding degree of extension through the bowel wall:
microscopic only (m); gross extension confirmed by microscopy (m&g); adherence to
or invasion of surrounding organs or structures ($B_3 + C_3$)

OPERATIVE FAILURES - IMPLICATIONS FOR ADJUVANT THERAPY

The term "failure" in relation to initial treatment is used to indicate later evidence of cancer. Incidence and patterns of operative failures have been analyzed
in moderate detail in both re-operative and clinical series.

TABLE 2   Patterns of Failure in Rectal Re-Operation Series After Curative Resection

Pattern of Failure**	Only Failure	Any Component
LF-RF	25-48.1%(33.8%)	48-92.3%(64.9%)
DM	4- 7.7%(5.4%)	26-50.0%(35.1%)
PS	0	3- 5.8%(4.1%)

* Modified from Gunderson and Sosin (1974) - Open % are of the 52 patients in the
failure group and in parentheses of the total group of 74
** See text.

Tables 2 and 4 present data from the University of Minnesota re-operative series
(Wangensteen, 1949) on a group of patients analyzed by Gunderson and Sosin (1974)
who were re-explored at varying intervals after the initial operation but before
the terminal event. Seventy-four patients with complete bowel wall penetration
and/or involved lymph nodes at the time of initial curative surgery had planned
single or multiple re-operations. Tumor due to recurrent and/or metastatic carcinoma was found in 52.

Patterns of failure in the re-operative series are shown in Table 2. Distant

metastasis (DM) alone was uncommon but occurred as some component of failure in
35% of the total group or 50% of the group with failure. Peritoneal seeding (PS)
was rare. Local failure and/or regional lymph node metastases (LF-RF) occurred
frequently as either the only failure or in combination with distant metastases
(approximately 1/3 of the entire group or 1/2 of the failure group had only this
pattern of failure through total follow-up).

TABLE 3   Operative Extent Vs. Local Failure (LF) - U. Chicago Rectal and Recto-
Sigmoid Series*

	Local Failure	
Extent (gross)	#	%
Within wall	14/122	11.4%
{A_1B_1, C_1, B_2 or C_2 (m)}**		
Through Wall	17/30	56.7%
{B_2 or C_2 (m&g), B_3C_3}**		
TOTAL	31/152	20.4%

*Modified from Moosa and others, 1975.
**Equivalent pathologic stage by modified Astler-Coller method (Table 1)

Subgroups have been defined in both clinical and re-operative analyses with differential survival rates and variable potential benefits from a local regional adjuvant such as radiation. The University of Chicago rectal series (Moosa and others,
1975) (Table 3) noted subsequent clinical evidence of pelvic recurrence in 56.7%
of patients with the operative finding_ of local spread (equivalent to modified
Astler-Coller B_2 or C_2 (m&g) or B_3 or C_3 lesions) vs. 11.4% if this were not
present. In the M.D. Anderson series (Withers and Romsdahl, 1977), the incidence
of local recurrence plateaued in patients with follow-up of 2-3 years at 50% for
the combined node negative and positive groups with adjacent organ involvement
(B_3 & C_3) 45% in the C_2 group (LN+, through wall) and 20% in the B_2 group (LN-,
through wall). (Table 4).

TABLE 4   Ca Colo-Rectum - Extent of Disease Vs. Later Local Failure (LF)*

Modified A-C Stage	Colorectum U Florida	Rectum and Rectosigmoid		
		MDAH	Portland (ME)	U Minn Re-Op'n**
Within Wall				
C_1	4/19 (21%)	--	1/5 (20%)	4/17 (23.5%)
Through Wall				
B_2 (± B_3)	20/58 (34%)	-- (20%)	13/37 (35.1%)	--
C_2 (± C_3)	33/64 (52%)	-- (45%)	24/37 (64.9%)	28/40 (70%)
B_3 + C_3	--	(50%)	--	--

* Curative series (clinical and re-operation) with minimum 2 year follow-up.
** If include all nodal failures including aortic then 33/40 or 82.5% have local-
regional failure (LF-RF)

The Gilbert (1978) Portland, Maine rectal-rectosigmoid and Cass, Pfaff and Million
(1976) University of Florida colorectal analyses yielded virtually identical results. The groups at highest risk for local recurrence were those with extension

of tumor through the entire bowel wall whether the nodes were uninvolved (B_2 & B_3: $\simeq$ 35%) or involved (C_2 or C_3: $\simeq$ 52-65%) as opposed to $\simeq$ 20% when nodes were involved but the lesions was confined to the wall (C_1). This latter finding correlated well with the University of Minnesota rectal re-operative series in which the incidence of local failure in the C_1 group was only 23.5% (4/17) as opposed to 70% (28/40) with the C_2 & C_3 group if the five patients with nodal failures outside the pelvis are excluded.

As the preceding and corroborating data (Polk and others, 1973) indicate, the use of radical operative procedures, while occasionally justifiable, does not uniformly prevent either local failures or regrowth (LF) in the tumor bed and regional lymph nodes or distant failures (DF) by hematogenous (DM) or peritoneal routes (PS). Progressive extension of operative procedures may yield slight gains in cure rates but these gains are often offset or minimized by a corresponding increase in operative morbidity or mortality. Many of the local regional failures that occur are predictable and are due to the presence of microscopic or subclinical residual disease left in spite of "curative operative attempts". Most of these failures should be preventable with the use of moderate doses of radiation in the range of 4500-5000 rad in accordance with the "subclinical disease radiation dose concept".

Radiation and/or chemotherapy may be logically used in combination with "curative resection" (operative removal of all known disease). Local regional failures (LF-RF) comprise a major problem in these malignancies but occur in combination with distant metastases (hematogenous or peritoneal) about half the time.

RADIATION THERAPY - PHILOSOPHY AND RESULTS

Differences of opinion exist regarding the preferred sequence of combining surgery and irradiation. (Gunderson and Sosin, 1974). A well devised combination of pre- and post-operative radiation therapy (Gunderson, 1976) (sandwich technique) could have the theoretical advantages of each.

Pre-Operative Irradiation

A number of centers have utilized pre-operative irradiation with a variety of dose and portal arrangements (Kligerman and others, 1972; Roswit and others, 1975; Stearns and others, 1974; Stevens and others, 1976, 1977) All have demonstrated proof of tumoricidal responsiveness at the time of surgery either by partial or total regression of the primary or the finding of a lower incidence of lymph node involvement than would ordinarily have been anticipated.

TABLE 5   Ca Rectum & Rectosigmoid - Incidence of Local Failure (LF) After Pre-Op Radiation & Curative Resection

Series	LF Incidence	
	RT + Op'n	Op'n
VAH- Autopsy (2000-2500/2-2½ wk)	17/58 (29%)*	26/64 (40%)*
U Oregon - Clinical (5000-6000/6-7 wk)	1/45 (2.3%)	-----

* Maximum incidence as an unspecified no. had extrapelvic failures

The two major pre-operative series have been the large randomized low dose 2000-2500 rad series from the Veterans Administration Hospital (VAH - Roswit and others,

1975) and the non-randomized high dose series from the University of Oregon (Stevens and Others, 1976, 1977). The former study showed a definite advantage in the irradiated group that underwent abdomino-perineal resection when compared with operative controls. This was reflected by an improvement in five year survival rates from 28.4 to 40.8% (0.02 > P < 0.01) and a decrease in local recurrence and distant metastases in an autopsy subgroup although both rates were still unacceptably high (29% and 47% respectively). The local failure incidence in that series is compared in Table 5 with that in the 5000-6000 rad high dose non-randomized Oregon series. In the latter series, only 1 of 45 patients or 2.3% with curative resection subsequently had a clinically evident pelvic component of failure.

Post-Operative Radiation

Three major prospective non-randomized series were undertaken in the early 1970's. The Salt Lake City (Gunderson, Votava and others, 1978) and Houston (Withers and Romsdahl, 1977) series were very similar utilizing moderately high doses of 4500-5000 rad in 5 to 6 weeks to extended pelvic fields and a dose of approximately 5500 rad in $6\frac{1}{2}$ weeks within a boost field if the lesion extended through the bowel wall. In the Salt Lake series, when residual disease was present, the dose within the boost field was raised to 6000-7000 rad in 7 to 8 weeks depending on findings of special small bowel films done to determine position and degree of mobility. In the Albert Einstein series (Turner and others, 1977), boost fields were not utilized unless there was proven residual disease and then 1500-2000 rad was given.

TABLE 6   Ca Rectum and Rectosigmoid, Post-Op Radiation - Incidence of Local Failure*

Series	Curative	Curative + Residual
MDAH (Houston, Texas)		
(4500/5wk L_5 + boost)	2/45 (4.4%)	---
LDS (Salt Lake City, Utah)		
(5100/6wk L_4 ± boost)	1/24 (4.2%)	2/29 (6.9%)
A Einstein (New York, NY)		
(4600/4½wk mid L_2 ± boost)	---	2/19 (10.5)

*After curative resection included modified A-C Stage $B_{2,3}$; $C_{2,3}$ ± C_1

Results from those series are shown in four separate tables. Table 6 shows that local recurrence rates to date have been exceedingly low whether analyzing those treated following curative resection but at high risk for local recurrence or when both curative resection and residual disease groups are combined.

TABLE 7   Ca Rectum and Rectosigmoid - Incidence of Local Failure After Curative Resection, Operation Vs. Operation and Radiation

Extent of Disease	Op'n Alone* U Florida, MDAH U Chicago, Maine	Op'n + Post-Op Rad'n (Sept '76 Analyses) MDAH	LDS-SLC
Through Wall			
LN- (B_2+B_3)	25-35%	0/20	0/5
LN+ (C_2+C_3)	45-65%	2/25 (8%)	1/13(7.7%)
LN Status Unk	---	---	0/4
(B_{2-3} vs C_{2-3})			

* See Tables 3 and 4

TABLE 8   Ca Colorectum - Incidence of Local Failure After Curative Resection, Operation Vs. Op'n + Radiation

| | Incidence of LF | |
Modified A-C Stage	Op'n Alone (U Florida)	Op'n + Rad'n (LDS-SLC; 9/77)
$B_2 + B_3$	20/58 (34%)	0/10
C_1	4/19 (21%)	0/2
$C_2 + C_3$	33/64 (52%)	*2/16 (12.5%)
B_{2-3} vs C_{2-3}	---	0/6
TOTALS	57/141(40%)	2/34 (6%)

*Both received a maximum dose $\approx$4500 rad/5 weeks (500-1000 rad less than perferred)

In Tables 7 and 8, local recurrence rates after "curative resection" and post-operative radiation are compared with the previously discussed operation alone series. They are markedly reduced for each extent of disease both for the rectal-rectosigmoid group as shown in Table 7 ($B_2 + B_3$ - 0/25 vs. 25-35%; $C_2 + C_3$ - 8% vs. 45-65% and also for the combined colorectal group (Table 8) in which both series had minimum two year follow-up. Such differences will hopefully persist in continued follow-up and in randomized trials. Results in the radiation series from Houston and Salt Lake City are virtually identical with the only local recurrences to date occurring in the group with both nodal involvement and extension through the entire wall. As shown in Table 9, distant metastases, however, occurred as a new manifestation via hematogenous or peritoneal routes in approximately 20-30% of patients depending on the series.

TABLE 9   Ca Colorectum, Post-Op Radiation - Distant Failures

Series	No. Pts.	DF* Alone	DF* Component
LDS-SLC (9/76 Analysis)			
Curative	32	5(15.6%)	7(21.9%)
Curative + residual	38	7(18.4%)	10(26.3%)
A. Einstein			
Curative + residual	40	7(17.5%)	12(30%)

*DF = DM (hematogenous) + PS (peritoneal) failures

Complications

Both moderate and high dose pre- and post-operative radiation might increase the rate of complications, but this possibility must be considered in perspective by weighing potential benefits against risks. At present, a significant portion of patients with the more advanced colorectal carcinomas (extension through the entire wall and/or lymph node involvement) suffer from the complications of recurrence, metastases and death if treated by operation alone. In the discussed pre- and post-operative series with doses in the range of 5000 rad in 6 weeks, the incidence of small bowel adhesions requiring operative intervention has been approximately 10%. Comparable information is not readily available in operation alone series with similar extent of disease and operative procedures and is needed before therapeutic ratio's of local control or cure vs. complications can be developed for each available method of treatment. Although radiation related complication rates are reported to be minimal in the VA Hospital low dose pre-op series, that series also reports a local recurrence rate of 29% in an autopsy subgroup which in itself is a major complication.

Therapeutic Ratio

A number of possibilities exist to achieve acceptable local control rates as found in the high dose pre- and post-op rectal radiation series and an acceptable complication rate. They are: 1) Improved tumor and normal tissue localization. 2) Operative attempts to decrease adhesions and/or displace normal tissues. 3) Optimize radiation equipment and techniques.

Improved tumor and normal tissue localization can be accomplished operatively with precise descriptions and good clip placement and/or perhaps with non-operative diagnostic techniques such as computerized body tomography (CT), ultrasound, lymphangiography, nuclear medicine scans, vessel studies, and barium studies including special small bowel films to determine position and degree of mobility (Green and others, 1975). While many physicians feel clips may interfere with subsequent diagnostic studies, especially CT, many, including this author, prefer and encourage this practice on surgically explored patients. With increasingly sophisticated ultrasound and CT techniques, these studies may become complementary to the use of clips or make clip placement unnecessary.

Further research attempts to decrease post-operative adhesions and displace normal tissues are indicated. In addition to the common sense approach of reperitonealizing traumatized soft tissue surfaces, research is needed into causes of adhesions and potential prevention by medication and/or mechanical manipulation (use of temporary inflationary devices, bladder distension, patient positional change post-op including Trendelenburg, alternating right and left side up, etc). Operative displacement of normal tissues may include pelvic floor reconstruction with residual peritoneum, an omental pedical flap or the use of pelvic organs such as the uterus or even the bladder (Gunderson, Doppke, and others, 1978).

Optimization of radiation equipment and techniques is also a necessary factor in accomplishing a favorable therapeutic ratio. This includes the use of shaped multiple field portals and shrinking field or precision radiotherapy techniques to decrease the volume of normal irradiated tissues. The increasing availability of high-energy supervoltage equipment results in improved dose-distribution and delivery in many more centers. Specialized beams (modulated protons, pi mesons, intra-operative electrons, etc) may allow an even more precise geographic distribution of radiation dose and effectiveness. Such sophistication is of value only if the means to define the tumor and normal tissue volumes are as precise as the methods of dose delivery. A lack in the former could lead to marginal recurrences.

In an effort to minimize both acute toxicity and chronic complications of pelvic and abdominal radiotherapy for colorectal malignancies, special small bowel series are utilized in our institution (Gunderson, Doppke, and others, 1978; Russell and others, 1978) to influence portal design and radiation doses. These studies demonstrate considerable variability in the localization and mobility of the small intestine following extensive intra-abdominal procedures. The advantage of 4-field extended (PA:AP and laterals) or 3-field boost portals (PA and laterals) over AP:PA techniques in sparing the small intestine becomes apparent when radiation portals are superimposed over small bowel films as shown in Figure 1.

Progressive field expansion to include more and more in the way of nodal chains by going from local pelvic fields to mid L4 or higher may merely increase the risk of complications to the small bowel or other normal tissues with little gain in tumor control. For pelvic lesions, the value of bladder distension to displace small bowel has been more useful than the Trendelenburg position. For extra-pelvic lesions, treatment of the tumor bed and/or para-aortic nodes with the patient on his side rather than supine can markedly shift small intestine.

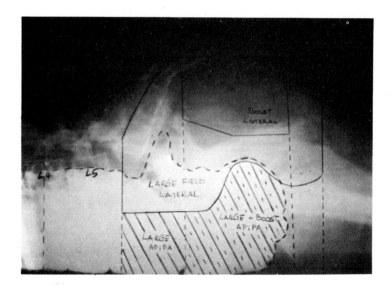

Fig. 1   Patient M.H. received post-op pelvic radiation after a low anterior resection for adenocarcinoma of the mid to high rectum (posterior wall lesion with gross extra-rectal extension and positive nodes).
Lateral large field portals were used in conjunction with PA-AP fields
to cover the tumor bed as well as internal iliac and presacral nodes
(4-field setup).   The tumor bed was "boosted" with 3-field PA and laterals.   Both large and boost field portals are shown in solid lines
superimposed over special small bowel films.   A small amount of small
intestine is seen within the antero-superior portion of the large lateral field but is totally out of the boost field portal (patient in
prone treatment position).   The interrupted lines extending anteriorly
from the lateral ports reveal the additional amount of small intestine
that would receive full radiation dosage if only PA-AP portals had been
utilized (shown in diagonal cross hatches).

CONCLUSIONS AND FUTURE POSSIBILITIES

In conclusion, operation alone is probably insufficient treatment for the large
group of patients with tumor extension grossly through the wall and/or nodal involvement.   The local-regional failure problem has been markedly reduced in the
moderate dose (4500-5000 rad) pre-operative and post-operative adjuvant radiation
series.   The lower dose pre-operative VA study (2000-2500 rad) has shown statistical improvement in survival of selected groups of patients and some, but not
adequate, improvement in local control.   Distant metastases continue to be somewhat
of a problem in both pre- and post-operative series and could possibly be decreased
with the use of effective systemic therapy.

Randomized prospective trials will be necessary to answer some of these questions.
The Veterans' Administration group is continuing its randomized study and has
raised the pre-operative dose in an attempt to further decrease the incidence of
failures.   Post-operative studies are under way in a number of national study
groups as well as localized institutions with some of the following options being
of interest-- 1) Operation alone (surgical control group); 2) Post-operative radiation; 3) Post-operative 5-FU plus nitrosourea; 4) Post-operative radiation plus

maintenance chemotherapy as in Arm 3; 5) Immunotherapy in combination with some of the above arms.

Areas of future treatment possibilities exist in the colorectal battlefield. Items 1-3 are in the Pilot study stage in individual institutions: 1) The addition of radiation to regimes for selected extra-pelvic colonic lesions at high risk for local-regional failure. For anatomically immobile or relatively immobile colon (ascending and descending colon, hepatic and splenic flexures and occasionally cecum) indications would be relatively the same as for rectum and rectosigmoid - ie. at least gross extension through the entire bowel wall and/or lymph node involvement ($B_{2,3}$; $C_{2,3} \pm C_1$). For the more mobile colon (mid sigmoid and transverse colon + cecum) indications would be adjacent organ or structure involvement (B_3 or C_3) with or without residual disease. 2) Optimization of radiation portals as previously discussed. 3) Alter routine radiation schemes - this might include a) well designed combination of pre- and post-operative radiation (sandwich technique) comparing results with either pre- or post-operative radiation or b) radiation of potential sanctuary sites such as liver if chemotherapy programs do not accomplish satisfactory results.

Ideas or concepts 4-7 are perhaps even further in the future: 4) More ideal sequencing of radiation with systemic chemotherapy and/or immunotherapy-questionable whether such optimization can be accomplished in human tumor systems. 5) For lesions 8-12 cm above the anal verge, extend the indications for low anterior resection by combining small distal margin with routine radiation instead of utilizing abdomino-perineal resection as the standard procedure and adding radiation only as indicated. 6) Treat lesions primarily with radiation, using photon beams for the extended fields and boosting the gross lesion with specialized beams (modulated protons, pi-mesons, etc), intracavitary techniques or intra-operative radiation (implants or electron beams) 7) Use conservation surgical techniques (fulguration, or excision of the entire gross lesion with sleeve resection or other technique) when technically applicable in lower 1/3 rectal lesions and combine routinely with radiation (#6).

REFERENCES

Astler, V.B., and F.A. Coller (1954). The prognostic significance of direct extension of carcinoma of the colon and rectum. Ann. Surg. 139:846.

Cass, A.W., F.A. Pfaff, and R.R. Million (1976). Patterns of recurrence following surgery alone for adenocarcinoma of the colon-rectum. Cancer 37:286.

Gabriel, W.B., C. Dukes and H.J.R. Bussey (1935). Lymphatic spread in cancer of the rectum. Br. J. Surg. 23:395.

Gilbert, S.B. (1978). The significance of symptomatic local tumor failure following abdomino-perineal resection. Intl. J. Radiat. Oncol. Biol. Phys. In Press.

Green, N., G. Ira and W.R. Smith (1975). Measures to minimize small intestine injury in the irradiated pelvis. Cancer 35:1633.

Gunderson, L.L. (1976). Radiation therapy: Results and future possibilities. Chapter 16 in Gastrointestional Malignancies, P. Sherlock, and N. Zamcheck, (Ed), Clin. Gastroenterol. 5:743.

Gunderson, L.L., K.P. Doppke, H.J. Llewellyn, and A.H. Russell (1978). Use of small bowel films in treatment planning for colorectal carcinoma: II. Residual, inoperable or recurrent disease. Submitted for publication.

Gunderson, L.L. and H. Sosin (1974). Areas of failure found at reoperation (second or symptomatic look) following "curative surgery" for adenocarcinoma of the rectum" Clinicopathologic correlation and implications for adjuvant therapy. Cancer 34:1278.

Gunderson, L.L., C. Votava, R. Brown, and H.P. Plenk, (1978) Colorectal carcinoma: Combined treatment with surgery and post-operative radiation - LDS hospital experience. Submitted for publication.

Kligerman, M.M., N. Urdaneta, A. Knowlton, R. Vidone, P.V. Hartman and R. Vera, (1972). Pre-operative irradiation of rectosigmoid carcinoma including its regional lymph nodes. Am. J. Roentgenol. Radium Ther. Nucl. Med. 114:498.

Moosa, A.R., P.C. Ree, J.E. Marks, B. Levin, and C.E. Platz (1975). Factors influencing local recurrence after abdomino-perineal resection for cancer of the rectum and rectosigmoid. Brit. J. Surg. 62:727.

Polk, H.C., W. Ahmad, and C.O. Knutson (1973). Carcinoma of the colon and rectum. Current Problems in Surgery. Year Book Medical Publishers, Inc. Chicago.

Roswit, B., G.A. Higgins, R.J. Keehn, (1975). Pre-operative irradiation for carcinoma of the rectum and rectosigmoid colon. Report of a National Veterans Administration randomized study. Cancer 35:1597.

Russell, A.H., L.L. Gunderson, K.P. Doppke, H.J. Llewellyn, and L. Kalisher, (1978). Use of small bowel films in treatment planning for colorectal carcinoma: I. Parallel opposed vs. multiple field in adjuvant pelvic irradiation. Submitted for publication.

Stearns, M.W., M.R. Deddish, S.H. Quan, and R.H. Leaming, (1974). Pre-operative roentgen therapy for cancer of the rectum and rectosigmoid. Surg. Gynecol. Obstet. 138:584.

Stevens, K.R., C.V. Allen, and W.S. Fletcher, (1976). Pre-operative radiotherapy for adenocarcinoma of the rectosigmoid. Cancer 37:2866.

Stevens, K.R., W.S. Fletcher, and C.V. Allen, (1978). Anterior resection and primary anastomosis following high dose pre-operative irradiation for adenocarcinoma of the rectosigmoid. Cancer 41:2065.

Turner, S.S., E.F. Vieira, P.J. Ager, S. Alpert, G. Efron, H. Ragins, P. Weil, and N.A. Ghossein, (1977). Elective post-operative radiotherapy for locally advanced colorectal cancer. Cancer 40:105.

Wangensteen, O.H., (1949). Cancer of the colon and rectum - With special reference to: (1) earlier recognition of alimentary tract malignancy, (2) secondary delayed re-entry of the abdomen in patients exhibiting lymph node involvement, (3) subtotal primary excision of the colon, (4) operation in obstruction. Wis. Med. J. 48:591

Withers, H.R. and M.M. Romsdahl. (1977). Post-operative radiotherapy for adenocarcinoma of the rectum and rectosigmoid. Int. J. Rad. Oncol. Biol. and Phys. 2:1069.

ACKNOWLEDGMENT

The author is indebted to Miss Ann Marie Burke for the preparation of this manuscript.

Intracavitary Irradiation of Limited Rectal Cancer for Cure

J. Papillon, J. F. Montbarbon, J. L. Chassard and J. P. Gerard

Early rectal adenocardinomas, as long as they are well or moderately differentiated and if their local spread is confined to the rectal wall, have a very low probability of lymphatic spread: less than 6 per cent in cases of polypoid tumors, less than 12 per cent in cases of ulcerative cancers.

In poor risk patients, these tumors may be suitable for a purely local treatment such as the intracavitary irradiation. This method has two modalities: 1) Contact X-ray therapy which is the chief one and consists of four applications carried out in the outpatient department; 2) Interstitial curietherapy which uses a steel fork with two Iridium 192 wires and can give a boosted dose of 2000 rads on the bed of the tumor, one month after completion of the contact X-ray therapy in cases of slightly infiltrating tumors.

Out of 174 patients followed for more than 5 years, the rate of death by cancer was 11 per cent, and the 5-year survival rate is 75 per cent.

If one compares local excision, electrocoagulation on one hand, and intracavitary irradiation on the other hand, stress may be placed on some of the advantages of irradiation.

Contact X-ray therapy is a true ambulatory treatment. Tolerace is excellent, even in high risk patients. There is no risk of recto-vaginal fistula in cases of tumor of the anterior wall of the rectum in female patients. There are very few complications with proper treatment, and no risk of mortality. After irradiation, the scar remains supple, without stenosis, and it is easy to appreciate the consistency of the irradiation area and of the adjacent rectal wall during the follow-up period. It is also possible to treat successfully some adenocarcinomas of the juxta-anal area.

As compared with local excision, which is essentially reliable for malignant polyps, irradiation is able to control not only exophytic lesions, but also some ulcerative carcinomas. After local excision, if the histological report suggests that there is doubt about the complete removal of the lesion, an intracavitary irradiation may be carried out in order to increase the chances of local control, without performing a bowel resection. In such conditions, a low dose of intracavitary irradiation is applied to the scar of local excision (6000 roentgen in three sessions over one month).

Intracavitary irradiation is a method by which a lot of limited carcinomas of the lower half of the rectum can be controlled and cured. The technique is easy to apply, but great care must be taken, before the decision (selection), during the treatment (dose, time of irradiation), and after the treatment (regular follow-up).

Under these circumstances, intracavitary irradiation deserves an appreciable place in the management of limited carcinomas of the lower two-thirds of the rectum as an alternative to radical surgery, which usually needs a permanent colostomy.

Therapy of Disseminated Colorectal Cancer with High Doses of 5-Fluorouracil

Angel O. Masotta

*Director of the National Bank of Antineoplasic Drugs,
Buenos Aires, Argentina*

ABSTRACT

The author proclaims treatment of colon carcinoma with high doses of fluorouracil administered by intravenous (leakage) and intramuscular via with a high percentage of improvement. A remarkably low rate of collateral effects is produced as compared to that reported by other authors, reason for which it is suspected that there might exist a difference not of a molecular type but in the industrial preparation of 5 FU used in the Argentine Republic and in other countries such as the United States.

KEYWORDS

5 FU - HIGH DOSES - COLON - EXCELLENT TOLERANCE - GOOD RESPONSE

The study group was selected according to the following conditions:

```
Patients under treatment .............. 72
Eldest age ........................... 82 years
Youngest age ......................... 36 years
Male ................................. 42
Female ............................... 30
Patients with peritoneum and regional
lymph node involvement ............... 53 (88%)
Patients with liver metastasis ....... 8 (13%)
Patients with other organs metastasis.. 10 (16%)
(some patients suffered from simultaneous organs
metastasis (i.e. bones and lungs, peritoneum and
liver, etc).
```

THERAPY

According to the classical studies by Ansfield and co-workers, fluorouracil was used in different types of cancer at a basic dose of 15 mg. per kilogram weight per day for 4-5 days (related to clinical status), with additional half doses given on alternate days to toxicity.   Thus, a patient whose

41

weight was 70 Kg. received 1 gr. daily for 4-5 days with additional
half doses (500 mg daily) until the appearance of toxicity in 3-4
weeks.

The dosage schedules of Ansfield and co-workers gave us little or no
success, but, on the other hand, we did not register their reported
toxicity signs. These findings called up our attention and we tried
higher doses according to the following therapy:

> a) For patients weighing more than 55 kg.: fluorouracil,
>   1 gr. intravenously daily (all were hospitalized
>   patients and the administration speed rate was 3-4
>   hours for the 500 cc. glucose or saline solution).

Fluorouracil was administered beginning 2-4 weeks after surgery,
according to clinical status. We usually followed the fluorouracil
1 gr. per day therapy for 15-20 days.

At the beginning, routine studies were taken as well as X-ray of
chest and painful zones for metastasis. Clinical control was made
daily, and blood count controls every 3-4 days. No patient had previously received pelvic irradiation therapy.

After this attack therapy, those patients with no toxicity signs
went on a maintenance therapy: 500 mg. per day, alternate days, intramuscular via which proved to be very useful and delivered no complications.

Maintenance therapy will last the whole patient's life with 2 therapy
weeks and a rest week, provided there are no toxicity signs. Whenever
evidence of illness appeared, patients were hospitalized for an intravenous attack therapy for 15-20 days.

Throughout the maintenance therapy, blood count controls were initial
ly taken once a week and thereon every 15 days plus a clinical control.

When no leukopenia or thrombocytopenia appeared, we asked for a blood
count control once a month.

The amount of drug received per patient and per year of survival was
200-300 ampules, that is, 50-75 grs.

RESULTS:

Patients under treatment	72
Patients showing improvement ...	60 (83%)
Patients with no response	12 (16%)
Maximum survival time	46 months (still alive)
Minimum survival time	8 months
Mean survival time	22 months
Total remission	42 (70%)
Partial remission	18 (30%)

First signs of improvement observed:

1) Increased appetite and reduced anemia
2) Attenuation or disappearance of pain
3) Objective improvement of the general condition and gain of weight.
4) Slowering sedimentation rate.

Though patients with severe liver metastasis and high blood bilirubin levels did not show a good evolution, this is not an adverse condition to receive the fluorouracil therapy, since they delivered real benefit demonstrated by the normalization of the liver function. In patients that did not reveal any progress or improvement, or in others that showed a regressive evolution, after a stationary period, it was administered some other chemotherapy, which never proved to bring better effects than fluorouracil.

Toxic reactions to 5-FU by Ansfield and co- workers and present report

Ansfield and co-workers	Symptoms	Present study
64%	Diarrhea	8%
48%	Stomatits	3%
30%	Nausea and vomiting	6%
20%	Alopecia	2%
8%	Dermatitis	1%
6%	Esophagopharingitis	0,5%
3%	Epistaxis	0%
22%	Leukopenia from 2000/ 3000	12%
32%	Leukopenia under 2000	3%
?	Thrombocytopenia below 100.000	2%

CONCLUSIONS:

Evidence of different behaviour is observed between U.S. classical reports of 5-FU administration and our studies. An exact or definite answer for this was not found. Nevertheless, it has been reported for some other drugs, like chloramphenicol.
Toxicity levels are also quite different.
A possible hypothesis explaining these observations should consider:

a) Different physico-chemical properties due to
   diverse industrialization processes;
b) Racial tolerance (very unlikely);
c) Diet.

REFERENCES

Ansfield, F.J., (1964) A less Toxic Fluorouracil dosage schedule .
J. Amer. Med. Ass. (USA) 190,686-87

Ansfield, F.J., Curreri (1959). Further Clinical Studies with
5-Fluorouracil. J. Nat. Cancer. Inst. 22,497-505

Lemon HM. Modzen PJ. Mirchandani R. et al (1963). Decreased intoxi-
cation by fluorouracil when slowly administered in glucose. JAMA 185
1012-1016.

Treatment of Hepatic Metastases from Colo-rectal Cancer

A. El-Domeiri

*Division of Oncology, Department of Surgery, Texas Tech University
School of Medicine, Lubbock, Texas, U.S.A.*

ABSTRACT

Treatment of hepatic metastases in 31 patients with cancer of the colon and rectum
consisted of wedge resection or partial hepatectomy in 2; systemic chemotherapy in
13; chemotherapy infusion of the hepatic artery in 9; and chemotherapy infusion combined with intermittent arterial occlusion in 7. Patients treated by hepatic resection and chemotherapy infusion were maintained on systemic 5 FU therapy for a
maximum period of two years. One patient who had resection of solitary lesion in
the liver had been living with no evidence of disease for over three years. None
of the patients who received systemic chemotherapy exhibited evidence of objective
response. Four of 9 patients who received chemotherapy infusion, and 4 of 7 having
a combination of arterial occlusion and chemotherapy infusion, survived for periods
ranging from 18 to 30 months. Clinical evaluation of individual patients indicated
that those having metastases confined to the liver (Stages II and III), who received
intermittent arterial occlusion and chemotherapy infusion enjoyed longer periods of
objective response and developed less complications than those treated by chemotherapy infusion alone.

Hepatic - Metastases - Colon - Cancer - Surgery - Infusion - Chemotherapy

INTRODUCTION

The liver is the commonest site for hematogenous spread from cancer of the colon
and rectum. The incidence of liver metastases in patients with malignant tumors of
the colon at the time of initial presentation ranges between 20% and 25% (Nielsen,
Balsley, Jensen, 1971; Stehlin, Hafstrom, Greeff, 1974). According to published
reports the survival time in patients with liver metastases who received no treatment varied from 5 to 11 months (Stearns, Binkley, 1954; Jaffe, and others, 1968;
Rapoport, Burleson, 1970; Flanagan, Foster, 1967). Various therapeutic modalities
have been employed in order to eradicate or retard the growth of the tumor within
the liver and hence ameliorate the patient's symptoms and prolong his life. In recent years Hepatic dearterialization and/or chemotherapy infusion have been frequently used in the treatment of patients with hepatic metastases (Almersjo, and
others, 1972; Nagasue, and others, 1976; Nagasue, and others 1977; Cady, Oberfield,
1974; Koudahl, Funding, 1972). This report describes various therapeutic approaches
that have been used in the management of patients with liver metastases from cancer
of the colon and rectum.

MATERIAL AND METHODS

During the four year period, 1973-1977, 71 (24% of a total of 293) patients who had adenocarcinoma of the colon and rectum were found to have intra-abdominal or distant metastases at the time of initial presentation. Of these 71 patients, 31 (11% of the total) had gross metastases that were confined to the liver (Table 1). This latter group provides the material for this study.

TABLE 1   Cancer of Colon and Rectum (293 Patients)

Site	No. of Patients	Distant Metastasis*	Liver Metastasis**
Colon	177	53 (30%)	23 (13%)
Rectum	116	18 (15%)	8 (7%)
Total	293	71 (24%)	31 (11%)

*Extra or Intra-abdominal Spread Including Liver
**Visceral Metastases Confined to Liver

The diagnosis and extent of the disease in these 31 patients was confirmed at laparatomy and all had palliative resection of the primary tumor. The method of staging outlined in Fig. 1 was used to group together patients with comparable extent of disease and provide a guideline in evaluating the effect of therapy (El-Domeiri, Mojab, 1978).

Stage	I	Limited to one lobe	50% of liver
Stage	II	In both lobes	50% of liver
Stage	III	One or both lobes	50% of liver
Stage	IV	A) I, II or III with diffuse cirrhosis, impaired function or ascites.	
		B) I, II or III with intra-abdominal spread to lymph nodes, other organs or peritoneum.	
		C) I, II or III with a non-resectable primary, extensive intra-abdominal spread or with extra-abdominal metastases.	

Fig. 1   Staging of liver cancer (primary and metastatic)

Treatment of the hepatic metastases consisted of wedge resection or partial hepatectomy in 2; systemic chemotherapy in 13; chemotherapy infusion of the hepatic artery in 9; and chemotherapy infusion combined with intermittent arterial occlusion in 7. Patients who had hepatic resection or chemotherapy infusion were maintained on systemic 5 FU therapy for a maximum period of 2 years. The dose and frequency of systemic chemotherapy was regulated according to the patient's tolerance. The response to treatment was evaluated by clinical examination and biochemical tests at monthly intervals. Liver scan was performed at 3 and 6 months and hepatic angiogram at 6 to 12 months intervals, in surviving patients.

TREATMENT

Surgical

Two patients who had disease confined to one lobe of the liver (Stage I) were treated by hepatic resection, with 1 having wedge excision of a solitary metastases and the second right hepatic lobectomy. Both patients received systemic 5 Fluorouracil for several months after operation.

Systemic Chemotherapy

Thirteen patients with multiple hepatic metastases (Stages II, III, and IV) received systemic chemotherapy. In 8 of these 13 patients systemic therapy was used as an alternative to intra-arterial chemotherapy infusion. Three of the remaining 5 patients had anatomic abnormalities of the hepatic arterial tree which precluded the placement of an arterial catheter. The other 2 patients had initially a hepatic artery catheter inserted intra-operatively but because of technical problems that ensued in the early postoperative period, the arterial catheter was removed before chemotherapy infusion was started. Seven patients in this group received intravenous 5 FU only. The remaining 6 patients received a combination of 5 FU and CCNU (2-Chloroethyl -3 cyclohexyl-1 nitrosourea).

Arterial Chemotherapy Infusion

Nine patients were treated by hepatic intra-arterial infusion with 5-FUDR (5 Fluorodeoxyuridine). This was accomplished by inserting a No. 14 polyvinyl catheter via the right gastroepiplois artery at laparotomy. The catheter was advanced into the hepatic artery and the tip was positioned distal to the bifurcation of the vessel. Correct positioning of the catheter was ascertained by palpation as well as by intra-operative angiogram. Continuous infusion of 5 FUDR, in doses ranging between 0.3 and 0.6 mg/Kgm/day, was carried out for an average period of 4 weeks.

Chemotherapy Infusion and Intermittent Arterial Occlusion

Seven patients were treated by a combination of chemotherapy infusion and intermittent interruption of the hepatic arterial flow (El-Domeiri, 1976). In this group an arterial catheter that has double lumen and fitted with a balloon near its tip was used for chemotherapy infusion with 1 to 1.5 cc of air. Heparine was administered intravenously prior to inflation of the balloon to prevent intra-arterial clotting. Occlusion of the artery was maintained for 45 to 60 minutes and repeated twice daily. Intermittent occlusion of the arterial flow and continuous infusion with 5 FUDR was carried out for a minimum period of three weeks.

RESULTS

Surgical

One patient having right hepatic lobectomy for 2 large metastatic nodules in the lateral aspect of the liver presented with recurrent disease 6 months after operation. The second patient, who had resection of a solitary lesion in the left lobe of the liver, had been living with no evidence of disease for 40 months.

Systemic Chemotherapy

None of the patients who received systemic chemotherapy exhibited evidence of objective response in the way of tumor regression or improvement of liver function. In this group the average length of survival in patients with Stages II and III disease was 16.5 and 10.5 months respectively.

Intra-arterial Chemotherapy

Four of 9 patients who received chemotherapy infusion, and 4 of 7 having a combination of arterial occlusion and chemotherapy infusion, survived for periods ranging between 18 and 30 months. Significant reduction of the size of the metastatic nodules was noted in subsequent hepatic scans in approximately half the patients. Marked decrease in the size of the liver and dramatic relief of pain occurred in 2 patients who presented with marked hepatomegaly. The length of survival in relation to the extent of disease in the different treatment groups is shown in Table 2.

TABLE 2   Liver Metastases from Colo-Rectal Carcinoma, Mode
of Therapy and Survival (31 Patients)

Stage	Art. Chemo + Occlusion (7)		Art. Chemo (9)		Syst. Chemo (13)	
	No.	Average Survival (Mo)	No.	Average Survival (Mo)	No.	Average Survival (Mo)
II (<50% both lobes)	2	26	2	27	4	16.5
III (>50% both lobes)	4	15	6	13.5	6	10
IV, A (Cirrhosis, Ascites)	1	5	1	6	3	5

DISCUSSION

The presence of hepatic metastases in patients with colo-rectal cancer is generally considered a sign of incurability. Nevertheless, significant palliation and prolongation of survival can be accomplished in these patients by the proper application of existing therapeutic modalities. Resection of a metastatic nodule, if feasible, is by far the most effective means of controlling the disease (Foster, 1978). The best results are achieved in patients having a small tumor volume that is confined to one lobe of the liver.

The longest survivor in this series had a solitary nodule excised from the left lobe of the liver. Wanebo, and others (1978) reported a five year survival rate of 28% in patients with solitary metastases which were resected at the time of colectomy. In contrast none of 20 patients reported by Wilson, and others (1976), who had resection of multiple tumors in the liver, survived five years.

In this series resection of the tumor was feasible in only 2 (7%) of the patients. This low incidence of resectability is comparable to that reported by other workers (Cady, Oberfield, 1974). The great majority of patients who have hepatic metastases, therefore, are treated by chemotherapy. Systemic chemotherapy, using a single or multiple cytotoxic agents, has produced little or no response and no appreciable increase in survival time (Rapoport, Burleson, 1970; Brennan, and others, 1963). Intra-arterial infusion of the liver with chemotherapy was used to deliver a high concentration of the drug directly to the tumor and hence improve the response rate. In this study a longer period of objective response and survival time was noted in

patients receiving chemotherapy infusion than in those treated by systemic chemotherapy. Similar results were reported by other workers who used arterial chemotherapy infusions (Ansfield, and others, 1971; Rochlin, Smart, 1966; Humphrey, 1973).
One study indicated that hepatic artery infusion with 5-FUDR more than doubled the
duration of survival and produced a clinical response rate of 71% of patients with
hepatic metastases from colon cancer (Cady, Oberfield, 1972).

Interruption of the arterial supply to the liver has been used as a means of de-
stroying hepatic metastases. This approach is based on the finding that the tumor
tissue receives its blood supply almost exclusively from the arterial circulation,
whereas normal liver parenchyma receives a dual blood supply (Breedis, Young, 1954;
Nilsson, and others, 1976). Hepatic dearterialization alone has not been effective
in controlling the tumor growth within the liver and has been associated with a
postoperative mortality of approximately 20% (Almersjo, and others, 1972). Hepatic
artery ligation was combined with chemotherapy infusion to potentiate the anti-tumor
effect of the post-ligation ischemic period (Fortner, and others, 1973). A major
objection to this approach, however, is that hepatic artery ligation produces throm-
bosis of the small blood vessels within the tumor, thus rendering these viable cells
inaccessible to the circulating drug.

The rationale for using intermittent occlusion of the hepatic artery is that a short
period of warm ischemia is more likely to affect the tumor cells adversely than the
normal liver parenchyma, which has a dual blood supply. With this technique, interruption of the arterial flow is complete since the time interval is too short for
the establishment of a collateral circulation. Also, the administration of heparin
during arterial occlusion preserves the integrity of the small vessels, which facilitates perfusion of the neoplasm with the cytotoxic drug with resumption of the
arterial flow. None of the patients who had intermittent occlusion of the hepatic
artery suffered from extensive liver damage nor showed evidence of deterioration of
hepatic function.

So far, the results of chemotherapy infusion alone, or a combination of infusion
and intermittent arterial occlusion, are comparable. However, clinical evaluation
of individual patients indicated that patients with metastatic disease, Stages II
and III, who had intermittent arterial occlusion and chemotherapy infusion, enjoyed
longer periods of objective response and developed less complications than those
treated by chemotherapy infusion alone. The response to therapy and survival time
in patients receiving chemotherapy infusion, or chemotherapy infusion and intermittent arterial occlusion, correlated with the extent of the tumor. Patients who had
tumor confined to the liver and normal hepatic function, tolerated the treatment
well, had a low incidence of drug related complications, and survived for a relatively long period of time.

REFERENCES

Almersjo, O., and others (1972). Evaluation of hepatic dearterialization in pri-
    mary and secondary cancer of the liver. Am. J. Surg., 104, 5-8
Ansfield, F. J., and others (1971). Intrahepatic arterial infusion with 5-fluoro-
    uracil. Cancer, 28, 1147-1151.
Breedis, C., G. Young (1954). The blood supply of neoplasms in the liver.
    Am. J. Path., 30, 969-977.
Brennan, M. J., R. W. Talley, E. H. Drake, and others (1963). 5-fluorouracil treat-
    ment of liver metastases by continuous hepatic artery infusion via cournand
    catheter. Ann. Surg., 158, 405.
Cady, B., and R. A. Oberfield (1974). Regional infusion chemotherapy of hepatic
    metastases from carcinoma of the colon. Am. J. Surg., 127, 220-227.
El-Domeiri, A. (1976). A method of intermittent occlusion and chemotherapy infusion
    of the hepatic artery. Surg. Gynecol. Obstet., 143, 107-109.

El-Domeiri, A., and K. Mojab (1978). Intermittent occlusion of the hepatic artery
    and chemotherapy infusion for carcinoma of the liver. Am. J. Surg., 135,
    771-775.
Flanagan, L., and J. H. Foster (1967). Hepatic resection for metastic cancer. Am.
    J. Surg., 113, 551-556.
Fortner, J.G., and others (1973). Treatment of primary and secondary liver cancer
    by hepatic artery ligation and infusion chemotherapy. Ann. Surg., 178, No. 2,
    162-172.
Foster, J. H. (1978). Survival after liver resection for secondary tumors. Am. J.
    Surg., 135, 389-394.
Humphrey, L. J. (1973). Prolonged intermittent arterial infusion for metastatic
    carcinoma of the liver. Am. Surg., August, 425-427.
Jaffe, B.M., and others (1968). Factors influencing survival in untreated hepatic
    metastases. Surg. Gynecol. Obstet., 127, 1-8.
Koudahl, G., and J. Funding. (1972). Hepatic artery ligation in primary and second-
    ary hepatic cancer. Acta. Chir. Scand., 138, 289-292.
Nagasue, N., and others (1976). Hepatic dearterialization for nonresectable primary
    and secondary tumors of the liver. Cancer, 38, 2593-2603.
Nagasue, N., and others (1977). Complete devascularization of hepatic lobe with
    nonresectable hepatoma. Am. J. Surg., 134, 650-655.
Nielsen, J., I. Balsley, and H. Jensen. (1971). Carcinoma of the colon with liver
    metastases. Acta. Chir. Scan., 137, 463-465.
Nilsson, A. V., and others (1967). Vascularisation of liver tumors and the effect
    of hepatic artery ligature. Bibl. Anat., 9, 425-431.
Rapoport, A. H., and R. L. Burleson (1970). Survival of patients treated with sys-
    temic fluorouracil for hepatic metastases. Surg. Gynecol. Obstet., 130,
    773-777.
Rochlin, D. B., and C. R. Smart (1966). An evaluation of 51 patients with hepatic
    artery infusion. Surg. Gynecol. Obstet., September, 535-538
Stearns, M. W., Jr., and G. E. Binkley (1954). Palliative surgery for cancer of the
    rectum and colon. Cancer, 7, 1016-1019.
Stehlin, J., L. Hafstrom, and P. J. Greeff (1974). Experience with infusion and re-
    section in cancer of the liver. Surg. Gynecol. Obstet., 138, 855-863.
Wanebo, H. J., and others (1978). Surgical management of patients with primary
    operable colorectal cancer and synchronous liver metastases. Am. J. Surg., 135
    81-85.
Wilson, S. M., and M. A. Adson (1976). Surgical treatment of hepatic metastases
    from colorectal cancers. Arch. Surg., 111, 330.

Anus and Anal Cancer

Maus W. Stearns

*Chief, Rectum and Colon Service, Memorial Sloan Kettering Cancer Center,
New York, U.S.A.*

ANAL CANCER

Anal cancer in the United States of America is a relatively infrequent tumor. The
usual malignant lesion in this region is epidermoid carcinoma. There are many
histologic variants giving rise to a profusion of terms — basaloid, cloacogenic,
muco-epidermoid, squamous, baso-squamous, transitional cell — to list the more
common. The usual treatment in the United States has been surgical resection.
Local excision has been used successfully for the peri-anal lesions which do not
invade the anal musculature. Lesions of the anal canal and lower rectum which
invade the musculature have been treated by a Miles' type of abdominoperineal resection. Prophylactic (elective) groin dissections have not been performed widely.
While therapeutic groin dissections when inguinal node metastases appear after the
primary tumour has been controlled have been quite successful, inguinal lymph-
adenectomy has rarely been curative when the inguinal nodes were present before the
primary tumor was treated.

There is great promise in combined treatment consisting of preoperative chemotherapy and radiation. This preoperative regimen has so altered the clinical
presentation that surgical resections of lesser magnitude are being considered in
many individuals. This regimen has also been extremely promising in the management
of recurrent lesions.

ANUS AND ANAL CANCER

The order of frequency of malignant tumour presenting in the anal canal is adenocarcinoma, epidermoid cardinoma and melanoma. We will not discuss adenocarcinoma
as the treatment is no different from those arising in the low rectum.

Melanoma

In our experience the prognosis of melanoma in this anatomic location is so poor
that it does not warrant a lengthy discussion. The basic reason for this poor
prognosis is that by the time these tumors cause symptoms leading to diagnosis
they are in an "advanced" stage, implying both depth of invasion and thickness of
the lesion. Fortunately, anal melanoma is relatively rare. At Memorial Sloan
Kettering Cancer Center we have a series of 49 patients as compared with a series

of 299 epidermoid carcinoma in the same anatomic site.

For many years accepted treatment of a patient with this lesion has been abdomino-perineal resection, frequently combined with abdomino-pelvic and inguinal lymph-adenectomy. We did not cure a single patient, although several lived more than five years.

At the present time my own personal approach, not necessarily shared by my colleagu is that if local excision can adequately encompass the primary tumor, I discuss alternatives and risks involved in local excision and abdomino-perineal resection. I will perform a local excision if the potential risks are acceptable to the patien If, on the other hand, they want everything possible done I will do an abdomino-perineal resection. In either course a careful follow-up should be instituted. If there is local recurrence amenable to local excision, this should be carried out. If the recurrence is extensive, then abdomino-perineal resection as a palliative procedure is usually indicated. Localized groin metastases should be excised. If painful metastases develop, particularly to bone, the pain may often be relieved by radiation therapy.

This grim outlook eventually may be altered by immunotherapy and/or chemotherapy. Currently our immunotherapists suggest injection of BCG into the tumor, or prepar-ation of vaccines derived from tissue culture of the tumor or its metastases. More effective chemotherapy hopefully will be developed.

Epidermoid Carcinoma

These tumors constituted 20% of all malignant tumors of the anal canal and distal 2 cm of the rectum seen at Memorial Sloan Kettering Cancer Center. Two hundred and ninety-nine patients with this neoplasm have been seen and treated by our Service through 1970. The evaluation of these patients provides the basis for our current management[4,5,6].

The nomenclature of these tumors has been confusing. Because of the variations in the histology of the cell type lining the anal canal, the presenting histologic variations have led to many terms: squamous, baso-squamous, transitional cell, cloacogenic, mucoepidermoid, basaloid, to mention a few. These terms have no meanir for the clinician as they are variants of epidermoid carcinoma and the clinical management is not influenced by the variant. There may be a somewhat better prog-nosis with pure "basaloid" lesions.

Clinical characteristics of these tumors are important in their management. They may be located in the distal anal canal and peri-anal skin (Figure 1). Here they may grow to considerable size without invading anal or sphincter muscles. These may be treated by local excision. However, tumors in this location do metastasize to the inguinal region. Thus the follow-up of these patients emphasizes detection of local recurrence or metastases to groin.

When the lesion is situated higher in the anal canal, comparable depth of invasion results in infiltration of sphincteric muscles quite early (Figure 2). Metastases from these lesions appear in the inguinal region or in the deep pelvic nodes. They may also metastasize into the meso-rectal nodes. Liver metastases are infrequent. For these reasons the accepted treatment of lesions with invasion of anal and sphincteric muscle has been abdominal perineal resection. Pelvic lymphadenectomy has been added in suitable good risk patients but in an obese patient it is tech-nically difficult and not very satisfactory. The regular follow-up examinations should include careful surveillance of the inguinal regions for early detection of metastases.

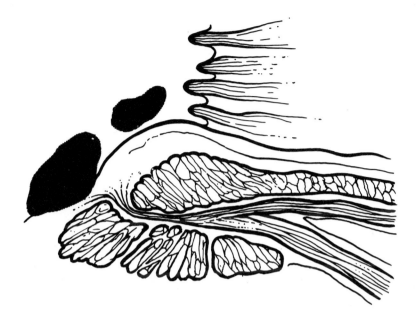

Figure 2

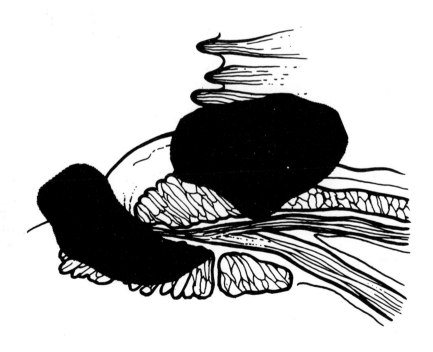

Figure 1

M. W. Stearns

Since inguinal metastases occur in up to 20% of these patients, some surgeons have advocated elective or prophylactic groin dissection. As a result of analysis of our own relevent data, which has been updated several times, we do not believe elective groin dissection is warranted. These data are contained in Tables I and II In summary, of 96 patients surgically treated 14 had groin metastases when first seen. These were all subjected to therapeutic groin dissection. None were cured, although two lived five years.

There were 82 candidates for elective bilateral radical groin dissection. No metastases developed in 61 patients. These then would not have benefited by elective dissection. In 21 groin metastases did occur. Twenty had unilateral radical groin dissection, of whom 15 lived five years, although three died later of carcinoma. Of the five who died before five years, three had multiple deep pelvic and mesenteri node metastases and probably were not salvageable. It was our conclusion that somewhat less than 10% of the potential candidates might have benefited from elective bilateral radical groin dissection. This possible benefit weighed against the morbidity associated with bilaterial radical groin dissections in the remaining 61 patients, led us to the conclusion that elective groin dissection was not justified, but therapeutic dissections were justified.

As indicated in Table III, the five-year survival following our treatment has worsened in our most recent group — 33% for patients treated surgically, as compared with 57% in those treated from 1944-1963. This appears to be attributable to the fact that for some reason patients are being referred to us with considerably more advanced disease than previously.

In view of our poor results we have adopted the program reported by Nigro and Vaitkevicius of combined preoperative radiotherapy, Mitomycin and 5'-Fluouracil, followed by surgical resection[1]. Initially we used this program for those who presented with advanced disease. The degree of regression of the lesion was so striking that we have extended its use to patients with lesions which we would previously

TABLE I

EPIDERMOID CARCINOMA '44 - '63
Groin Metastasis

Surgically treated	96
Groin metas. when first seen	14*
Candidates elective groin dis.	82
Groin metas. subsequently	21**
Groin dissection no value	61

* All had groin dissection. All DOD
   — two lived over 5 years
**One treated by x-ray only

TABLE II

EPIDERMOID CARCINOMA '44 - '63

Groin Metas - 2

Possible salvage by elect. groin	20
DOD less than 5 years	5 *
Living over 5 years	15 **
Overall 5 year survival	75%
Determinate NED	60%
Deaths possibly attributable to failure to do elective bilat rad. groin	5
or 6% of 82	

* 3 had pelvic and / or mesenteric node metas - probably not salvageable
** 3 DOD after 5 years - potentially salvageable by initial elective groin dissection

TABLE III

EPIDERMOID CANCER OF THE ANORECTUM

MSKCC, N.Y., N.Y.

Five Year Survival Rates

	Patients	Overall	Surgery
Prior to 1944	125	29 %	41 %
1944 - 1963	109	53 %	57 %
1964 - 1970	65	25 %	33 %

have treated by abdomino-perineal resection. Here again regression has been so striking that we have substituted local excision in a number of instances. While this combined approach has been of too short a duration to allow definitive evaluation, preliminary results are most encouraging[3].

This program has been more effective for recurrent lesions than any other regimen we have previously employed.

It is uncertain at this time as to the relative role of chemotherapy and radiation. Radiotherapy has not been widely used in the United States. Relatively few of our patients have been treated initially by radiation therapy for cure. However, of seven who did receive a full course of radiation, four lived five or more years without evidence of recurrence. Roentgen therapy has been more widely used in Europe as the primary treatment for epidermoid carcinoma with comparable survival. The results in selected patients reported by Papillon of combined Cobalt 60 and Curie therapy are considerably better than our series[2].

CONCLUSION

To date the treatment of melanoma of the ano-rectum has been unsatisfactory. It should be directed at wide removal of local disease. Recurrence and metastases should be resected where feasible. Additional treatment in the form of immunotherapy including vaccines and chemotherapy should be actively investigated.

Epidermoid carcinoma which is primarily peri-anal and does not involve anal canal musculature can be treated effectively by wide local excision or by well-planned radiotherapy. Treatment by either modality requires careful follow-up surveillance for local recurrence or inguinal metastases.

Invasive epidermoid carcinoma of the anal canal traditionally has been managed by abdomino-perineal resection with or without limited pelvic lymphadenectomy. It appears evident, as reported by Papillon, that selected lesions may be treated as effectively by carefully planned Curie therapy and external cobalt when these modalities and the expertise to use them are available. Following either method, follow-up surveillance for local recurrence or inguinal metastases is essential. If inguinal metastases appear, prompt inguinal dissection should be done.

Preoperative chemotherapy and radiotherapy should be tried with advanced tumors to improve the chance of operative control. The same regimen for more favorable lesions may permit excision of lesser magnitude to be substituted for abdomino-perineal resection, although this should be considered experimental at this time.

REFERENCES

1. Nigro, N.D., Vaitkevicius, V.K., Considine, B.J.   Combined therapy for cancer of the anal canal: a preliminary report. *Dis. Colon and Rectum* 17, 354 (1974).

2. Papillon, J. Radiation therapy in the management of epidermoid carcinoma of the anal region. *Dis. Colon and Rectum* 17, 181-187 (1974).

3. Quen, S.H.Q., Magill, G.B., Leaming, R.H. and Hajdu, S.I.   Multidisciplinary preoperative approach to the management of epidermoid carcinoma of the anus and anorectum. *Dis. Colon and Rectum* 21, 89-91 (1978).

4. Stearns, M.W., Jr. Epidermoid carcinoma of the anal region: Inguinal metastases. *Amer. J. Surg.* 90, 727-733 (1955).

5. Stearns, M.W., Jr. Epidermoid carcinoma of the anal canal. *Surg., Gyn. and Obst.* 106, 92–96 (1958).

6. Stearns, M.W., Jr. and Quan, S.H.Q. Epidermoid carcinoma of the anorectum. *Surg., Gyn and Obst.* 131, 953–957 (1970).

Pancreatic and Liver Tumors

Epidemiology of Liver Cancer

C. A. Linsell

International Agency for Research on Cancer, Lyon, France

ABSTRACT

Of the two types of primary liver cancer, one arising from the liver cells and the other from cells lining the bile ducts, only the former will be considered, as research on this cell type has advanced markedly in recent years. The global incidence and aetiological factors of liver cell cancer will be reviewed. Particular attention will be paid to the possible role of aflatoxin and hepatitis, including the prospects for primary prevention.

Key Words: Liver cell cancer; Epidemiology; Aflatoxin; Hepatitis.

The global pattern of the incidence of this cancer is still to a large extent incomplete, as the areas of high incidence are found in Africa and the Far East and it was only recently that cancer registries there have offered reliable data for comparison with reports from Europe and North America. Research on liver cell cancer has advanced markedly in recent years, particularly with regard to aetiology, and this may lead one to wonder whether primary prevention may be a practical possibility.

The exact definition of liver cell cancer for use in epidemiological studies has presented many difficulties, as the precise definitions used by histologists are rarely reflected in the collection of morbidity and mortality data; and even at the histological level the difficulties are often made worse by the acinar or adenoid type of liver cell cancer being classified as mixed liver cell and bile duct cell cancers. To aid standardization the World Health Organization has established an internationally accepted histological classification of tumours and the publication on the classification of liver tumours is in press. Using this, it is hoped that a more precise histological identification of tumours on a global basis may be possible. This is essential, as there is consistent evidence that liver tumours of different cell types have differing aetiologies.

The cancer is more frequent in developing countries where it is difficult to collect accurate data, as the range of medical care is often uneven and a low autopsy rate is usual. However, one can be more confident about a frequent occurrence than be certain that a reported scarcity is accurate. Where the cancer is reported as rare in technically developed countries, medical facilities and cancer registration are of course more sophisticated. The frequency of this cancer is generally considered to be low in Europe, North America and Japan (see Table 1). There are exceptions in countries, such as Switzerland, with well developed services, but it is thought that this is a relatively recent phenomenon and probably based on the improved treatment and longer survival of cirrhotics.   It appears that the remarkable incidence reported from Mozambique has not been maintained since the reports in the early 1960s and, in fact, evidence from hospitals in South Africa treating mainly gold miners from Mozambique shows that the incidence is decreasing there, as indeed it is in most parts of southern Africa.

The high frequency in the Far East appears to have been maintained and, in fact, if preliminary reports from China, Philippines and Indonesia, very populous areas, are confirmed, liver cancer may be one of the most frequent human cancers in the world.

Males are much more prone to develop liver cell cancer than females, particularly in areas of high incidence where too the patients present at an earlier age.

Those of African or Asian descent who emigrate to countries of lower incidence tend to acquire the risk for liver cancer of their adopted country.   In Singapore it was at one time felt that there was a higher risk among China-born Chinese than among Singapore-born Chinese, but more recent studies have shown no relation between cancer frequencies, birth in Singapore, the duration of residence in Singapore, the province of birth in China, or indeed between different Chinese dialect groups.   In Hawaii, however, the risk for Chinese immigrants appears to be even lower than among the indigenous Hawaiians, whereas among the Japanese it appears to have increased.   On the other hand, Europeans who leave areas of low incidence for those where the tumour is common, such as in southern Africa, appear to retain their low rate.   It is suggested that those migrating from a high to a low incidence area usually adopt much of their new environment, whereas the European migrants have taken most of their habits and customs with them to Africa. An evaluation of all this evidence points to environmental factors rather than to racial or genetic predisposition.

In Latin America cancer registration and relative frequency studies indicate a low incidence in this continent.

A number of diseases have been associated with the aetiology of liver cancer.   It appeared likely that infantile malnutrition and its effects on the liver were involved in the induction of cirrhosis and cancer when the protein calorie deficiency liver disease was first examined by pathologists.   However, an almost complete recovery of the liver after these insults in infancy has been demonstrated, and the lack of an increased frequency of liver cancer in countries such as India, where malnutrition is as great a problem as it is in Africa, have enabled us to exclude this as a major factor in the aetiology of cancer.   For many years bile duct cancer has been associated with distomiasis, the commonest species affecting man being Clonorchis sinensis.   However, with this particular cancer an association with cirrhosis is rare, and the sex and age distribution differ markedly from the liver cell type.   Bilharzia is also common in areas of Africa with a high frequency of the cancer and the parasites do indeed cause impressive 'pipestem' fibrosis in the liver.   A low risk for liver cancer in Egypt, where bilharzia infection is so common, again excludes this as a major aetiological factor.

There is a marked association of cirrhosis and liver cancer, but much still needs to be learned about the sequence of events leading to these conditions.   The main facts of this complex story can be summarized as follows:

1.   Liver cell cancer is usually associated with cirrhosis worldwide.

2.   There is still some doubt that the incidence of liver cell cancer without unequivocal cirrhosis parallels an increased frequency of the cancer.   In

Uganda and Rhodesia this does not appear to be so, whereas in South Africa, where a high frequency has been reported, 40% of liver cell cancers show no signs of cirrhosis.

3.   The macronodular type of cirrhosis is the one usually associated with this cancer, and this is the type which is anyway found more commonly in areas of high and medium incidence of the cancer.   This is the so-called nutritional, or post-hepatic, cirrhosis which now has a close relationship with hepatitis B infection.

4.   Other diseases, such as hepatitis, are common in areas of medium and high incidence, but there are countries such as Egypt where we think that a high incidence of hepatitis is not paralleled by an increased risk for liver cancer.

The possibility that chemicals and viruses might be involved in this cancer was suggested 20 years ago and it is these which remain the principal aetiological candidates.

Of the long list of chemicals which produce liver cancer in animals, we can extract those to which man is exposed, as opposed to those which are purely laboratory carcinogens, and when we do this, one group of chemicals, the mycotoxins, now implicated both by experimental and epidemiological evidence, stand out as the prime suspects.   The mycotoxins which have attracted most attention are the afla-toxins.   They came into prominence following the death of a large number of poul-try in Britain in 1966.   The so-called Turkey X Disease was traced to mould con-tamination of South American peanuts, as indeed was the death of trout from liver cancer in California.   The fungi responsible and the toxins they produce and analytical methods for their estimation were soon established.   The fungi which are known to give rise to the aflatoxins are found worldwide, and are most likely to invade cereals and nuts during storage.   The production of aflatoxin depends on the micro-climate surrounding and within the cereals and it is critically related to humidity.

Many commodities were examined for the aflatoxins and it was soon realized that they represented a global problem, particularly in the humid tropics.   The toxic and carcinogenic properties were studied in a wide range of animals and marked differences in species susceptibility were detected.   Males were more generally sensitive than females, as indeed were new-born and young animals.   Although it was soon realized that the aflatoxins were probably the most potent hepatocarcinogens known to the experimentalists, it required six years feeding to produce unequivocal liver tumours in monkeys.   While all this experimental work was going on, field studies were established to assess the relationship with human liver cell cancer and early studies showed a correlation between the contamination of food available to African and Asian farmers and the frequency of the cancer.   It was then shown that these levels of contamination did not necessarily correspond to those found in food ready for ingestion, as housewife selection of foodstuffs by rejecting obviously damaged material greatly reduces the level of the aflatoxins in food.   The field studies which compare the analysis of food ready for ingestion in Africa and Asia are shown in Table 2.   The association demonstrated by these studies is con-sidered to be sufficiently strong to justify the consideration of an intervention programme aimed at lowering the aflatoxin exposure and observing the trend of liver cancer incidence.   The basis of this programme would be the improvement of harvesting, drying and storage.   Much will be learnt, even at an early stage of such studies, about the methods of achieving this in developing countries.   These studies will not only act as a definitive epidemiological proof, but will, even if negative, improve local agricultural practices.   Such intervention programmes are planned, and it is hoped will soon be under way, but as the latent period of the induction of cancer is unknown, a number of years must elapse before we can obtain the final proof of causality.

It has been suspected for many years that viral hepatitis might be associated with the type of cirrhosis frequently seen with liver cancer in high incidence areas, and the discovery of the hepatitis B antigens gave us the means to assess the association, at least with one type of hepatitis. Several case control studies have indeed demonstrated an association, which is specific for the active infection with hepatitis B virus when this is defined as the presence of hepatitis B surface antigen with or without antibodies to the surface antigen, or by the presence of antibody to the core antigen. The four studies illustrated in Table 3 and 4 were selected because the control populations are representative. Few risk factors associated with human cancer give relative risks of this magnitude, heavy smoking and lung cancer being only 10. That this association, besides being strong, is also specific is suggested by the lack of association of HBV with other cancers and with metastatic liver cancer. Table 5 shows that when a mother is a carrier of hepatitis B the relative risk for the offspring is 15 and when the father does not have anti-HBS the relative risk for liver cell cancer is 59. These data suggest that the maternal transmission of hepatitis B may be a factor in the development of the cancer and that there may be an additional factor which affects the immunological response to the virus of the fathers of patients with this cancer.

We now have two agents, one chemical and the other viral, associated with liver cell cancer and we must now consider the complex interplay between these factors, always bearing in mind that these may not indeed be the only ones.

The evidence for the involvement of aflatoxin is at present based on a group or population association and can be considered merely a refinement of the general statement that the cancer is more common when a mycotoxin contamination is more likely. We have no evidence on individual exposure or dose response in man, although the general characteristics of the evidence from field studies is compatible with experimental evidence in animals. For example, the algebraic expression of the values in Table 2 is similar to that in dose response experiments in rats. We need refined techniques to detect small quantities of mycotoxins in biological fluid and work is going on in this field. We have of course the problem, as with all suspect dietary carcinogens, that ingestion may precede the cancer by many years. However, in the populations which we have studied, diets are simpler and more stable than perhaps in the so-called developed countries. The intervention studies I have mentioned may offer reliable confirmation of our hypothesis provided we can be confident of the assessment of the involvement of the hepatitis B virus.

The prospects of prevention of the viral component of the aetiology may be even more difficult. If we assume that perinatal infection is the vital issue, we can treat the expectant mother, the carrier of the virus, protect the baby at birth, and treat at the same time horizontal contacts if they have no antibodies to the virus. Studies are proceeding along these lines. The production of vaccines is under way and although the direct part they may play in cancer prevention is far from clear, as the rate of natural infection is so high in Africa and Asia, they will be useful to protect those at high risk in hospital treatment units. So again our intervention, if not effective as a preventive measure against cancer, may well be so against a virulent, often severe, infectious disease. Another line of investigation which will provide valuable information is the following of cohorts of carriers to assess their risk for liver disease and cancer. These are again long term studies, but we know that some are already in operation and I am sure carriers are being followed in many parts of the world.

I would like to summarize the most important gaps in our knowledge at the present time and indicate some ways in which we may try to fill these.

1. The introduction of a universally accepted nomenclature and classification will

greatly aid future registration of cases of this disease, and we may avoid some of the errors of earlier studies. Reports from Africa in the 1950s that both bile duct cell cancer and liver cell cancer were increased were based erroneously on the assumption that the adenoid type of liver cancer was derived from the bile duct cells. The classification of cirrhosis has itself, apart from an association with liver cancer, also had a confused history and there is still a plethora of individual classifications. Recent reviews, however, concentrating on simplicity of criteria, should prove most helpful.

2. The definition of the problem as a global one still has many deficiencies. More detailed national and regional data will allow us not only to pinpoint more accurately areas of high and low incidence, but allow us to proceed to analytical studies on a firm basis. Cancer registration of a high standard will certainly be necessary to monitor the benefits of any preventive measures.

3. We have discussed in some detail the possible role of the aflatoxins and hepatitis in the aetiology of the disease. With regard to the former it is now considered appropriate to proceed to primary prevention by trying to remove these hazards from the environment and assess the trend of cancer rates. If the order of magnitude of the decrease is significant and we can be sure that there are not major biases, then this will be strong evidence of a causal nature. It was not until the demonstration of a fall in risk among British doctors who stopped smoking was observed, that we could speak of cigarettes as a cause of, rather than association with, lung cancer. Even strong associations have to be viewed in the light of biological likelihood of cause and effect. Here for aflatoxin we appear to be on strong ground, as experimental evidence provides us with information on the metabolism and cellular biology which makes aflatoxin a good candidate as a human carcinogen. The recent studies which have been possible, using the hepatitis B marker, have reinforced the possible sequence of events of chronic hepatitis, cirrhosis and cancer, which were suggested many years ago, and this certainly appears an important aetiological factor, particularly for cancers occurring in areas of low incidence, such as North America and Europe. The elucidation of the interaction, if it exists, of these two factors, both common in areas of high incidence, is likely to be complex, but with the sophisticated techniques now available in both spheres, a reappraisal or a repetition of early studies may be required. We may recall that both the aflatoxin and hepatitis hypotheses arose from work unrelated to human cancer; the former from disasters in animal husbandry followed by extensive laboratory experimentation, and the latter from genetic studies in Australia and Polynesia. In fact, as you know, the hepatitis B antigens were known as the Australian antigens, as they were detected initially in Australian indigenous peoples. There may still be unidentified factors, and we must be prepared to continue to monitor the whole field of biological research and, in particular, experimental research on animal liver cancer, to characterize these.

4. We do not seem to have biological markers which can currently be recommended as mass screening techniques for liver cancer. Even the alpha-fetoprotein estimations, which are so helpful in diagnosis, and perhaps in the early diagnosis of liver cancer in established liver disease, have not been successfully applied to mass screening. Again, the whole principle of secondary prevention is complex, particularly as we are dealing with a cancer which, if the experience in South Africa is general, may be of very rapid onset.

I would suggest, therefore, that liver cancer, perhaps one of the most frequent cancers in global terms, may present unique opportunities for research and that indeed possibilities for prevention may exist.

C. A. Linsell

TABLE 1   Incidence of Primary Liver Cancer
          in Selected Countries - Annual age
          standardized rates per 100 000
          population

Site	Males	Females
Lourenço Marques, Mozambique	103.8	30.8
Bulawayo, S. Rhodesia	47.5	34.2
Singapore (Chinese)	33.5	7.8
Dakar, Cap Vert, Senegal	24.5	10.0
Hawaii, USA, (Hawaiians)	15.2	4.0
Singapore (Malay)	14.4	6.6
Singapore (Indian)	11.2	6.5
Geneva, Switzerland	9.7	1.3
Alameda, California, USA (blacks)	8.8	1.2
Romania	5.7	4.8
Alameda, California, USA (whites)	2.4	0.6
S.W. Region, United Kingdom	1.7	0.6

TABLE 2   Summary of Available Data on Aflatoxin Ingestion
          Levels and Primary Liver Cancer Incidence in
          Adults

Country	Area	Aflatoxin	Liver Cancer	
		Estimated average daily intake in adults: ng/kg body weight/day*	No. of cases	Incidence per 10^5 of total population/ year
Kenya	High altitude	3.5	4	1.2
Thailand	Songkhla	5.0	2	2.0
Swaziland	High veld	5.1	11	2.2
Kenya	Middle altitude	5.9	33	2.5
Swaziland	Mid-veld	8.9	29	3.8
Kenya	Low altitude	10.0	49	4.0
Swaziland	Lebombo	15.4	4	4.3
Thailand	Ratburi	45.0	6	6.0
Swaziland	Low veld	43.1	42	9.2
Mozambique	Inhambane	222.4	460	13.0**

*Excludes any aflatoxin present in native beers

**Revised incidence estimate taken from Van Rensburg

TABLE 3 Association Between Hepatitis B Virus (HBV)
Infection and Primary Liver Cancer (PLC)

Country	No. of patients		Present or past HBV infection*		Active HBV infection**		
	PLC	Control	PLC %	Control %	PLC %	Control %	RR
Greece[1]	80	206	80.0	57.3	48.8	9.2	11.3
Zambia[2]	19	40	100.0	62.5	68.4	12.5	15.2
Uganda[2]	47	50	93.6	76.0	72.3	8.0	30.1
USA[2]	27	200	74.1	5.0	40.7	1.0	68.1

*Positive for one or more HBV marker
**Positive for HBsAg (with or without anti-HBS) or for anti-HBc (without anti-HBs)

[1]Trichopoulos and others, (in press)
[2]Tabor and others, 1977.

TABLE 4 Association between Hepatitis B surface antigen
(HBsAg) and Primary Liver Cancer (PLC)

Country	No. of patients		Presence of HBsAg or Anti-HBsAg		Presence of HBsAg		
	PLC	Control	PLC %	Control %	PLC %	Control %	RR
Senegal[1]	165	328	79.4	53.4	61.2	11.3	12.4
S.Africa[2]	158	200	72.9	42.4	59.5	9.0	14.9
Kenya[3]	42	450	59.5	28.7	54.8	4.7	24.7
Japan[3]	215	10738	42.3	21.2	36.7	2.7	20.6

[1]Prince and others, 1975
[2]Macnab and others, 1976
[3]Nishioka and others, 1975

TABLE 5 Hepatitis B virus (HBV) Infection in the Parents
of Liver Cancer and Control Patients

	Mothers			Fathers		
	PLC	Control	RR	PLC	Control	RR
Total No.	28	28		27	27	
Positive for HBsAg (%)	71.4	14.3	15	18.5	18.5	
Positive for Anti-HBsAg (%)	19.7	53.6		0	48.1	59
Present or past HBV infection	75.0	67.9		18.5	66.6	

Larouze and others, 1976

Larouzé, B., Blumberg, B.S., London, W.T., Lustbader, E.D., Sankalé, M. and Payet, M
    (1977). Forecasting the development of primary hepatocellular carcinoma by the
    use of risk factors: Studies in West Africa.   J. natl Cancer Inst., 58,
    1557-1561.
Macnab, G.M., Urbanowicz, J.M., Geddes, E.W. and Kew, M.C. (1976). Hepatitis-B
    surface antigen and antibody in Bantu patients with primary hepatocellular
    cancer. Br. J. Cancer, 33, 544-548.
Nishioka, K., Levin, A.G. and Simons, M.J. (1975). Hepatitis B antigen, antigen
    subtypes, and hepatitis B antibody in normal subjects and patients with liver
    disease.   Bull. Wld Hlth Org., 52, 293-300.
Prince, A.M., Szmuness, W., Michon, J., Demaille, J., Diebolt, G., Linhard, J.,
    Quenum, C. and Sankalé, M. (1975). A case/control study of the association
    between primary liver cancer and hepatitis B infection in Senegal. Int. J.
    Cancer, 16, 376-383.
Tabor, E., Gerety, R.J., Vogel, C.L., Bayley, A.C., Anthony, P.P., Chan, C.H. and
    Barker, L.F. (1977). Hepatitis B virus infection and primary hepatocellular
    carcinoma. J. natl Cancer Inst., 58, 1197-1200.
Trichopoulos, D., Tabor, E., Gerety, R.J., Xirouchaki, E., Sparros, L., Muñoz, N.
    and Linsell, C.A. (1978). Evidence of a causal relationship between Hepatitis
    B virus and primary hepatic carcinoma in a European population. (In press).

Liver and Pancreatic Tumours, Liver Tumours - Oncogenesis

M. J. Simons* and S. H. Chan**

**Immuno-Diagnostic Centre, 20 Collins Street, Melbourne, Victoria, Australia
and Immunology (Pathology) Laboratories, 19 Tanglin Road, Singapore 10,
Republic of Singapore
**Department of Microbiology and WHO Immunology Research and Training
Centre, Faculty of Medicine, University of Singapore, Republic of Singapore*

ABSTRACT

Epidemiological and serological studies have revealed that aflatoxin ingestion and exposure to hepatitis B virus (HBV) are risk factors for hepatocellular carcinoma (HCC). Several questions concerning aflatoxin intake, HBV infection and their possible interaction as cofactors cannot be resolved in the absence of in vitro cell culture systems or experimental animal models. However, some information of an immunological and a molecular biological nature is emerging which is relevant to the possible oncogenic role of HBV. Whether HBV genome is present in tumour cells as required by a direct oncogenic hypothesis can be tested by DNA hybridization studies. HBV immune subgroups based on the presence or absence of surface antigen and antibody have been identified. The occurrence of HB_s antigenaemia is thought to reflect an immunodeficiency to HBV infection. The relative risk for HCC associated with the non-immune subgroup HB_s antigenemic patients (sAg+/sAb-) was two-three fold higher than that of the total HB_sAg positive group (approximately 22 and 9 respectively). This suggests that immunodeficiency to HBV is a high risk factor for HCC. HLA patterns of Singapore Chinese HCC patients reveal differences between patients, normals and other Chinese subjects with the HLA-associated nasopharyngeal carcinoma, as well as differences between HB_sAg positive and HB_sAg negative subgroups. These preliminary findings are consistent with the hypothesis of an HLA-genetically influenced immunodeficiency to HBV underlying the development of HCC in at least some patients. If the immunogenetic-immunovirologic strategy for HCC case-control studies is extended to include aflatoxin exposure it should be possible to establish whether the risk for HCC accompanying aflatoxin intake is interrelated with, or is independent of, the risk associated with HBV infection. Intervention studies for lowering aflatoxin intake that take account of HBV immune status may also provide information on any cofactor effect.

KEYWORDS

Liver tumours - oncogenesis - aflatoxin - hepatitis B virus - HBV immunity - HLA genetics.

ONCOGENESIS OF LIVER TUMOURS

A discussion of the oncogenesis of human liver tumours can only begin if factors
have been identified which are associated with risk for tumour development. In
the case of hepatocellular carcinoma, aflatoxin ingestion and exposure to hepatitis
B virus (HBV) have been identified as risk factors. Epidemiological data relating
HCC to aflatoxin intake will have been discussed by Dr. Linsell in the previous
paper (see also Peers and Linsell, 1973; Linsell, 1977). Evidence for a relation
between HBV infection and HCC, and proposals for an aetiological basis to the
association have been the subject of numerous meetings and publications (eg.
Cameron, Linsell and Warwick, 1976; Okuda and Peters, 1976; Shanmugaratnam, Nambiar,
Tan and Chan, 1976; Zuckerman, 1977; Shikata, 1977). By striking contrast, very
little attention has been given to the possible interaction of chemical and viral
mechanisms. In view of the limited knowledge concerning cellular and subcellular
events following HBV infection and aflatoxin assimilation it may be premature to
expect answers to questions such as the following:

1.   Can aflatoxin induce those changes which lead to HCC in the absence of
     HBV infection?

2.   Is the sequence of events leading to malignancy accelerated by HBV
     infection?

3.   Conversely, can HBV infection set the stage for HCC development in the
     absence of toxic liver damage?

4.   Does aflatoxin-induced damage promote any oncogenic potential of HBV?

5.   Is it HBV infection per se, or chronicity of infection that predisposes
     to HCC development?

6.   Does some form of immunodeficiency underlie chronicity of HBV infection
     through a failure of immune-associated mechanisms which normally terminate
     acute hepatocellular infection?

7.   Are genetic factors involved in any immunodeficiency-based chronicity?

8.   What environmental events around the time of primary HBV infection
     precipitate any immunogenetic predisposition to immunodeficiency, or
     result in progression of infection to chronicity, irrespective of
     genotype?

9.   Is the time sequence of exposure to HBV and aflatoxin ingestion important
     in any cofactor process which may lead to HCC?

10. What is the molecular basis of any cofactor process, and what determines
     whether the interactive effect results in HCC?

At the present time there is no established in vitro system for cell culture of HBV
and hence no means of assessing any cell-transforming properties of the virus.
Similarly, there is at present no experimental animal model in which HCC can be
regularly induced by HBV. Thus it is not presently possible to answer questions 1
to 4, 9 and 10. However, there are two areas where some comment is possible.
Firstly, some information of an immunological and a molecular biological nature is
emerging which is relevant to the possible role of HBV infection in HCC. Secondly,
in the absence of an in vitro cell culture systems and experimental animal models,

some clues about the oncogenesis of HCC may be obtained from carefully designed studies of populations selected on the basis of the three major variables of HCC incidence, HBV infection rates and aflatoxin intake amounts.

1.   ROLE OF HBV IN HCC

Seroepidemiological studies of markers of HBV infection, including surface antigen (HB_sAg), antibody to HB_sAg (HB_sAb), antibody to core antigen (HB_sAg), e antigen (HBe) and antibody to HBe (HBeAb) have established that, in general, HCC patients have a higher frequency of exposure to HBV, and a higher frequency of HB_sAg. (Nishioka, Levin and Simons, 1975).

Geographical differences have been observed in that the endemicity of HBV infections amongst certain tropical African peoples results in almost 100% exposure. Using the same markers, exposure rates are of the order of 60-80% in many Asian tropical populations. Nevertheless, in high incidence populations in both tropical zones, the relative increase in HB_sAg frequency in HCC patients is similar, being 6-7 times higher than controls (eg. HCC patients 60-70%, controls 10%). The reason why serum titres tend to be lower in Asian populations is not clear. Among HCC patients living in temperate zone countries HBV exposure rates are lower and HB_sAg frequencies in normal subjects in these populations is in the range of 0.1% to 1% so, although HBV infection does not appear to be as common a characteristic in temperate country HCC patients, the risk for HCC associated with HB_s antigenaemia is 10-100 fold greater than where HBV is ubiquitous and infection endemic. Strictly, the use of the term "risk" for HCC development implies that HB_s antigenaemia exists prior to HCC, that there is a progression from chronic HBV infection manifesting as HB_s antigenaemia to HCC, and that HCC patients with HB_s antigaemia arise from those individuals with chronic HB_s antigenaemia. In addition to suggestive circumstantial evidence that HB_sAg positivity is associated with pre-malignant states such as macronodular cirrhosis, prospective studies are confirming that at least in some patients the presence of HB_sAg precedes the onset of clinical HCC by several years.

The introduction of more sensitive assays of markers of HBV infection has resulted in the detection of higher rates of HBV exposure. In order to characterize HCC patients into those in whom HBV infection has occurred and those in whom no evidence of infection can be detected it will be necessary to use even more sensitive and direct tests. Molecular biological approaches to the detection of viral DNA integrated into the genome of infected cells can be expected to reduce the size of the subgroup of "no detectable HBV serological markers" and hence define more precisely, albiet by exclusion, those patients in whom a role for risk factors other than HBV should be sought.

DNA hybridization studies are beginning to be applied to the question of whether any oncogenic role of HBV is direct or indirect. A direct role is more likely to involve viral genomic integration. Using liver tissue, Lutwick and Robinson (1977) have reported evidence consistent with viral DNA being integrated into host DNA. Continuation of these studies can be expected to answer the question of whether HBV genome is present in the malignant cells of HCC.

The hypothesis of a direct oncogenic role for HBV would seem to require malignant transformation of infected cells and therefore require the presence of HBV genome in tumour cells. It should be noted that the presence of HBV genome may be

necessary but not sufficient for a direct oncogenic effect. Other genetic phen-
omena, including activation of latent C-type RNA viral genes, may also be required
for hepatocyte transformation.

By contrast to a direct oncogenic hypothesis, the presence of viral genome in
tumour cells is not a necessary requirement for an indirect action hypothesis since
the malignant cells may arise as a result of chronic HBV infection but not from
infected cells per se. A major question that this hypothesis raises is why some
individuals fail to terminate acute HBV infection and eventually suffer with HCC
as a consequence of protracted infection. Based on the demonstration that the
majority of asymptomatic Singapore Chinese, Malay and Indians who were found to be
positive HB_sAg also had HB_sAb in their serum, detectable by counterelectrophoretic
radioimmunoassay screen, called radioelectrocomplexing (REC), my colleagues and I
have proposed that the immunodeficiency underlying chronic infection may involve
persisting HB_sAg/HB_sAb immune complexaemia. (Simons, Yu and Shanmugaratnam, 1973,
1975, 1976). Although the deficiency is frequently described as immunological
tolerance, in the sense of immunological unresponsiveness, this cannot be the case
since the presence of HB_sAb reflects some degree of immune response. The presence
of specific immune complexes in HB_sAg positive patients with acute hepatitis B
infection was an early observation by several groups. However, our claim that
HB_sAg/HB_sAb immune complexes was a common feature of the chronic carrier state has
had a slower acceptance. Using REC, four immune subgroups of HBV can be identified
based on HB surface antigen and antibody.

Of relevance to the oncogenesis of HCC was the finding that the proportion of
HB_sAg positive HCC patients who lacked HB_sAb detectable by REC was much higher
than in asymptomatic carriers. In the first study (Simons, Yu and Shanmugaratnam,
1975), a minimum of 113 (75%) of 150 HB_sAg positive Chinese blood donors had HB_sAb,
while only 19 (37%) of 51 HCC patients had specific immune complexes. The proportion of those subjects in the total normal and HCC groups who were HB_sAg positive,
but lacked detectable HB_sAb was 37 (2%) of 1875 and 32 (27%) of 117 respectively.

The relative risk for HCC associated with the "non immune antigenaemic" subgroup
(Ag+/Ab-) was three-fold higher than that of the total group of HB_sAg positives,
being 22.4 and 8.9 respectively. A second study confirmed these results (Simons,
Yu and Shanmugaratnam, 1976). One interpretation of these observations is that
the immunodeficiency state may involve an inability to produce high avidity
HB_sAb. If so, there may be abnormalities of T and B lymphocyte function including
alteration of T-B lymphocyte interactions. This possibility is of interest
because the regulation of immune responses conferred in mice by H2 gene products,
and presumably also in man by HLA gene products, appears to occur at the level of
lymphoid cell interaction and T lymphocyte subset activation. By HLA typing of HCC
cases and controls, and by comparing HLA patterns between HBV immune subgroups as
well as between patients and controls, HLA differences may be recognized. Preliminary results presented later in this paper indicate that HLA differences do
exist.

The differences in risk for HCC associated with the HBV immune subgroups provides
an answer to question 5. It is the mode of immune response following exposure to
HBV that is important. There is evidence to suggest that a major route of
infection is maternal transmission to newborn babies. If the mother is HBe
antigen positive there is greater likelihood that infection will ensue and
chronicity follow. However, if mother has HBeAb, transmission is less likely to

HBV IMMUNE STATUS SUBGROUPS OF
SINGAPORE CHINESE BLOOD DONORS AND HCC PATIENTS

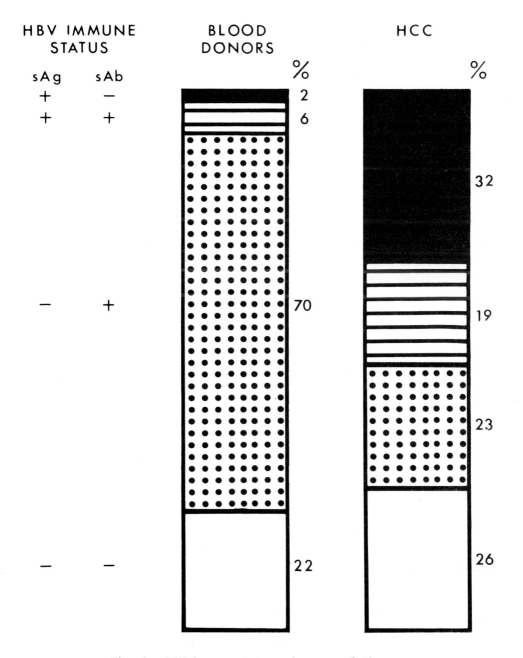

Fig. 1.   HBV immune status subgroups of Singapore
Chinese blood donors and HCC patients.

occur. It has been established that $HB_s Ab$ protects against re-infection. However, 10-30% of HCC patients appear to have only $HB_s Ab$, although the existence of anti-body excess soluble complexes, while unlikely, has not been rigorously excluded. Are these patients immune in that they do not have chronic HBV infection? Have they recently converted from $HB_s Ag$ positivity, or can chronic infection continue despite the presence of $HB_s Ab$ unassociated with $HB_s Ag$?

Clues about immune processes may also be gleaned from studies of those liver diseases which do not proceed to HCC. There is no evidence of hepatitis A virus (HAV) infection proceeding to chronicity and no suggestion of an oncogenic role for HAV. Malignancy is a very uncommon complicstion of the autoimmune form of chronic active hepatitis (CAH). Perhaps CAH represents the other end of the spectrum from immunodeficiency-based chronic HBV hepatitis in that immune responses are over-reactive leading to autoimmunopathy. However, the immune hyperresponder state may provide increased resistance to HCC development. The possible assoc-iation of CAH with the HLA 1, 8 haplotype (Mackay and Morris, 1972) provokes the thought that those HCC patients who have $HB_s Ag$, and particularly those who lack $HB_s Ab$, may have a lower frequency of commonly occurring haplotypes such as A1, B8; A2, B12 and A3, B7.

2.   APPROACHES TO UNDERSTANDING ONCOGENIC MECHANISMS IN HCC

2.1   In vitro culture assays and in vivo experimental models.
A complete understanding of oncogenic mechanisms will have to await the development of in vitro cell culture assay systems and of animal models of HBV and aflatoxin-associated hepatocarcinogenesis. At this stage it is not clear whether there is a cofactor effect. If there is, the epidemiological evidence that HBV infection commonly occurs in the new-born period would favour the view that establishment of infection precedes exposure to aflatoxin. Perhaps the increased rate of hepatocyte turnover increases susceptibility to carcinogenic action of agents like aflatoxin (Craddock, 1976), and other toxic materials such as alcohol and iron in haemachromatosis. (Anthony, 1977). There seems to be a paucity of models of liver carcinogenesis interrelating viral infection and chemical irritation.

2.2   Intervention studies.
The case for an intervention study directed to lowering aflatoxin intake has been advocated by Peers and Linsell (1977). In relation to HBV infection, subunit vaccines are being prepared and evaluated. If clinical trials are not already taking place, they soon will be. The task is now to design studies that will enable the effect of vaccination on acute infection and chronic liver disease rates to be assessed, and any change in HCC incidence to be recognized. If both chemical and viral intervention approaches were undertaken in a population of high HCC incidence it should be possible to obtain information pertaining to questions 1 to 4 and 9 and 10.

2.3   HCC case-control studies
Whether the risk for HCC accompanying aflatoxin intake is interrelated with, or is independent of, the risk related to HBV infection can also be investigated by HCC case-control studies. The strategy is to diminish the heterogeneity of patients with risk factors that have already been identified and then to compare the patterns of distribution of factors

within the subgroups by multifactorial discriminant analyses. Our experience has been with an immunogenetic-immunovirologic strategy for analysis
of the possible relation between HLA genetic type, immune responsiveness
following exposure to HBV, and development of HCC. We have established
that HLA genes A2 and BW46, and also AW19 and B17, occur as pairs more
commonly than expected among Chinese. (Simons and colleagues, 1978b). They
are equivalent to caucasian haplotype pairs A1, B8 (mentioned previously in
connection with chronic active hepatitis), A2, B12 and A3, B7. At the time
of the first report on HLA and HCC in Chinese (Simons and colleagues, 1978a),
the 29 patients studied were too few to subgroup. No differences in A2,
Sin2 or in AW19, B17 frequencies were evident. However, there was evidence
of an altered pattern of A locus gene frequencies, due mainly to an
increased frequency of A9. To date, 79 patients have been studied, including the original 29. Forty-two (42) patients were positive for HB_sAg by

RIA, leaving 37 patients in whom HB_sAg was not detected. These two sub-

groups were further subdivided into AFP positive by immunodiffusion
(ID- >1000 ng/ml), AFP positive by RIA (>10 ng/ml) and no AFP detectable
by RIA. The previously reported association of HB_sAg positivity and

elevated AFP level in Singapore Chinese patients (Simons, 1973) was again
confirmed (by ID, 30 (71%) of 42 and 14 (38%) of 37; by RIA, 38 (90%) of
42 and 22 (59%) of 37; $\chi^2 \doteq 9$ and 10.4 respectively).

The HLA results are of interest in that three approaches indicated differences in
HLA pattern between HCC patients who were HB_sAg positive and those who lacked

HB_sAg. Table 1 shows the distribution of the two patient subgroups according to

the number of detected HLA antigens.

TABLE 1   Frequencies (%) of Detectable HLA Antigens in HCC
          patients subgrouped according to HB_sAg status

		HLA antigens				
		0	1	2	3	4
Normal subjects (389)		0	0	6	36	58
HCC (79)	sAg+ (43)	0	0	0	33	62
	sAg- (37)	0	0	5	52	43

Comparing HCC subgroups for 4 and <4 HLA antigens;
$\chi^2 = 4.4$; p <0.05

It can be seen that the sAg+ subgroup has a frequency distribution of detectable
HLA antigens similar to that of normal subjects. By contrast, HCC patients lacking HB_sAg appear to have a higher frequency of blank antigens (ie. less than 4

detectable antigens). The distribution of the blanks between the A and B loci
were similar for the two groups (sAg+ 8A and 6B; sAg- 10A and 9B). Whether the
higher frequency of <4 antigens in the sAg- patients reflects antigens yet to be
identified, homozygosity of known antigens, or both, remains to be established.

A second approach is to compare the frequencies of combinations of antigens. In the addendum to our first report (Simons and colleagues, 1978a) we noted the occurrence of A9-associated interactions including A9, A11, BW40, B.Blank. In this expanded series of 79 patients this combination occured six times (8%) compared with 3 (1%) of 238 controls. Of the 6 patients with the gene combination, 5 were with HB$_s$Ag negative.

Another important category of gene combination is those genes which show linkage disequilibrium. Table 2 shows the frequencies of the two joint phenotypes showing strongest linkage disequilibrium in Chinese.

TABLE 2 Frequencies (%) of A2, BW46 and A19/A.Blank, BW17
         in Singapore Chinese subjects

HLA antigens	Singapore Chinese Subjects				
	Normal (238)	Total (79)	HCC[1]		NPC[2] (141)
			Ag+ (42)	Ag- (37)	
A2, BW46	17	19	24	14	29
AW19/A.Blank, BW17	11	13	7	19	26

[1] HCC = Hepatocellular Carcinoma

[2] NPC = Nasopharyngeal Carcinoma

The conclusion drawn from the study of the first 29 of these patients was that the HLA pairs A2, BW46 and AW19/A.Blank, BW17 that show an association with nasopharyngeal carcinoma in Chinese do not show an association with HCC. When the 79 patients are grouped together this remains the case. However, subgrouping raises the possibility that differences exist in that A2, BW46 is relatively more common in sAg+ HCC patients, whereas the reverse is seen for AW19/A.Blank, BW17.

A third approach is to examine the frequencies of individual genes. This is the least satisfactory form of data analysis since biological function probably resides in combinations of genes. Nevertheless, for the limited objective of assessing whether differences between two groups are likely to exist, gene frequency determination may be helpful. Frequencies of some genes which are relatively common in Chinese are shown in Table 3.

Two points can be made. Firstly, taking the HCC patients in total, there appears to be differences from normal subjects in that A9 and BW15 are more frequent while A11 and BW40 are less frequent. Secondly, between the subgroups there appear to be differences even for antigens that show no difference in the total patient group from normal, eg. A2, B5, BW16, BW17, BW46 and B.Blank. No statistical analyses have so far been attempted but it seems very likely that the two subgroups are dissimilar in HLA gene pattern. Further studies are needed to clarify these patterns and to determine whether differences exist between the non-immune antigenaemic (Ag+/Ab-) and immune complexaemic (Ag+/Ab+) subgroups of the patients. If HLA patterns characteristic of one or both subgroups were also present in the same subgroups of asymptomatic HB$_s$Ag-positive carriers the case for an HLA gene-associated immune deficiency would be strengthened. The finding would also be compelling evidence in support of an oncogenic role for HBV. Since HLA genotype is an unchangeable characteristic existing prior to the development of malignancy, the HLA genetic similarity of the HBV infection subgroup having the highest risk for HCC would be perhaps the strongest evidence in support of the hypothesis that the HCC subgroup derived from the carrier subpopulation which could be achieved without a prospective study.

TABLE 3   HLA Antigen frequencies (%) in Singapore Chinese HCC patients

	HLA antigens												
	A2	A9	A11	A19 A.B1	B5	B13	BW15	BW16	BW17	BW22	BW40	BW46	B.B1
Normal subjects (238)	53	27	61	52	13	20	22	11	14	12	41	23	24
HCC sAg+ (42)	64	38	52	40	19	12	33	26	10	17	26	29	14
sAg- (37)	51	32	54	51	8	8	41	5	32	16	35	14	30
TOTAL (79)	58	35	53	46	14	10	37	16	20	16	30	22	22

The ideal situation would be to extend the immunogenetic-immunovirologic strategy to include aflatoxin exposure, and decrease patient heterogeneity by subgrouping according to histopathological evidence of chronic liver disease, age at diagnosis, and duration of survival. The major problem in such case-control studies is the number of patients necessary for analysis. For example, studies of HLA A and B locus gene type according to HBV immune and AFP subgroups (total 12) requires around 100 patients for satisfactory analysis, and a similar number would be required in a second series to test any hypothesis that results of the first study may warrant. The organizational and logistic problems are considerable, especially when recourse has to be taken to patients in more than one location. Nonetheless, multifactorial case-control studies may be the least difficult approach to establishing whether the risk for HCC accompanying aflatoxin intake is associated with, or is independent of, the risk related to HBV infection.

REFERENCES

Anthony, P.P. (1977). Cancer of the liver : pathogenesis and recent aetiological factors. Trans. Royal Soc. Trop. Med. Hyg., 71, 466.
Craddock, V.M. (1976). Cell proliferation and experimental liver cancer. In Liver Cell Cancer, Cameron, H.M., Linsell, C.A. and Warwick, G.P. (Editors) Elsevier, Amsterdam, 153.
Linsell, C.A. (1976). The field studies designed to test a possible association between the ingestion of aflatoxin and liver cell cancer. In Liver Cancer, Cancer Problems in Asian Countries, Proc. 2nd. Asian Cancer Conference Shanmugaratnam, K., Nambiar, K., Tan, L.K. and Chan, L.K.C. (Editors) Singapore Cancer Society, pp.43-44.
Linsell, C.A. and Peers, F.G. (1977). Aflatoxin and liver cell cancer. Trans. Royal Soc. Trop. Med. Hyg., 71, 471.
Lutwick, L.I. and Robinson, W.S. (1977). DNA synthesized in the hepatitis B Dane particle DNA polymerase reaction. Virol. J., 21, 96.
Mackay, I.R. and Morris, P.J. (1972). Association of autoimmune active chronic hepatitis with HL-A1, 8. Lancet, ii, 793.
Okuda, K. and Peters, R.L. (1976). Eds. Hepatocellular Carcinoma, Wiley, New York.

Nishioka, K., Levin, A.G. and Simons, M.J. (1975). Hepatitis B antigen, antigen subtypes and hepatitis B antibody in normal subjects and liver disease patients in Asian, Pacific and African countries. Bull. Wld. Hlth. Org., 52, 293-300.

Peers, F.G. and Linsell, C.A. (1973). Dietary aflatoxin and liver cancer - a population based study in Kenya. Brit. J. Cancer, 27, 473.

Shikata, T. (1976). Hepatitis B virus and hepatocellular carcinoma. In Liver Cancer, Cancer Problems in Asian Countries, Proc. 2nd. Asian Cancer Conference. Shanmugaratnam, K., Nambiar, R., Tan, L.K. and Chan, L.K.C. (Editors) Singapore Cancer Society, pp. 67-72.

Simons, M.J. (1973). Detection of hepatitis B antigen by radioelectrocomplexing. Bull. Wld. Hlth. Org., 49, 107-109.

Simons, M.J., Yu, M. and Shanmugaratnam, K. (1973). HB antigenaemia, specific immunodeficiency and hepatocellular carcinoma. Tumour Research, 8, 120.

Simons, M.J., Yu, M. and Shanmugaratnam, K. (1975). Immunodeficiency to hepatitis B virus infection and genetic susceptibility to development of hepatocellular carcinoma. Annals New York Acad. Sciences, 259, 181-195.

Simons, M.J. (1978). HLA antigen profiles and malignancy. In Proc. XII International Cancer Congress, Symposium No. 17.

Simons, M.J., Chan, S.H., Wee, G.B. and Mathews, J.D. (1978a). HLA and hepatocellular carcinoma. In Hepatitis Symposium, T. Oda (Ed.), University of Tokyo Press.

Simons, M.J., Chan, S.H., Wee, G.B., Shanmugaratnam, K., Goh, E.H., Ho, J.H.C., Chan, J.C.W., Darmalingam, S., Prasad, U., Betuel, H., Day, N.E. and de Thé, G. (1978b). Nasopharyngeal carcinoma and histocompatibility antigens. In Nasopharyngeal Carcinoma : Etiology and Control. de Thé, G and Ito, H. (Editors). IARC Scientific Publications, Lyon, France, pp. 271-282.

Simons, M.J., Yu, M. and Shanmugaratnam, K. (1976). Immunodeficiency to hepatitis B viral infection and hepatocellular carcinoma. In Liver Cancer, Cancer Problems in Asian Countries, Proc. 2nd. Asian Cancer Conference. Shanmugaratnam, K., Nambiar, R., Tan, L.K. and Chan, L.K.C. (Editors). Singapore Cancer Society, pp. 61-66.

Zuckerman, A.J. (1977). Hepatocellular carcinoma and hepatitis B. Trans. Royal Soc. Trop. Med. Hyg., 71, 459.

Liver Tumors—Pathology

Wataru Mori, Rikuo Machinami and Kaoru Tanaka

*Department of Pathology, Faculty of Medicine, University of Tokyo,
Tokyo, Japan*

ABSTRACT

Primary liver cancer, especially hepatocellular carcinoma, shows
remarkable geographic differences in incidence, epidemiologically.
Pathologically, hepatocellular carcinoma is closely related to liver
cirrhosis, among which types A and B (postnecrotic and posthepatitic)
are considered to be significant and almost exclusive. From our
histopathological study, only these two types of cirrhosis can be
assumed to be the result of hepatitis or hepatic necrosis, most of
which are of viral origin, and the above described geographic
difference is also caused by the differences in the commonest type
of cirrhosis in respective areas of the world. On the other hand,
high detectability of Hepatitis-B antigen in the liver tissue
bearing hepatocellular carcinoma is confirmed histopathologically.
Besides, familal accumulation of hepatocellular carcinoma cases is
reported not uncommon in Japan and a high positivity of Hepatitis-B
antigen is also detected in these families. Thus, existence of some
relation between hepatitis virus and hepatocellular carcinoma is
definite, from histopathological and epidemiological evidences, but
it is still very difficult to decide whether the relationship is the
direct one or not.

INTRODUCTION

Primary cancer of the liver is known as the malignant tumor which shows
remarkable difference in incidence according to geographical areas of
the world. For example, its incidence is very high showing more than
60 per 100,000 population per year in some parts of Africa, while it
is very low and only less than 1 in some countries of North America
and Europe. In our country, Japan, it is around 4, and occupies 8.5%
of all malignant neoplasms, according to the statistical analysis based
on autopsy records covering the whole country (Table 1).
As so is the fact in the other organs of the body, there are more than
one kind of primary malignant tumors which originate in the liver; the
most common examples are hepatocellular carcinoma, cholangiocellular
carcinoma, hemangioendothelial sarcoma, malignant mesenchymoma, rhabdo-

---

This study was supported, in part, by a research grant from the
Japanese Ministry of Education, Science and Culture.

or leiomyosarcoma, etc. Among these, hepatocellular carcinoma seems
to be the most important and interesting from every view-point of
etiology, epidemiology, morphology, and clinical features. And actually, the geographical difference in incidence of primary hepatic cancer
above mentioned, is mostly due to that of hepatocellular carcinoma.

TABLE 1. Malignant Tumors in Japan
(From: Annual of the Pathological
 Autopsy Cases in Japan, 1974)

Total No. of Malignant Tumors 12,336

Gastric ca.	2,288
Pulmonary ca.	1,712
Hepatic ca.	1,051 (8.5%)
Leukemia	1,101
Colorectal ca.	673
Malignant lymphoma	658
Pancreatic ca.	623
Gall bladder, bile ductal ca.	567
Esophageal ca.	447
Brain tumor	347
Breast ca.	291
Uterine ca., corpus & cervix	280

On the other hand, tremendous new findings in recent studies on hepatitis viruses and carcinofetal proteins have provided us much progress
in the study of hepatocellular carcinoma. Therefore, because of these
reasons, and considering its importance not only in the field of
pathology but also in other fields of medical sciences, I would like
to utilize the limited space here for the discussion with main focus
on hepatocellular carcinoma.

GENERAL INCIDENCE

TABLE 2. Age Distribution of Primary
Hepatic Cancer in Japan (From: Annual
of the Pathological Autopsy Cases in
Japan, 1974)

Age (Years)	No. of cases (Male)	(Female)
0 - 9	7	0
10 - 19	2	1
20 - 29	3	1
30 - 39	33	3
40 - 49	135	20
50 - 59	241	44
60 - 69	249	85
70 - 79	143	58
80 - 89	12	7
90 - 99	0	0
Total	825	219

Hepatocellular carcinoma in our country is far more common among the
male. In the annual of the pathological autopsy cases in Japan, 1974,

there listed 825 male and 219 female cases of primary hepatic cancer
most of which are hepatocellular carcinoma, and their age distribution
shows that the highest incidence is seen in the 7th decade of life in
the both sexes (Table 2). As to be discussed later, hepatocellular
carcinoma is very commonly associated by cirrhosis of the liver. And
when two groups are compared with each other, one hepatocellular carcinoma with liver cirrhosis and the other without, there seems to
exist some difference in the age distribution between the two. Namely,
a remarkable peak-formation between 50 and 70 years of age is seen in
the former, while rather equal incidence is seen through all age groups
in the latter (Table 3).

TABLE 3. Age Distribution of Hepatocellular Carcinoma
(Dept. Path. Univ. Tokyo, 76 cases)

Age (Years)	No. of cases (Hepato. ca. with liver cirrhosis)	(Hepato. ca. without liver cirrhosis)
- 20	0	2
21 - 30	0	5
31 - 40	1	4
41 - 50	7	7
51 - 60	13	6
61 - 70	14	5
71 - 80	5	6
81 - 90	1	0
Total	41	35

MORPHOLOGICAL CLASSIFICATION

Grossly, hepatocellular carcinoma is devided, as in other malignant
neoplasms of the liver, into three major forms; massive, nodular, and
diffuse.
Histologically, there have been proposed many ways of classification.
But usually, thin-trabecular, wide-trabecular, solid or medullary are
the commonest terms used for this purpose. Tubular formation is not
rare, some of which are apparently bile-producing evidenced morpho-
logically by bile-thrombi in the tubule. Fatty infiltration of tumor
cells is not rare either, and appearance of giant cells can sometimes
be observed. Some hepatocellular carcinomas are quite desmoplastic
and the epithelial tumor cell nests are surrounded by dense fibrous
tissue.

METASTASIS

Concerning its metastasis, hepatocellular carcinoma is understood usually as a malignant tumor which shows rather limited metastasis to the
other organs of the body. Although its local, intravascular spread is
very common, and sometimes it grows by continuity even up to the heart
through the vein, but its real metastasis is rather rare, and the lung,
adrenal, bone marrow, spleen, regional lymph nodes, etc. are the common
sites of affection. Here again, some differences are seen between hepatocellular carcinoma with cirrhosis and without cirrhosis, the latter
usually shows a little more extensive metastasis than the former,
probably in relation to the fact that hepatocellular carcinoma occurring in non-cirrhotic liver is of lower differentiation than that in

cirrhotic liver (Table 4).

TABLE 4.   Metastasis of Hepatocellular Carcinoma
(Dept. Path. Univ. Tokyo, 76 cases)

	Hepato. ca. with liver cirrhosis (41 cases)	Hepato. ca. without liver cirrhosis (35 cases)
Lung metastasis	18 (44%)	22 (63%)
Lymph node metastasis	12 (29%)	11 (31%)
Other metastasis	10 (24%)	11 (31%)
Peritoneal dissemination	8 (20%)	10 (27%)
No metastasis	14 (34%)	8 (23%)

RELATIONSHIP BETWEEN LIVER CIRRHOSIS AND HEPATOCELLULAR CARCINOMA

As mentioned several times already, hepatocellular carcinoma and liver cirrhosis are quite closely related each other. For example, as far as our cases in Tokyo, Japan, are concerned, about 35% of cirrhosis cases are associated by hepatocellular carcinoma at the time of autopsy, and about 80% of hepatocellular carcinoma is associated by cirrhosis. However on the other hand, with cases of Cambridge, United Kingdom checked under the same standard, only 7% of cirrhotic liver were found developing hepatocellular carcinoma at autopsy. In this instance too, however, frequency of cirrhosis association in hepatocellular carcinoma is quite the same as in Japan, about 75%. We were quite interested in this fact and tried to see the reason of such difference, and obtained the solution rather soon and easily, which was quite simple. In the Japanese cases there were much more cirrhosis which was considered to be the sequela of viral hepatitis than in British cases, and hepatocellular carcinoma occurred mainly from this type of cirrhosis in the both places (Mori and Shah, 1972).

TABLE 5.   Causes of Liver Cirrhosis

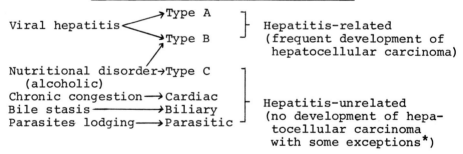

* Budd-Chiari's cirrhosis
Schistosoma-induced cirrhosis

In Japan, liver cirrhosis of common type has been classified traditionally into three types, A, B, and C. Type A is almost similar to the postnecrotic type of Dr. Gall, U. S. A., B to posthepatitic, and C to nutritional. Namely, type A is cirrhosis with wide fibrous septa and nodules of various sizes, type B with multilobular nodules and thin septa, and type C is micro-nodular and usually with fatty change. And according to our experiences, type A seems to be the result of viral

hepatitis, type B is also the result of viral hepatitis mostly in
Japan, but is mixed considerably by the terminal stage of type C cirrhosis in Britain, and type C seems to be almost exclusively resulted
from nutritional disorder, alcoholic. Through the above reason, Mori
called cirrhosis of type A and B "heatitis-related", and type C and
other specific forms of cirrhosis such as cardiac, biliary, parasitic,
etc. "hepatitis-unrelated". Quite interestingly, as mentioned before,
hepatocellular carcinoma occurs almost constantly from hepatitis-
related cirrhosis, and actually, hepatitis-related cirrhosis occupies
more than 2/3 of all cirrhosis in Tokyo, while it is less than one half
in Cambridge. This kind of difference between Japan and western countries has also been demonstrated clearly between cases of Tokyo and these
of Cincinnati, Ohio, U. S. A. (Mori, 1967). Like this, the relationship, either direct or indirect, between viral hepatitis and hepatoma
had been strongly suggested already on the routine, histological basis
of study with a parameter of liver cirrhosis as an intermediate stage
(Table 5).

HBs ANTIGEN DETECTION IN HISTOLOGICAL SPECIMEN

Since many years ago, some feature with ground glass appearance had
been noticed histopathologically by various staining methods in the
liver, and this was proved to be the Hepatitis B surface antigen ---
HBs antigen --- by the fluorescence antibody technique. And now, this
can be demonstrated very sensitively by orcein and other staining
methods even on the formalin-fixed, paraffin-embedded, and thin-
sectioned specimen. This time, we checked the mode of HBs antigen
existence in the liver of various conditions by means of orcein staining. Table 6 shows the result with liver cirrhosis which had no hepatocellular carcinoma occurrence in it. Orcein positivity was 25% as
a whole, and only types A and B ----- hepatitis-related cirrhosis ----
showed positive result.

TABLE 6.   Result of Orcein Staining of the Liver
(Cirrhosis without hepatocellular carcinoma cases)

Type of cirrhosis	Number of cases	Orcein positivity
Type A	11	2 (18.2%)
Type B	27	9 (33.3%)
Type C	3	0
Biliary	3	0
Total	44	11 (25.9%)

On the other hand, there were 39 recent cases of hepatocellular carcinoma
with cirrhosis in our department, among which 15 cases, namely 38%,
showed orcein positivity. To make a comparative study, we collected
hepatocellular carcinoma cases without cirrhosis, the total number of
which reached 34. Among these, orcein positive feature was found in
the liver of 8 cases, incidence of which was 24%, and all the positive
picture was obtained in non-tumorous area of the liver, except for
one case which showed suspicious positivity also in tumor tissue.
From the data introduced above, it is confirmed that previously defined
hepatitis-related or unrelated cirrhoses are really so at least HBs
antigen is concerned, and it is also assumed that coexistence of HBs
antigen is revealed not rarely in the liver bearing hepatocellular
carcinoma, but its incidence is not differ significantly from that of
simply cirrhotic liver which does not show hepatocellular carcinoma

occurrence at all (Table 7).

TABLE 7.   Result of Orcein Staining of the Liver
(Hepatocellular carcinoma cases)

Type of lesion	No. of cases	Orcein positivity
Cirrhosis without hepatocellular ca.	44	11 (25%)
Cirrhosis with hepatocellular ca.	39	15 (38%)
Hepatocellular ca. without cirrhosis	34	8 (24%)

Table 8 shows HBs-Antigen detectability in the serum with cases of
cirrhosis and hepatocellular carcinoma, incidence seems to be a little
higher in the latter.

TABLE 8.   Result of HBs-Ag Test of the Serum

	HBs-Ag in the serum	
	(+)	(−)
Cirrhosis only	12(32.4%)	25(67.6%)
Hepatocellular ca. with or without cirrhosis	19(45.2%)	23(54.8%)

When the incidence of orcein-positivity of the liver tissue is compared with that of HBs antigen detectability in the serum with the
same patients group, the result came out as shown in Table 9. It is
interesting that some discrepancy can be seen between the results of
two observations. Here, it seems to be worthy to add that HBs-antigen
positivity in the serum of normal individuals in Japan is around 2%.

TABLE 9.   HBs-Antigen in the Serum and
Orcein Staining of the Liver (Cases of
cirrhosis and/or hepatocellular carcinoma)

		Orcein staining of liver	
		(+)	(−)
HBs-Ag in serum	(+)	21	9
	(−)	4	44

FAMILIAL ACCUMULATION OF HEPATOCELLULAR CARCINOMA

It is not rare to see familial accumulation of hepatocellular carcinom
patients in our country, most of which are usually associated by liver
cirrhosis. Table 10 is an example of a family tree, where all of the
5 siblings in this family died from hepatocellular carcinoma with
liver cirrhosis. Such a phenomenon is considered to be the result of
vertical transmission of HB antigen in one family, and here, some
relationship between hepatocellular carcinoma and hepatitis virus is
strongly suggested again.

TABLE 10. A Family Tree Showing Accumulation of
Hepatocellular Carcinoma Patients

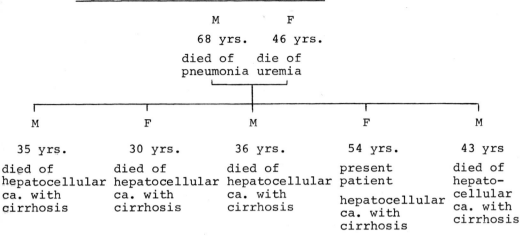

ALPHA-FETOPROTEIN IN HEPATOCELLULAR CARCINOMA

Another recent finding of big importance with hepatocellular carcinoma
is a carcinofetal protein, alpha-fetoprotein. We collected 47 cases
of hepatocellular carcinoma with which the result of alpha-fetoprotein
test of the serum was clarified. As a whole, 36 cases out of the 47,
namely 82%, showed positive result, more than 200ng/ml of the serum.
The relationship between HBs antigen positivity in the liver tissue
and alpha-fetoprotein test of the serum, in cases of hepatocellular
carcinoma, is shown in Table 11. There was a slight tendency that
orcein-positivity was a little higher in cases which did not show
alpha-fetoprotein elevation of the serum, clinically.

TABLE 11. Alpha-fetoprotein and HBs-Antigen
in Hepatic Tissue
(Hepatocellular ca.: 47 cases, checked by
orcein-stain)

		Alpha-Fetoprotein		
		(+)	(-)	Total
HBs-Ag	(+)	9	4	13
HBs-Ag	(-)	27	7	34
Total		36	11	47

As far as the relation between tissue type of hepatocellular carcinoma
and its alpha-fetoprotein production is concerned, positivity of the
serum test is higher in cases of rather well-differentiated tumors
which show tubular structure or bile production. This fact has been
almost accepted widely, but too far differentiated hepatocellular
carcinoma is said not to produce alpha-fetoprotein any more. Other
changes in morphology, such as fatty change of tumor cells, appearance
of giant cells, etc., would not cause any difference in alpha-
fetoprotein positivity at all.

TABLE 12. Alpha-Fetoprotein and Morphological
Type of Tumor (Hepatocellular ca.: 46 cases)

| | | Alpha-Fetoprotein | | |
		(+)	(−)	Total
Tubular structure	(+)	18(50%)	3(30%)	21
	(−)	18(50%)	7(70%)	25
Bile production	(+)	18(50%)	3(30%)	21
	(−)	18(50%)	7(70%)	25
Total		36	10	46

The fact that rather differentiated type of hepatocellular carcinoma
produces alpha-fetoprotein seems to have some relation to the mode of
its metastasis. Table 13 indicates that alpha-fetoprotein producing
tumors show rather less metastasis than non-producing ones. But, thi
is probably not the influence of carcinofetal protein itself, but
because of the undifferentiated character of tumor cells.

TABLE 13. Alpha-Fetoprotein and Tumor Metastasis
(Hepatocellular carcinoma: 46 cases)

| | | Alpha-Fetoprotein | | |
		(+)	(−)	Total
		(36 cases)	(10 cases)	(46 cases)
Metastasis (+) to	Lung	16(44%)	5(50%)	21
	Lymph node	7(19%)	5(50%)	12
	Others	10(28%)	7(70%)	17
Metastasis (−)		12(33%)	2(20%)	14

SUMMARY AND CONCLUSION

Here, a very rapid and brief over-view of the pathology of hepatocell
lar carcinoma is made, the connection between morphology and virology
or biochemistry seems to be the main focus of pathology at present.
Thus, existence of some relation between hepatitis virus and hepatocellular carcinoma seems to be definite for us, from the view-point
of pathology in a wide sense. But, it is still very difficult to
decide whether the relationship is a direct one or indirect one, and
high incidence of hepatocellular carcinoma also in Budd-Chiari's
cirrhosis or schistosoma induced cirrhosis may suggest of the high
risk type of cirrhosis for hepatocellular carcinoma development,
irrespective of the cause of cirrhosis itself, although HBs antigen
may also be playing some role in these cases especially in the latter

REFERENCES

Mori, W. (1967). Cirrhosis and primary cancer of the liver ----
    comparative study in Tokyo and Cincinnati. Cancer, 20, 627-631.
Mori, W. and M. Shah (1972). A comparative geo-pathological study
    of liver cirrhosis and primary hepatic cancer between Cambridge
    and Tokyo. Gann, 63, 765-771.

Blood Gas Changes in Hepatic
Artery Ligation

R. E. Madden, H. de Blasi and J. Zinns

New York Medical College, 1249 Fifth Avenue, New York, New York 10029

ABSTRACT

Hepatic artery ligation (HAL) is widely used in the treatment of metastatic and primary liver tumors. Significant morbidity has been frequently encountered. In this study, alterations in oxygen content with HAL have been used in selecting those patients who will safely tolerate the procedure. Six patients with liver metastases were studied intraoperatively. PO_2 and O_2 saturations were simultaneously determined in arterial (HA) portal (PV) and hepatic vein (HV1) blood. Hepatic vein blood was then restudied after clamping the hepatic artery (HV2). Oxygen content was calculated in blood from each of the three sample sites by standard methods. Percent relative drop in oxygen content of the liver ($\triangle\%$) was then estimated by the formula. Four patients underwent HAL. In these patients, $\triangle\%$s were 11, 19.9, 13 and 15. Two patients were denied HAL because of low HV2 oxygen saturation after clamping. $\triangle\%$s in these were 26 and 36. There were no surgical mortalities and no significant morbidity due to HAL in this series. Intraoperative blood gas determinations may be of value in selecting those patients who will tolerate HAL and those in which an alternate strategy should be used.
Keywords: Artery, ligation, blood gases, metastases, liver, safety.

INTRODUCTION

Hepatic artery ligation has been used to palliate metastatic disease to the liver.[1,2,3,4] The basis for this treatment is the belief that hepatic tumors probably derive their nutrition from the arterial circulation.[5,6] In addition, angiographic and histologic evidence of induced tumor necrosis secondary to interruption of hepatic arterial flow has been reported.[7,8,9]

The morbidity, mortality, and therapeutic benefits have been recorded previously.[1,2,10] Notwithstanding the anatomic variation and adaptability of the blood supply to the liver,[5,11,12] the morbidity following common hepatic artery ligation depends on the subsequent alteration in oxygen availability to the liver after ligation. In some cases a drastic drop might occur and prove significantly injurious to the normal hepatic parenchyma. In many others, however, common hepatic artery ligation may be safely employed.[1,2,3]

We have developed a facile method for quick estimation of the safety of common

87

hepatic artery ligation. This involves the calculation of the percent drop in blood oxygen content produced by temporary clamping of the artery. An operative decision is then made to ligate the artery, or, if deemed unsafe, to employ other therapeutic approaches.

Material and Methods

Six patients with hepatic metastases were studied. Five patients had liver disease secondary to colonic carcinoma, while one patient had metastatic breast disease. There were four males and two females in the group. The youngest patient was 54 years old, while the oldest was 76 years old.

Pre-operative diagnosis of hepatic metastasis was made by clinical assessment, liver enzymes, liver scan, and angiographic data. In all cases the diagnosis was confirmed intraoperatively.

On the morning of surgery the patients were first taken to the angiographic suite where a catheter was placed percutaneously in the femoral vein and, under fluoroscopic control, into an hepatic vein. After securing the catheter in place, the patients were transferred to the operating room.

Following operative confirmation of the metastatic disease, samples of blood were taken from the hepatic artery (HA), portal vein (PV) and the hepatic vein (HV_1). The oxygen tension and saturation of these specimens were determined. A vascular clamp was then applied to the common hepatic artery and its flow temporarily occluded. The liver was observed over the next fifteen to twenty minutes and changes in color noted. In two patients, the liver became cyanotic, while in the others no significant color changes occurred. After this period of arterial occlusion, another sample of hepatic venous blood (HV_2) was obtained and its oxygen tension and saturation determined.

It was decided empirically that if the hepatic venous saturation dropped below fifty-five percent or the oxygen partial pressure below 30 mm of mercury, hepatic artery ligation would be abandoned. The mitochondrial oxygen gradient could be too low below these levels and jeopardize hepatocyte viability.[13,14,15] In two out of the six patients, this proved to be the case.

RESULTS

The two patients who developed an hepatic venous saturation below fifty-five percent were those two in whom cyanosis of the liver was noted (Case 1 and 5 - Table 1). The other four patients underwent hepatic artery ligation for their metastatic disease (Table 2).

TABLE 1   Two Patients Developing Liver Cyanosis

	HV1 SATURATION	HV_1	HV2 SATURATION	HV_2	PERCENT OXYGEN CONTENT CHANGE
Case 1	81%	16.4	48%	9.71	26.2%
Case 5	68%	12.4	43%	7.80	36.2%

Definitions: HA=Hepatic Artery; PV=Portal vein; HV_1=Hepatic vein, pre-clamp; HV_2=Hepatic vein, post-clamp;   [ ]=Oxygen content/100 ml.

TABLE 2   All Patients Studied, Hepatic Artery Clamping

CASE	AGE	DIAGNOSIS	OXYGEN CONTENT CHANGE	HEPATIC ARTERY LIGATION
1	64	Rectosigmoid carcinoma	26.2%	No
2	76	Carcinoma left colon	19.9%	Yes
3	67	Carcinoma left colon	11.2%	Yes
4	62	Rectosigmoid carcinoma	15.1%	Yes
5	54	Breast carcinoma	36.2%	No
6	64	Carcinoma left colon	10.7%	Yes

There were no surgical mortalities and no significant morbidity in this group.

Post-operatively, the six cases were reviewed and alterations in oxygen content were calculated. Oxygen content was calculated for each blood sample using the formula:

$$\text{Content} = 1.34 \times \text{Hgb} \times \text{Sat } \% \, O_2 = 0.0031 \times \text{partial pressure } O_2 \qquad (1)$$

The precent drop in oxygen content to the liver was then based on the premise that in the original pre-ligation state the hepatic oxygen content was equal to the sum of that delivered by the hepatic artery and portal vein minus the content of the hepatic vein: HA   +   PV   - HV_1

In the post-ligation state, hepatic oxygen content was equal to that delivered by the portal vein minus the amount calculated in the hepatic vein, $PV - HV_2$. The ratio of the status of the post-ligation state to that of the pre-ligation state x 100 is defined as the percent change in oxygen content.

$$\frac{PV - HV_2}{HA + PV - HV_1} \times 100 = \quad \% \text{ change in oxygen content.} \qquad (2)$$

Oxygen availability, which would necessitate flow measurements of the major vessels, and quantitation of arterial collateralization, were not determined. The hepatic vein oxygen saturation and tension signify tolerable oxygen gradients since these levels are greater than cellular levels.[13,11,14,15]

In the four patients who underwent and tolerated common hepatic artery ligation, the percent changes in oxygen content were 19.9%, 11.2%, 15.1%, and 10.7%. Two patients were denied hepatic artery ligation because of low venous saturation and cyanotic livers. The percent changes in oxygen content in these cases was 26.2% and 36.2%, representing significant alterations. (Table 2)

Discussion

It is recognized that the blood gas status at any time in a particular hepatocyte or tumor cell strongly depends upon its own metabolism as well as upon the nature of the microcirculation.[14] Nonetheless, certain trends in overall blood gas alterations can be interpreted as able to portend these effects. With this in mind, if one were able to calculate the oxygen content supplied to the liver, and then measure again the amount after ligating the common hepatic artery, the safety of the procedure might be predicted. If the difference in oxygen content is relatively small. i.e. less than 20%, assuring continued normal hepatic parenchymal supply, then interrupting the hepatic artery is a safe procedure.[16] On the other hand, if the drop in oxygen content to the liver is drastic enough to jeopardize normal cellular function, then the risk of the procedure must be questioned. The determination of blood gases intraoperatively appears to be useful in selected cases in which arterial interruption is contemplated as a mode of therapy.

REFERENCES

1. Fortner, J., R. J. Mulcure, A. Solis, R. C. Watson, R. B. Golbey. Treatment of Primary and Secondary Liver Cancer by Hepatic Artery Ligation and Infusion Chemotherapy. Annals of Surgery, 178: 2, 162, 1973.

2. Lien, W., N. Ackerman. The Blood Supply of Experimental Liver Metastases. Surgery, Vol. 68, No. 2, 334, 1970.

3. Mori, W., M. Masuda and T. Miyanaga. Hepatic Artery Ligation and Tumor Necrosis in the Liver. Surgery, Vol. 59, No. 3, 359, 1966.

4. Nagasue, N., K. Inokuchi, M. Kobayashi, Y. Ogawa, A. Iwaki, and H. Yukaya. Hepatic Dearterialization for Nonresectable Primary and Secondary Tumors of the Liver. Cancer, 38: 2593, 1976.

5. Healey, J. Jr. Vascular Patterns in Human Metastatic Liver Tumors. Surgery, Gynecology & Obstetrics, 120: 6, 1187, 1965.

6. Krogh, A. The Number and Distribution of Capillaries in Muscles with Calculation of the Oxygen Pressure Head Necessary for Supplying the Tissue. The Journal of Physiology, 52: 409-415, 1919.

7. Madding, G. F., P. A. Kennedy, S. Sogemeier. Hepatic Artery Ligation for Metastatic Tumor in the Liver. The American Journal of Surgery, Vol. 120: 95, 1970.

8. McDermott, W. Jr., T. Hensle. Metastatic Carcinoid to the Liver Treated by Hepatic Dearterialization. Annals of Surgery, 180: 3, 305, 1973.

9. Michaels, N. Newer Anatomy of Liver-Variant Blood Supply and Colateral Circulation, JAMA, 172: 2, 125, 1960.

10. Madding, G. F., P. Kennedy. Hepatic Artery Ligation. Surgical Clinics of North America, Vol. 52: 3, 1972.

11. Imamura, M., T. Suzuki, A. Nakase, and I. Honjo. Hemodynamic Changes in the Liver of the Rabbit After Hepatic Dearterialization. Surgery, Gynecology & Obstetrics, 140: 412, 1975.

12. McDermott, W. Jr., A. L. Parris, M. R. Clouse, W. A. Meissner. Dearterialization of the Liver for Metastatic Cancer: Clinical, Angiographic and Pathologic Observations. Annals of Surgery, Vol. 187, No. 1, 1978.

13. Davis, P. W., and D. W. Bronk. Oxygen Tension in Mammalian Brain. Federation Proceedings, 16: 689-692, 1957.

14. Kety, S. S. Determinates of Tissue Oxygen Tension. Federation Proceedings, 16: 666-670, 1957.

15. Sparks, F. C., M. B. Mosher, W. C. Hallauer, M. J. Silverstein, D. Rangel, J. E. Passaro and D. L. Morton. Hepatic Artery Ligation and Post operative Chemotherapy for Hepatic Metastases. Cancer 35: 1074, 1975.

16. Van Liew, H. D. Tissue Gas Tensions by Microtonometry: Results in Liver and Fat. Journal of Applied Physiology, 17: 359-363, 1962.

Eight Years' Experience with the Surgical Management of 321 Patients with Liver Tumors

J. G. Fortner, D. K. Kim, M. K. Barrett, S. Iwatsuki, D. Papachristou, C. McLaughlin and B. J. Maclean

Gastric & Mixed Tumor Service, Department of Surgery,
Memorial Sloan-Kettering Cancer Center, New York, N.Y., U.S.A.

ABSTRACT

Three hundred twenty-one individuals with liver tumors have undergone exploratory laparotomy during the past eight years. Surgical procedures included hepatic lobectomy or segmentectomy (108 patients), hepatic vascular ligation and/or cannulation (134 patients), hepatic wedge resection (10 patients), unroofing of hepatic cyst (5 patients), isolation-chemoperfusion of the liver (4 patients), liver transplantation (8 patients), and liver biopsy only (52 patients). Ninety percent of these procedures were performed for malignant disease. The resectability rate for malignant disease was 33%.

This study focuses on the two most frequently performed operations- hepatic resection and vascular ligation and/or cannulation. One hundred eight individuals underwent resection : extended hepatic lobectomy (27), lobectomy (57), and segmentectomy (24). Primary liver cancer was present in 36, metastatic colorectal cancer in 25, miscellaneous other cancers in 27, and benign tumor, principally giant hemangioma, in 20. Forty-one resections utilized the isolation-perfusion technique. Standard resections employ an abdominal approach except when resection of the diaphragm is included. The 30-day operative mortality rate was 9% after resection. Three-year actuarial survival for all patients with malignant tumor undergoing resection was 46% being 81% for curative resection but only 18% for palliative resection.

Vascular cannulation and/or ligation was performed when there was diffuse hepatic involvement. Sites of primary tumor in this treatment group were liver in 37, colorectum in 55, and miscellaneous in 42. Individuals with vascular tumors, as determined by preoperative angiography, usually underwent hepatic artery ligation and cannulation (HALC); those with hypovascular tumors generally underwent HALC and portal vein cannulation. Eight of the nine postoperative deaths were early in the series and resulted from hepatorenal failure. This complication has been avoided in more recent cases by performing cannulation alone without ligation if tumor involvement encompasses 70% or more of the liver. Postoperative intrahepatic chemotherapy was administered according to one of three protocols for each of the primary site tumor groups. Individuals receiving at least two cycles of intrahepatic treatment had an improved one-year actuarial survival rate (33%) over those receiving fewer treatments (0%).

KEYWORDS

Hepatic resection
 Curative
 Major
 Palliative
 Wedge
Hepatic artery ligation/cannulation
Portal vein cannulation

This paper focuses on the two hepatic surgical procedures most frequently performed during the past eight years - hepatic resection and vascular ligation and/or cannulation. One hundred eight individuals underwent hepatic resection (Fortner and others, 1978). Eighty-eight (81%) of these resections were for malignant tumors. Of 36 primary liver cancers, 26 were hepatocellular, four were mixed hepatocellular and cholangiocarcinoma, three were sarcoma, one was cholangiocarcinoma, one was carcinoid, and one was unclassified. Additionally, there were five children with hepatoblastoma who were evaluated as a separate group. The majority of the metastatic tumors, 25 of 40, were colorectal in origin. Fifteen were of other types: melanoma in three, sarcoma in three, breast in two, carcinoid of the rectum in two, embryonal carcinoma in two, islet cell carcinoma of the pancreas in one, adenocarcinoma of the kidney in one, and adenocarcinoma of the stomach in one. There were four patients with primary gall bladder cancer and three with major bile duct cancer. Twenty of the resections were performed for benign disease: giant hemangioma of the liver in seven, focal nodular hyperplasia in five, cyst in three, hamartoma in three, adenoma in one, and Carroli's disease in one.

The thirty-day operative mortality rate for hepatic resection was 9% overall with a rate of only 4% for the standard type of resection. The operative mortality rate with the isolation-perfusion technique was 17% reflecting the advanced stage of disease in many individuals who underwent resection prior to 1975 (Fortner and others, 1974). The operative mortality rate with extended right hepatic lobectomy was 14%(4/27), right lobectomy 3%(1/36), left lobectomy 24%(5/21), and segmentectomy 0%(0/24). The rates were similar for curative and palliative resection being 10% and 12.5%, respectively. Cause of death for the ten patients dying within 30 days of surgery is shown in Table 1.

TABLE 1 30-Day Operative Mortality After Hepatic Resection

Cause of death	Number of patients
Coagulopathy with hepatic failure	4
Portal vein thrombosis (indwelling catheter)	1
Warm ischemia(40 min); postnecrotic cirrhosis	1
Unrecognized operative hemorrhage	1
Uncontrollable operative hemorrhage	1
GI bleeding, hepatorenal syndrome	1
Pulmonary embolus	1
Total	10

Several postoperative complications often occurred in the same patient. The most common was subphrenic abscess which developed in one-fifth of the patients. This has been virtually eliminated during the past two years following the introduction of a closed system of drainage.

Forty-six percent of the resections for malignant disease were termed curative. A resection was termed palliative if there was regional spread (23 patients) or distant metastasis (19 patients). The most common type of regional spread was vascular, either invasion of the intrahepatic vessels or of the vena cava (Fortner, Kallum, and Kim, 1977). Lymph node metastasis was the most frequent type of extrahepatic metastasis.

Actuarial survival rates were calculated for the first three postoperative years. The ten thirty-day operative deaths are excluded. Of the 36 individuals undergoing curative resection, 100% were alive at one year and 81% at three years (Table 2).

TABLE 2 Actuarial Survival in Individuals Undergoing Hepatic Resection

Curative resection	Number of patients	Actuarial survival	
		One year	Three years
Liver	13	100%	88%
Colorectal	17	100%	72%
Other	6	100%	83%
Total	36	100%	81%
Palliative resection			
Liver	16	78%	31%
Colorectal	6	56%	0%
Other	20	70%	0%
Total	42	71%	18%

Primary liver cancer had the highest survival rate, 88%, at three years. Approximately two-thirds of patients lived one year after palliative resection and 18% lived three years. Survival rates were similar for those with regional spread and with distant metastasis being 17% and 21% at three years.

The three-year survival rate was 48% for individuals with metastatic colorectal cancer undergoing either curative or palliative resection. This can be compared with a report by Attiyeh, Wanebo, and Stearns (1978) of 19 patients treated over a 26-year period who underwent wedge resection for metastatic colorectal cancer to the liver. The median size of the metastasis was 1.5 cm with 84% being solitary. This compares with a median size of 6.5 cm in this series, with 52% being solitary. The three-year actuarial survival rate was not significantly different for the two procedures: 56% after wedge resection and 48% after major hepatic resection. Thus, lobectomy is not an obligatory procedure. Resection of the metastasis with a margin of normal liver tissue can be a satisfactory procedure. The extent of surgical resection depends on the size and location of the tumor. A large mass of metastatic cancer need not preclude cure.

Survival rates for patients with primary hepatoma undergoing curative resection were high. Even patients undergoing a palliative resection had a good result. These results reflect, in part, the type of cancer being treated. Cirrhosis was considered a contraindication for major hepatic resection with only three such patients in this series. The survival rate for individuals with metastatic colorectal cancer undergoing curative resection also was excellent. Palliative resection for colorectal metastasis appears not to be indicated as no individuals have survived two years. The number of resections performed in individuals with the various other primary cancers is too small to provide meaningful survival figures.

Extensive liver involvement by primary or metastatic tumor precluded hepatic resection in 134 patients who underwent ligation and/or cannulation of the hepatic vessels. The primary tumor arose in the liver in 37 patients, in the colorectal area in 55, and at miscellaneous other sites in 42. The prognosis after hepatic artery ligation has been shown to correlate with the degree of tumor vascularity: patients with hypervascular lesions demonstrated the longest survival (Kim and others, 1977). It appears that hypervascular tumors derive their blood supply from the hepatic artery while hypovascular tumors receive blood from the portal vein. Thirty-six livers were classified as Grade I, II, or III in order of increasing vascularity as judged by preoperative arteriography. Over two-thirds of hepatomas were Grade III lesions while only 14% of metastatic colorectal carcinomas were hypervascular. Thus, individuals with vascular tumors usually underwent hepatic artery ligation and cannulation. Those with hypovascular tumors generally were subjected to hepatic artery ligation and cannulation with portal vein cannulation. Of 134 patients, 78 received hepatic artery ligation and cannulation, 24 hepatic artery ligation and cannulation combined with portal vein cannulation, 15 hepatic artery ligation alone, 8 portal vein cannulation alone, 5 hepatic artery ligation alone, and 4, other combinations. Eight of the nine 30-day operative deaths were early in the series and resulted from hepatorenal failure (Kim and others, 1976). The best treatment in such cases is prevention since renal failure following hepatic artery ligation was associated with a 78% mortality rate. This complication has been avoided in more recent cases by performing cannulation alone without ligation if tumor involvement encompasses 70% or more of the liver. A program of mannitol diuresis has practically eliminated renal failure as a postligation complication in this series.

Intrahepatic chemotherapy was administered according to one of three protocols depending on the primary site of the tumor (Fortner, 1977; Fortner and Pahnke, 1976). Heparinized saline is injected in the catheter following each infusion. If the catheter becomes occluded by thrombi, treatment is continued by peripheral intravenous route. Adequate treatment arbitrarily was defined as the administration of at least two cycles of drugs during the first three postoperative months. Adequate intrahepatic chemotherapy was administered to 65% of patients undergoing hepatic artery or portal vein cannulation. The actuarial survival rates in individuals receiving adequate intrahepatic chemotherapy are shown in Table 3.

TABLE 3 Adequate Intrahepatic Chemotherapy After Ligation/Cannulation

Primary tumor	Number of patients	Actuarial survival	
		One year	Two years
Liver	20	39%	28%
Colorectal	32	32%	12%
Other	23	26%	16%
Total	77	33%	18%

One-third of patients lived one year and 18% a second year. Survival was highest in the primary liver tumor group both at one and two years. In addition to a prolongation of life, patients receiving intrahepatic infusion of chemotherapy experienced significant relief from symptoms attributed to liver enlargement such as epigastric pain and fullness and right shoulder pain. Most patients were ambulatory and, with a few exceptions, were able to live a useful life with their families. No individuals receiving inadequate chemotherapy have survived one year.

An additional eleven patients received adequate doses of chemotherapy via the intravenous route. Their survival rates were somewhat poorer than those treated intrahepatically, being 27% at one and 8% at two years. A trial is underway at the present time in which individuals are randomized to receive chemotherapy via either the intrahepatic or the systemic route.

Ligation/cannulation proved most successful in individuals with primary liver tumors, expecially if adequate chemotherapy was given. Patients with metastatic colorectal or other metastatic neoplasms did more poorly perhaps because most of them had already been failures from systemic chemotherapy.

REFERENCES

Attiyeh, F., H. Wanebo, and M.W. Stearns, Jr. (1978). Hepatic resection for metastases from colorectal cancer. Dis Colon & Rectum, 21, 160-162.

Fortner, J.G. (1977). Current management of tumors of the liver. In G.F.Madding and P.A.Kennedy (Eds.), Symposium on Hepatic Surgery, Surgical Clinics of North America, Saunders, Philadelphia. pp.465-472.

Fortner, J.G., B.O.Kallum, and D.K.Kim (1977). Surgical management of hepatic vein occlusion by tumor. Arch Surg, 112, 727-728.

Fortner, J.G., D.K.Kim, B.J.Maclean, M.K.Barrett, S.Iwatsuki, A.D.Turnbull, W.S. Howland, and E.J.Beattie, Jr.(1978). Major hepatic resection for neoplasia. Personal experience in 108 patients. Ann Surg, 188,363-371.

Fortner, J.G. and L.D.Pahnke (1976). A new method for long-term intrahepatic chemotherapy. Surg Gynecol Obstet, 143, 979-980.

Fortner, J.G., M.H.Shiu, D.W.Kinne, D.K.Kim, E.B.Castro, R.C.Watson, W.S.Howland, and E.J.Beattie, Jr. (1974). Major hepatic resection using vascular isolation and hypothermic perfusion. Ann Surg, 180, 644-652.

Kim, D.K., R. Penneman, B.O.Kallum, M.Carillo, E.Scheiner, and J.G.Fortner (1976). Acute renal failure after ligation of the hepatic artery. Surg Gynecol Obstet, 143, 391-394.

Kim, D.K., R.C.Watson, L.D.Pahnke, and J.G.Fortner (1977). Tumor vascularity as a prognostic factor for hepatic tumors. Ann Surg, 185, 31-34.

Experimental Pancreatic Carcinogenesis

J. K. Reddy, D. G. Scarpelli and M. A. Rao

*Department of Pathology, Northwestern University Medical School,
Chicago, IL 60611, U.S.A.*

ABSTRACT

A number of different chemical substances, many of them unrelated, are capable of
inducing the neoplastic transformation of ductal and acinar cells of pancreas. Re-
producible models for the study of pancreatic carcinogenesis have been developed
in a variety of rodent species, several of the tumors induced have been successfully transplanted as solid tumors and one has been converted to an ascites tumor.
The histogenesis of ductal adenocarcinoma is complex and appears to involve modulation and perhaps dedifferentiation of acinar epithelial cells (i.e. progressive
proliferation with loss of zymogen maturation and ductular transformation) in addition to the proliferation and neoplastic transformation of preexisting ductular
and ductal cells. Biochemical studies have demonstrated that both acinar and ductal epithelium of pancreas are capable of metabolically activating carcinogens. The
activity of drug metabolizing enzymes responsible for carcinogen activation in pancreas can be increased significantly following treatment with appropriate compounds.

KEYWORDS Azaserine; 4-hydroxyaminoquinoline-1-oxide; N-nitrosobis(2-oxopropyl)
amine; methylnitrosourea; N-nitroso-2,6-dimethylmorpholine; histogenesis of pancreatic carcinoma, transplantable pancreatic carcinomas, acinar cell regeneration,
drug metabolism by pancreas.

INTRODUCTION

Epidemiological studies indicate an alarming increase in the incidence of pancreatic carcinoma in several countries during the past three decades. This is now
the fourth commonest cancer causing death in the U.S. and accounts for approximately 22,000 deaths this year. The reasons for this rising incidence are not readily apparent. Difficulty in early diagnosis, as well as lack of adequate knowledge
of its biological behavior appear to be major factors contributing to the poor prognosis. Under the auspices of the National Cancer Institute Pancreatic Carcinogenesis
Program concerted efforts are being made to reproduce the induction and development
of pancreatic carcinomas in experimental systems for integrated studies of its pathogenesis by morphological and biochemical methods (Pledger, Bates and Saffiotti, 1975;
Cohn, 1976). It is highly significant to emphasize that within five years of the
inception of this program a number of models for pancreatic carcinogenesis, including two transplantable pancreatic carcinomas, have been developed and are now being
used for detailed studies on the histogenesis, biological behavior and of modifying
factors involved in pancreatic carcinogenesis. The present report briefly reviews
recent progress in experimental pancreatic carcinogenesis.

Supported, in part, by Grant CA23055 from the National Institutes of Health.

REGENERATION OF THE EXOCRINE PANCREAS

Several studies have now established that the so-called non-dividing pancreatic
acinar cells (Pelc, 1964) can be stimulated to proliferate under appropriate conditions (Table 1). The pioneering work of Fitzgerald and co-workers clearly demonstrated that the rat pancreatic acinar cells divide following partial pancreatectomy (Lehv and Fitzgerald, 1968), or after an ethionine-protein free diet regimen (Fitzgerald and co-workers, 1968). The effectiveness of ethionine-protein
free diet in inducing pancreatic acinar cell regeneration has been subsequently
confirmed in guinea pigs (Wenk, Reddy and Harris, 1974). A model of pancreatic
acinar cell regeneration, dependent upon a single application of the stimulus, has
been described by Reddy and co-workers (1975). In this study, a single intravenous
injection of 4-hydroxyaminoquinoline-1-oxide (4-HAQO), in a dose of 22.5 mg/kg body
weight, induced marked necrosis of the exocrine pancreas in inbred strain 13 guinea
pigs within 48 hours. The necrotic phase was followed by a striking regenerative
response of pancreatic acinar and ductal epithelium (Fig. 1). If regenerating pancreas proves to be as vulnerable as regenerating liver to carcinogenic stimuli
(Craddock, 1971), these models of pancreatic regeneration may be of considerable
importance in delineating the role of cell division in the enhancement of initiation and/or promotion of pancreatic carcinogenesis. Indeed, recent studies suggest
that the regenerating pancreas is sensitive to the induction of pancreatic acinar
cell nodules as well as acinar cell carcinoma by 4-HAQO or azaserine (Longnecker
and co-workers, 1977; Konishi and co-workers, 1978).

TABLE 1 Experimental Models of Pancreatic Regeneration

Species	Stimulus	Reference
Rat	Partial Pancreatectomy	Cameron (1927); Lehv and Fitzgerald (1968)
Rat	Ethionine injections with protein-free diet for 10 days	Fitzgerald and co-workers (1968)
Rat	Cyclopropenoid fatty acids in diet	Scarpelli (1975)
Rat	Puromycin injection	Longnecker, Crawford and Nadler (1975)
Guinea Pig	Ethionine injections with protein-free diet for 10 days	Wenk, Reddy and Harris (1974)
Guinea Pig	4-Hydroxyaminoquinoline-1-oxide single dose intra-venously	Reddy and co-workers (1975)

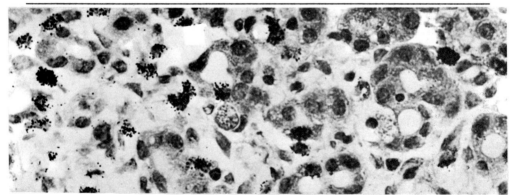

Fig. 1. 4-HAQO-induced regeneration of the guinea pig pancreatic acinar cells. H^3-
thymidine autoradiography reveals numerous labeled acinar cells (H&E 580).

SPONTANEOUS TUMORS OF THE PANCREAS

The incidence of spontaneously occurring exocrine pancreatic tumors in mice, rats and guinea pigs is quite low (Slye and co-workers, 1935; Rowlatt and Roe, 1967). In contrast however, Syrian hamsters (Takahashi and Pour, 1978) and mastomys (Hosoda, Suzuki and Suzuki, 1976) appear to develop a variety of proliferative, dysplastic and neoplastic lesions in pancreas spontaneously with advancing age. For example, ductular proliferation and dilatation were encountered in 41% female and 36% male Syrian hamsters over the age of 90 weeks (Takahashi and Pour, 1978). To what extent these spontaneously developing pancreatic lesions contribute to the unique susceptibility of the hamster to the successful induction of pancreatic carcinoma by β-oxidized derivatives of diisopropanolnitrosamine (Krüger, Pour and Althoff, 1974) remains to be determined, since these carcinogenic agents failed to induce pancreatic neoplasms in rats (Mohr and co-workers, 1977a), guinea pigs (Rao and Reddy, 1977; Rao and Pour, 1978), mice (Konishi and co-workers, 1977) and tree shrews (Rao and Reddy, unpublished data).

ANIMAL MODELS OF PANCREATIC CARCINOMA

Druckrey and co-workers (1968) reported the development of pancreatic tumors in random bred guinea pigs following prolonged treatment with the carcinogens methyl-nitrosourea and methylnitrosourethane. During the past five years, a number of promising models of pancreatic carcinoma have been developed (Table 2).

TABLE 2 Experimental Models of Pancreatic Carcinoma

Species	Carcinogen	Mode of Administration	Reference
Guinea pig (outbred)	Methylnitrosourea	Drinking water	Druckrey and co-workers (1968)
	Methylnitrosourethane	Drinking water	Druckrey and co-workers (1968)
Guinea pig (inbred strain 13)	Methylnitrosourea	Stomach tube	Reddy and Rao (1975)
Hamster (Syrian)	N-Nitrosobis(2-hydroxypropyl)amine	Subcutaneous	Krüger and coworkers (1974); Pour and co-workers (1974)
	N-Nitrosobis(2-acetoxypropyl)amine	Subcutaneous	Pour and coworkers (1976)
	N-Nitrosobis(2-oxopropyl)amine	Subcutaneous	Pour and coworkers (1977a)
	N-Nitroso-2,6-dimethylmorpholine	Stomach tube	Mohr and coworkers (1977b)
Rabbit	Dimethylhydrazine	Implants in pancreatic duct	Elkort and coworkers (1975)
Rat	4-Hydroxyamino quinoline-1-oxide	Intravenous	Hayashi and Hasegawa (1971)
	Azaserine	Intraperitoneal	Longnecker and Curphey (1975)
	Methylnitrosourea amino acid	Intraperitoneal	Longnecker and co-workers (1978)
	7-12-dimethylbenz(a)anthracene	Implants in pancreas	Dissin and coworkers (1975)
	Nafenopin	Dietary	Reddy and Rao (1977b)

At present, the models for chemical induction of pancreatic carcinoma involve three species: guinea pig, rat and hamster. Although inbred strain 13 guinea pigs appeared somewhat more susceptible to the rapid induction of pancreatic carcinoma by methylnitrosourea (Reddy, Svoboda and Rao, 1974; Reddy and Rao, 1975) than did the outbred strain, the high mortality rate during the first six months and less than 30% incidence of tumor significantly diminish the value of this model. Nevertheless, the guinea pig provided important insights into the histogenesis of methylnitrosourea induced pancreatic carcinoma (Reddy and Rao, 1975).

In the rat, either systemic administration of 4-HAQO (Hayashi and Hasegawa, 1971), azaserine (Longnecker and Curphey, 1975), nitrosated amino acids (Longnecker and co-workers, 1978) and nafenopin (Reddy and Rao, 1977b), or local implantation of 7-12, dimethylbenz(a)anthracene (DMBA) in pancreas (Dissin and co-workers, 1975) results in the development of pancreatic neoplasms of varying degrees of differentiation. All tumors that have been induced in rat pancreas by these structurally unrelated carcinogens appear to be derived from acinar cells. The reasons for the increased susceptibility of rat pancreatic acinar cells and not of ductal epithelium to neoplastic transformation remain to be elucidated.

Experimental evidence to date indicates that only the Syrian hamster is highly susceptible to the induction of pancreatic neoplasms by the β-oxidized derivatives of N-N-dipropylnitrosamine (DPN). The late Prof. Krüger synthesized N-nitrosobis(2-hydroxypropyl)amine, a derivative of DPN, which was found to induce a very high incidence of pancreatic neoplasms in Syrian golden hamsters (Krüger, Pour and Althoff, 1974; Pour and co-workers, 1974). During the last four years Pour and co-workers (1975, 1976, 1977a) have investigated the effects of several other β-oxidized derivatives of DPN, in an attempt to refine the hamster model, especially to minimize the incidence of simultaneously occurring non-pancreatic tumors. Of the three potent pancreatic carcinogens for the Syrian hamster (Table 2), N-nitrosobis(2-oxopropyl)amine (BOP) displayed the highest affinity for the pancreas (Pour and co-workers, 1977a). A single subcutaneous injection of this carcinogen has also been found to induce a high incidence of tumors in hamster pancreas (Pour and co-workers, 1978). Despite the additional development of an occasional tumor of the biliary tract, kidney, and lung in a few hamsters, the single dose BOP hamster model of pancreatic carcinogenesis may prove to be of special value in elucidating the influence of various factors on the initiation, promotion and/or biological behavior of this cancer.

N-nitroso-2,6-dimethylmorpholine (DMNM), a cyclic nitrosamine administered intragastrically to Syrian golden hamsters, induced pancreatic adenomas and adenocarcinomas in approximately 71% of animals (Mohr and co-workers, 1977b; Reznik, Mohr and Lijinsky, 1978). These animals also developed a variety of neoplasms of other organs, somewhat similar to the broad tumor spectrum observed in animals treated with β-oxidized derivatives of DPN (Pour and co-workers, 1974, 1975, 1976, 1977a). This similarity in tumor distribution may be attributable to the fact that DMNM as well as BOP form the same metabolites: N-nitrosobis(2-hydroxypropyl)(2-oxopropyl) amine and N-nitrosobis(2-hydroxypropyl)amine (Gingell and co-workers, 1976a, 1976b).

HISTOGENESIS OF PANCREATIC CARCINOMAS

The histogenesis of chemically induced pancreatic carcinomas is complex and a subject of current controversy based on recent experimental results which are in conflict with a long-established dogma concerning the embryological development of pancreas and the assumption that the majority of pancreatic carcinomas in humans are derived from preexisting ductules and ducts (Cubilla and Fitzgerald, 1975; Morgan and Wormsley, 1977; Webb, 1977).

The controversy centers around the interpretation of the fact that pancreatic acini of rats, guinea pigs and hamsters treated with a variety of compounds which induce predominantly adenocarcinoma undergo cell division and shed their apical cytoplasm converting the acinus into ductal-like structures as shown in Figs. 2

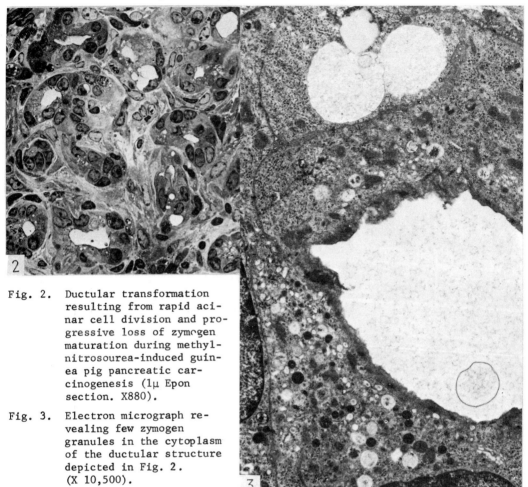

Fig. 2. Ductular transformation
resulting from rapid aci-
nar cell division and progressive loss of zymogen
maturation during methyl-
nitrosourea-induced guin-
ea pig pancreatic car-
cinogenesis (1μ Epon
section. X880).

Fig. 3. Electron micrograph re-
vealing few zymogen
granules in the cytoplasm
of the ductular structure
depicted in Fig. 2.
(X 10,500).

and 3. Such structures along with ductules and ducts appear to be the sites of
early development of ductal adenocarcinoma. The foregoing suggests that carcinogen induced proliferation and dedifferentiation of acinar cells leads to formation
of ductal cells (Reddy and Rao, 1975; Bockman and co-workers, 1978), a notion that
is counter to the sequence of developmental events believed to occur during normal
embryogenesis of the pancreas. Embryological studies suggest that pancreatic acini
and islets differentiate from the ductal system which appears early in the development of the organ. However, the fact that the acinar cell changes have been described by various authors utilizing different pancreatic carcinogens in a variety
of rodent species suggests that modulation of acinar cells into ductular ones is a
valid pathway (Reddy and Rao, 1975; Longnecker and Curphey, 1975; Shinozuka and co-
workers, 1976; Bockman and co-workers, 1978; Scarpelli and Rao, 1978). On the
other hand, it is maintained that in hamsters treated with the potent pancreatic
carcinogens preexisting peri- and intralobular ducts proliferate and serve as predominant sites of adenocarcinoma formation (Pour and co-workers, 1977b; Takahashi
and co-workers, 1977; Levitt and co-workers, 1977, 1978). However, in none of the
many photomicrographs showing ductules in islets does one find evidence of mitotic
activity. It is entirely probable that both pathways (i.e., ductular transformation of acinar cells and preexisting peri- and intrainsular ductules) may be operative in the histogenesis of chemically induced ductal adenocarcinoma of pancreas

in the hamster. The possibility that the peri- and intrainsular ductules in the
BOP treated hamster are derived from rapidly proliferating acinar cells in this
region can not be excluded.

Carcinomas of acinar cell origin have been induced in the rat and their histogenesis appears reasonably straightforward. Such neoplasms can either be well differentiated containing a full complement of zymogen granules, or poorly differentiated
with sparse to absent cytoplasmic secretory granules. These histogenetic pathways
are depicted in Fig. 4.

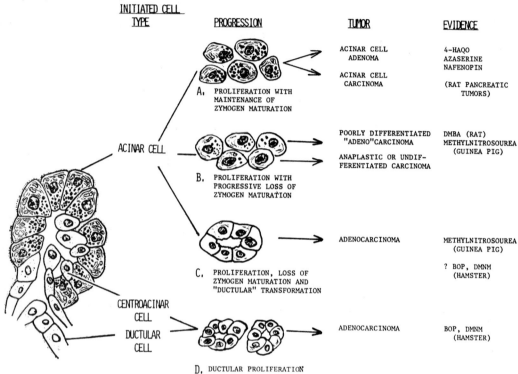

Fig. 4.   Proposed histogenetic pathways of pancreatic carcinogenesis.

CARCINOGEN METABOLISM AND ENZYME INDUCTION IN PANCREAS

The distribution pattern of pancreatic tumor development in various segments of
rat, guinea pig and hamster pancreas, as well as the result of other manipulations
such as diversion of bile flow, strongly suggest that the carcinogens and/or their
metabolites reach the pancreas via the ciruclation rather than through the bile.
The capacity of pancreas to metabolically activate carcinogens has been demonstrated
in a variety of rodent species, rat (Lilja and co-workers, 1977); hamster (Scarpelli
and co-workers, 1979), and guinea pig (Iqbal and co-workers, 1976, 1977, 1978). Enzymes in hamster pancreas capable of metabolically activating BOP and DMNM, can be
significantly increased by induction with β-nephthoflavone and 2,3,7,8-tetracholoro-
dibenzo-p-dioxin, both of which are potent inducers of cytochrome P-450-linked drug
metabolizing enzymes in extrahepatic tissues (Scarpelli and co-workers, 1979). The
demonstration of drug metabolizing enzymes capable of activating polycyclic hydro-
carbon carcinogens by epithelium of pancreatic ducts (Harris and co-workers, 1977)
suggests that all cellular components of pancreas may be implicated in the pathogenesis of pancreatic carcinoma.

IN VITRO MODELS OF PANCREATIC CARCINOMA

Development of appropriate in vitro systems should enable investigation of the differential role of acinar and ductal epithelium of the pancreas in the metabolic
activation of potential pancreatic carcinogens, and in the histogenesis of pancreatic carcinoma. In addition, such in vitro systems should also prove to be of importance for the investigation of various factors that modify pancreatic carcinogenesis
as well as for screening of potential pancreatic carcinogens.

A highly promising in vitro model of pancreatic carcinoma has been developed by
Parsa and Marsh (1976). This system utilizes pancreatic rudiments obtained from 13
day rat embryos, which are then cultured in a chemically defined medium for up to
10 weeks. Explants exposed to a single or multiple doses of the carcinogens di-
methylnitrosamine (Parsa and Marsh, 1976) or methylnitrosourea (Parsa and Sonchai,
1978) displayed morphological characteristics of adenocarcinoma. Upon xenotrans-
plantation into nude mice these transformed explants developed into adenocarcinomas.
Since the embryonic explants contain both acinar and ductal elements it is not certain if the transformation involves the acinar or ductal components. Despite the
uncertainty of histogenesis, this in vitro model system of Parsa appears highly
promising for screening the effects of promotors and inhibitors of pancreatic carcinogenesis. Long-term explant culture of human, bovine and rat pancreatic ducts
has recently been accomplished (Jones and co-workers, 1977; Githens and co-workers,
1978).

TRANSPLANTABLE PANCREATIC CARCINOMAS

Two transplantable pancreatic carcinomas have been established for the first time
during the last two years. These are 1) an acinar cell carcinoma of the rat pancreas (Reddy and Rao, 1977a), which has been transplanted in F-344 rats and athymic
nude mice through 15 successive passages (Rao and Reddy, 1979), and 2) a well-differentiated ductal adenocarcinoma of the hamster pancreas (Scarpelli and Rao, 1979)
which is currently in its tenth transplant generation in Syrian golden hamsters and
in nude mice. The transplantable acinar cell carcinoma of the rat pancreas (Fig.
5), displays substantial amylase and lipase activity and the tumor cells (Fig. 6)
contain variable numbers of zymogen granules (Reddy and Rao, 1977; Rao and Reddy,
1979). The transplantable adenocarcinoma of the hamster pancreas (Fig. 7) produces
mucin and rapidly and specifically binds secretin (Scarpelli and Rao, 1979). This
well-differentiated ductal adenocarcinoma has recently been converted into an
ascites form (Fig. 8) (Rao and Scarpelli, manuscript in preparation). These transplantable pancreatic carcinomas provide an unique opportunity to investigate the
biological (Reddy and co-workers, 1979) and biochemical properties of tumor cells
(which retain differentiated acinar or ductal characteristics) and their response
to various experimental manipulations.

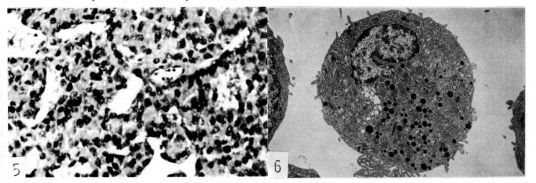

Fig. 5.   Pancreatic acinar cell carcinoma transplant (H&E X 220).   Fig. 6. Electron
          micrograph of a dissociated tumor cell from transplantable acinar cell car-
          cinoma reveals several zymogen granules (X 3000).

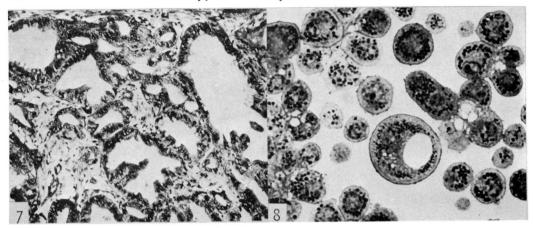

Fig. 7.   Transplantable ductal adenocarcinoma of the hamster pancreas (H&E 360).
Fig. 8.   Semi-thin section of a suspension of the ascites form of the tumor shown
          in Fig. 7; note the large signet tumor cell in the center (toluidine blue
          X 900).

CONCLUSION

In the present review we have outlined the developments that have occurred during
the past five years in the relatively new field of experimental pancreatic carcinogenesis,with the anticipation that the available models of pancreatic carcinogenesis and transplantable pancreatic carcinomas will serve as useful and important tools for the further investigation of various aspects of the induction and
biological behavior of pancreatic carcinoma.

REFERENCES

Bockman, D.E., O. Black, Jr., L.R. Mills, and P.D. Webster (1978). Origin of tu-
    bular complexes developing during induction of pancreatic adenocarcinoma by
    7,12-dimethylbenz(a)anthracene. Am. J. Pathol., 90, 645-658.
Cameron, G.R. (1927). Regeneration of the pancreas. J. Path. Bact. 30, 713-728.
Cohn, I. (1976). Cancer of the pancreas. Detection and diagnosis. Cancer, 37,
    582-588.
Craddock, V.M. (1971). Liver carcinomas induced in rats by single administration
    of dimethylnitrosamine after partial hepatectomy. J. Natl. Cancer Inst., 47,
    899-905.
Cubilla, A.L., and P.J. Fitzgerald (1975). Morphological patterns of primary
    nonendocrine human pancreas carcinoma. Cancer Res., 35, 2234-2248.
Dissin, J., L.R. Mills, D.L. Mainz, O. Black, Jr., and P.D. Webster III (1975).
    Experimental induction of pancreatic adenocarcinoma in rats. J. Natl. Cancer
    Inst., 55, 857-864.
Druckrey, H., S. Ivankovic, J. Bücheler, R. Preussmann, and C. Thomas (1968).
    Erzeugung von Magen-und pankreas-krebs beim meerschweinchen durch methyl-
    nitroso-harnstoff und-uretan. Z. Krebsforsch, 71, 167-182.
Elkort, R.J., A.H. Handler, and P.J. Mozden (1975). Preneoplastic changes in rab-
    bit pancreatic duct cells produced by dimethylhydrazine. Int. J. Cancer, 16,
    810-818.
Fitzgerald, P.J., L. Herman, B. Carol, A. Roque, W.H. Marsh, L. Rosenstock, C.
    Richardson, and D. Perl (1968). Pancreatic acinar cell regeneration 1. Cyto-
    logic, cytochemical and pancreatic weight changes. Am. J. Pathol., 52, 983-
    1011.

Gingell, R., L. Wallcave, D. Nagel, R. Kupper, and P. Pour (1976a). Common metabolites of N-nitroso-2,6-dimethylmorpholine and N-nitroso-bis(2-oxopropyl)amine in the Syrian hamster. Cancer Letters, 2, 47-52.

Gingell, R., L. Wallcave, D. Nagel, R. Kupper, and P. Pour (1976b). Metabolism of the pancreatic carcinogens N-nitroso-bis(2-oxopropyl)amine and N-nitro-bis(2-hydroxypropyl)amine in the Syrian hamster. J. Natl. Cancer Inst., 57, 1175-1178.

Githens, S., D.R.G. Holmquist, J.F. Whelan, and J.R. Ruby (1978). Carcinogenesis of isolated rat pancreatic ducts in rats. (Abstract) Proceedings of the American Pancreatic Study Group, Chicago.

Harris, C.C., H. Autrup, G. Stoner, S.K. Yang, J.C. Lentz, H.V. Gelboin, J.K. Selkirk, R.J. Connor, L.A. Barrett, R.T. Jones, E. McDowell, and B.F. Trump (1977). Metabolism of benzo(a)pyrene and 7,12-dimethylbenz(a)anthracene in cultured human bronchus and pancreatic duct. Cancer Res., 37, 3349-3355.

Hayashi, Y., and T. Hasegawa (1971). Experimental pancreatic tumor in rats after intravenous injection of 4-hydroxy-aminoquinoline 1-oxide. Gann, 62, 329-330.

Hosoda, S., H. Suzuki, and M. Suzuki (1976). Spontaneous tumors and atypical proliferation of pancreatic acinar cells in Mastomys (praomys) natalensis. J. Natl. Cancer Inst., 57, 1341-1346.

Iqbal, Z.M., M. Majdan, and S.S. Epstein (1976). Evidence of repair of DNA damage induced by 4-hydroxyaminoquinoline-1-oxide in guinea pig pancreatic slices in vitro. Cancer Res., 36, 1108-1113.

Iqbal, Z.M., M.E. Varnes, A. Yosyida, and S.S. Epstein (1977). Metabolism of benzo(a)pyrene by guinea pig pancreatic microsomes. Cancer Res., 37, 1011-1015.

Iqbal, Z.M., and S.S. Epstein (1978). Evidence of DNA repair in the guinea pig pancreas in vivo and in vitro following exposure to N-methyl-N-nitrosourethane. Chem-Biol. Interact., 20, 77-87.

Jones, R.T., L.A. Barrett, C. Van Haaften, C.C. Harris, and B.F. Trump (1977). Carcinogenesis in the pancreas. 1. Long-term explant culture of human and bovine pancreatic ducts. J. Natl. Cancer Inst., 58, 557-565.

Konishi, Y., H. Kondo, S. Inui, A. Denda, T. Ikeda, and K. Kojima (1977). Carcinogenic effect of N-bis(2-hydroxypropyl)nitrosamine by oral administration in mice. Cancer Letters, 3, 255-257.

Konishi, Y., A. Denda, S. Inui, S. Takahashi, N. Ueda, and M. Namiki (1978). Production of pancreatic acinar cell carcinoma by combined administration of 4-hydroxyaminoquinoline 1-oxide and azaserine in partial pancreatectomized rats. Cancer Letters, 4, 229-234.

Krüger, F.W., P. Our, and J. Althoff (1974). Induction of pancreas tumors by di-isopropanolnitrosamine. Naturwissenschaften, 61, 328.

Lehv, M., and P.J. Fitzgerald (1968). Pancreatic acinar cell regeneration IV. Regeneration after surgical resection. Am. J. Pathol., 53, 513-534.

Levitt, M.H., C.C. Harris, R. Squire, S. Springer, M. Wenk, C. Mollelo, D. Thomas, E. Kingsbury, and C. Newkirk (1977). Experimental pancreatic carcinogenesis. I. Morphogenesis of pancreatic adenocarcinoma in the Syrian golden hamster induced by N-nitrosobis(2-hydroxypropyl)amine. Am. J. Pathol., 88, 5-28.

Levitt, M., C.C. Harris, R. Squire, M. Wenk, C. Mollelo, and S. Springer (1978). Experimental pancreatic carcinogenesis. II. Lifetime carcinogenesis studies in the outbred Syrian golden hamster with N-nitroso-bis(2-hydroxypropyl)amine. J. Natl. Cancer Inst., 60, 701-705.

Lilja, H.S., E. Hyde, D.S. Longnecker, and J.D. Yager, Jr. (1977). DNA damage and repair in rat tissues following administration of azaserine. Cancer Res., 37, 3925-3931.

Longnecker, D.S., and T.J. Curphey (1975). Adenocarcinoma of the pancreas in azaserine-treated rats. Cancer Res., 35, 2249-2258.

Longnecker, D.S., B.G. Crawford, and D.J. Nadler (1975). Recovery of pancreas from mild puromycin-induced injury. A histologic and ultrastructure study in rats. Arch. Pathol., 99, 5-10.

Longnecker, D.S., J. French, E. Hyde, H.S. Lilja, and J.D. Yager, Jr. (1977). Effect of age on nodule induction by azaserine and DNA synthesis in rat pancreas. J. Natl. Cancer Inst., 58, 1769-1775.

Longnecker, D.S., T.J. Curphey, H.S. Lilja, J.I. French, and D.S. Daniel (1978). Carcinogenicity of a methylnitrosourea amino acid in rats. Fed. Proc., 37, 231.

Mohr, U., G. Reznik, and P. Pour (1977a). Carcinogenic effects of diisopropanol-nitrosamine in Sprague-Dawley rats. J. Natl. Cancer Inst.,58, 361-366.

Mohr, U., G. Reznik, E. Emminger, and W. Lijinsky (1977b). Induction of pancreatic duct carcinomas in the Syrian hamster with 2,6-dimethylnitrosomorpholine. J. Natl. Cancer Inst., 58, 429-432.

Morgan, R.G.H., and K.G. Wormsley (1977). Cancer of the pancreas. Gut, 18, 580-596.

Parsa, I., and W.H. Marsh (1976). An in vitro model of pancreatic carcinoma. Morphology and in vivo growth. Am. J. Pathol., 84, 469-478.

Parsa, I., and P. Sonchai (1978). The effects of DIPN on organ-cultured embryonic rat pancreas. Fed. Proc., 37, 232.

Pelc, S.R. (1964). Labeling of DNA and cell division in so-called non-dividing tissues. J. Cell Biol., 22, 21-28.

Pledger, R.A., R.R. Bates, and U. Saffiotti (1975). Introduction: National Cancer Institute Pancreatic Carcinogenesis Program. Cancer Res., 35, 2226-2227.

Pour, P., F.W. Krüger, J. Althoff, A. Cardesa, and U. Mohr (1974). Cancer of the pancreas induced in the Syrian golden hamster. Am. J. Pathol., 76, 349-358.

Pour, P., F.W. Krüger, J. Althoff, A. Cardesa, and U. Mohr (1975). A new approach for induction of pancreatic neoplasms. Cancer Res., 35, 2259-2268.

Pour, P., J. Althoff, R. Gingell, R. Kupper, F.W. Krüger, and U. Mohr (1976). N-nitrosobis(2-acetoxypropyl)amine as a further pancreatic carcinogen in Syrian golden hamsters. Cancer Res., 36, 2877-2884.

Pour, P., J. Althoff, F.W. Krüger, and U. Mohr (1977a). A potent pancreatic carcinogen in Syrian hamsters: N-nitrobis(2-oxopropyl)amine. J. Natl. Cancer Inst., 58, 1449-1453.

Pour, P., J. Althoff, and M. Takahashi (1977b). Early lesions of pancreatic ductal carcinoma in the hamster model. Am. J. Pathol., 88, 291-308.

Pour, P.M., S.Z. Salmasi, and R.G. Runge (1978). Selective induction of pancreatic ductular tumors by single dose of N-nitrosobis(2-oxopropyl)amine in Syrian golden hamsters. Cancer Lett., 4, 317-323.

Rao, M.S., and J.K. Reddy (1977). Induction of malignant vascular tumors of the liver in guinea pigs treated with 2,2'-diydroxy-ei-n,propylnitrosamine. J. Natl. Cancer Inst., 58, 387-392.

Rao, M.S., and P. Pour (1978). Development of biliary and hepatic neoplasms in guinea pigs treated with N-nitrosobis(2-oxopropyl)amine. Cancer Lett., 5, 31-34.

Rao, M.S., and J.K. Reddy (1979). Transplantable acinar cell carcinoma of the rat pancreas. Morphologic and biochemical characterization. Am. J. Pathol. (in press).

Reddy, J.K., D.J. Svoboda, and M.S. rao (1974). Susceptibility of an inbred strain of guinea pigs to the induction of pancreatic adenocarcinoma by N-methyl-N-nitrosourea. J. Natl. Cancer Inst., 52, 991-993.

Reddy, J.K., and M.S. Rao (1975). Pancreatic adenocarcinoma in inbred guinea pigs induced by N-methyl-N-nitrosourea. Cancer Res., 35, 2269-2277.

Reddy, J.K., M.S. Rao, D.J. Svoboda, and J.D. Prasad (1975). Pancreatic necrosis and regeneration induced by 4-hydroxyaminoquinoline-1-oxide in the guinea pig. Lab. Invest., 32, 98-104.

Reddy, J.K., and M.S. Rao (1977a). Transplantable pancreatic carcinoma of the rat. Science, 198, 78-80.

Reddy, J.K., and M.S. Rao (1977b). Malignant tumors in rats fed nafenopin, a hepatic peroxisome proliferator. J. Natl. Cancer Inst., 59, 1645-1647.

Reddy, J.K., M.S. Rao, J.R. Warren, and O.T. Minnick (1979). Concanavalin A ag-
glutinability and surface microvilli of dissociated normal and neoplastic pancreatic acinar cells of the rat. Exp. Cell Res. (in press).

Reznik, G., U. Mohr, and W. Lijinsky (1978). Carcinogenic effect of N-nitroso-2,
6-dimethylmorpholine in Syrian golden hamsters. J. Natl. Cancer Inst., 60,
371-378.

Rowlatt, U., and F.J.C. Roe (1967). Epithelial tumors of the rat pancreas. J.
Natl. Cancer Inst., 39, 18-32.

Scarpelli, D.G. (1975). Preliminary observations on the mitogenic effect of cyclo-
propenoid fatty acids on rat pancreas. Cancer Res., 35, 2278-2283.

Scarpelli, D.G., and M.S. Rao (1978). Pathogenesis of pancreatic carcinoma in hamsters induced by N-nitrosobis(2-oxopropyl)amine (BOP). Fed. Proc., 37, 231.

Scarpelli, D.G., and M.S. Rao (1979). Transplantable ductal adenocarcinoma of
Syrian hamster pancreas. Cancer Res., 39, 452-458.

Scarpelli, D.G., M.S. Rao, V.S. Rao, and P.H. Hollenberg (1979). Nitrosamine activation by hamster pancreas and revertant mutation of Salmonella typhimurium
TA-1535. Cancer Res. (submitted).

Shinozuka, H., J.A. Popp, and Y. Konishi (1976). Ultrastructures of atypical acinar cell nodules in rat pancreas induced by 4-hydroxyaminoquinoline-1-oxide.
Lab. Invest., 34, 501-509.

Slye, M., H.F. Holmes, and H.G. Wells (1935). The comparative pathology of carcinoma of the pancreas with report of two cases in mice. Am. J. Cancer, 23, 81-
86.

Takahashi, M., and P. Pour (1978). Spontaneous alterations in the pancreas of the
aging Syrian golden hamster. J. Natl. Cancer Inst., 60, 355-364.

Takahashi, M., P. Pour, J. Althoff, T. Donnelly (1977). Sequential alterations of
the pancreas during carcinogenesis in Syrian hamsters by N-nitrosobis(2-oxo-
propyl)amine. Cancer Res., 37, 4602-4606.

Webb, J.N. (1977). Acinar cell neoplasms of the exocrine pancreas. J. Clin.
Pathol., 30, 103-112.

Wenk, M.L., J.K. Reddy, and C.C. Harris (1974). Pancreatic regeneration caused by
ethionine in the guinea pig. J. Natl. Cancer Inst., 52, 533-538.

Morphological Types of Pancreas (Non-endocrine) Cancer

Antonio Cubilla and Patrick J. Fitzgerald

Department of Pathology, Memorial Hospital, Memorial Sloan-Kettering Cancer Center, New York, New York, U.S.A.

ABSTRACT

The clinical records and pathological tissues of 508 patients with pancreas cancer treated at Memorial Hospital during the years 1949 through 1972 were studied. Eleven distinctive morphologic types were delineated and in a 12th group were placed tumors yet to be classified. The types with their relative distribution were: Duct cell adenocarcinoma, 75%; giant cell adenocarcinoma, 4%; giant cell carcinoma (epulis with osteoid type), <1%; adenosquamous carcinoma, 4%; microadenocarcinoma, 3%; mucinous ("colloid") carcinoma, 2%; cystadenocarcinoma (mucinous), 1%; acinar cell carcinoma, 1%; pancreaticoblastoma, papillary and cystic tumor, and mixed acinar, islet and duct cell tumor, each <1%; and unclassified carcinoma, 10%. Pertinent demographic data and survival figures were obtained. Only 3 patients, all with duct adenocarcinoma of the head of the pancreas, survived 5 years (<1%) and they died of the disease 60, 63 and 90 months after surgical resection of the cancers. It is hoped that a type might be associated with an etiologic agent, a response to a particular chemotherapy regimen, or to some molecular event giving rise to the characteristic pattern.

Pancreas, cancer, adenocarcinoma, giant cell cancer, adenosquamous cancer, cystadenocarcinoma, acinar carcinoma, carcinosarcoma.

INTRODUCTION

Pancreas cancer causes the death of over 20,000 patients a year, it is increasing (Krain, 1975) and the number surviving for 5 years after diagnosis is only a few percent (Biometry Branch, NCI, 1972, 1974; Silverberg, 1978). Pathologists in general identify only a few distinctive morphological types and use the designations, "adenocarcinoma," or "carcinoma" for most pancreas cancers.

Ductal carcinoma, squamous cell carcinomas, acinar cell carcinomas, mucinous carcinoma and cystadenocarcinoma were well known in 1951 (Miller, Baggenstoss and Comfort). Sommers and Meissner (1954) described giant cell carcinoma and adenoacanthoma (adenosquamous). More recently a few tumors in childhood (Taxy, 1976) and a distinctive type in young females have been delineated (Oertel, 1975). Our classification contains these types and an additional one - the microadenocarcinoma (Table 1) (Cubilla and Fitzgerald, 1975).

111

From a survey of the records of 757 patient with cancer of the pancreas at Memorial Hospital during the years 1949 through 1972, we found adequate clinical data and pathological tissue for the study of 508 patients (Cubilla and Fitzgerald, 1978).

TYPES OF PANCREAS (NON-ENDOCRINE) CARCINOMA

DUCT CELL ADENOCARCINOMA (Adenocarcinoma, Carcinoma)(380 patients)

This was the most common type of pancreas cancer and will be considered the prototype (Cubilla and Fitzgerald, 1978). Because of the presence of mucin in most cases, an absence of zymogen granules and an incidence of carcinoma in situ in ductal epithelium of at least 24% (Cubilla and Fitzgerald, 1976), it is assumed that these cases arose from duct (or ductular) epithelium.

TABLE 1   Carcinoma of the Pancreas (Non-Endocrine)

	No. of Patients (%)
Carcinomas of Duct (Ductular) Cell Origin	
Duct cell adenocarcinoma	380 (75)
Giant cell carcinoma	22 (4)
Giant cell carcinoma (Epulis with Osteoid)	1 (-)
Adenosquamous carcinoma	18 (4)
Microadenocarcinoma	15 (3)
Mucinous ("Colloid") carcinoma	9 (2)
Cystadenocarcinoma (Mucinous)	3 (1)
Carcinoma of Acinar Cell Origin	
Acinar cell adenocarcinoma	6 (1)
Carcinomas of Uncertain Histogenesis	
Pancreaticoblastoma	1 (-)
Papillary cystic tumor	1 (-)
Mixed type: acinar, duct, and islet cell carcinoma	1 (-)
Unclassified carcinoma	51 (10)
Large cell	44 (9)
Small cell	7 (1)
Total	508 (100)

Our duct adenocarcinomas occurred predominantly in elderly (sixth and seventh decade), male (male/female ratio of 1:5), white (92%) patients who were heavy smokers (68%) and some (31%) were diabetic.

The cancer was localized to the head of the pancreas in 60% of patients, to the body in 13%, to the tail in 5% and in the remaining 20 to a combination of sites. Stage I (cancer confined to gland) patients made up 14%, Stage II (regional lymph nodes involved) comprised 21% and Stage III (metastases present) occurred in 65% of patients. The size of the cancers varied; in cancers of the head of the pancreas the largest diameter was less than 3 cm in only 13% of patients and in 60% of patients it was more than 5 cm. Body and tail lesions averaged about 10 cm.

Lymph node involvement of cancers of the head of the pancreas was commonest in the superior head and posterior pancreaticoduodenal groups but also occurred in the superior body, inferior head and anterior pancreaticoduodenal nodes (Cubilla, Fortner and Fitzgerald, 1978). Metastases were to the liver, and regional nodes primarily, then became widespread (Cubilla and Fitzgerald, 1977).

Pancreas adenocarcinoma resembled adenocarcinoma of the intestinal tract, lung, uterus and other organs, but occasionally it had the appearance of the epithelium of the biliary tract.   Large and small glands, poorly or well differentiated, were present.   Some glands resembled normal ducts or ductules, and other parts of the tumor showed considerable anaplasia.   Most tumor glands were formed by tall columnar cells or by cuboidal cells with a cytoplasm varying from watery clear to deeply eosinophic.   Nuclei were seen to vary in size and shape, polarity and distribution of chromatin.   Occasionally goblet cells were present and the mucin stains indicated the presence of mucin in the apex of cells or in extracellular pools in most tumors.   Papillary, cystic, and other histologic patterns were present, but always in less than 20% of the tissue.   Electron microscopy revealed mucigen granules in most cases but no zymogen granules in any case.

Desmoplastic response was very prominent in most tumors and foci of hemorrhage, necrosis and fat necrosis were also frequently present but they made up a very small portion of the tissue.   Atrophy of acinar cells was marked in most cases, as was ductule and duct ectasia, in association with duct obstruction.

Marked atypia of ductal epithelium and carcinoma in situ were present only in pancreas cancer cases and not in the controls (Cubilla and Fitzgerald, 1976).

Survival, without regard to type of therapy, varied with the site (head longest), size (longer with smaller lesions), and stage (the lower the stage the longer the survival).   Median overall survival was 4 months.   "Curative" surgery gave a survival rate of 21% at 1 year; at 5 years there were 3 survivors (1%) and these died of disease at 60, 63, and 90 months.

GIANT CELL CARCINOMA   (Pleomorphic cancer, sarcomatoid cancer) (22 patients).

In our cases of this distinctive group (Alguacil and Weiland, 1977; Guillan, 1968) the male/female ratio was 1:4, and the median age was 62 years.   The tumor occurred in the head of the pancreas in 10 patients and in the body and/or tail in 12 patients.   The median diameter was 8 cm.

Large polyploid, often bizarre, mono- or multi-nucleated tumor giant cells and malignant spindle cells were present.   The huge giant cells with many very large nuclei, often vacuolated, contained a large prominent nucleolus, deeply staining chromatin and abundant, dense, heavily stained cytoplasm.

The spindle cells, usually mononucleated, but sometimes multinucleated, were obviously malignant and resembled mesenchymal spindle cells but some appeared to be giving rise to gland formation and were thereby epithelial.   Cytoplasm was sparse, fusiform and often fibrillar in shape.   A third type of small round uniform-sized cell with a small amount of pale staining cytoplasm was present in sheets or clusters of cells in most cases.   Mitoses, often bizarre, were relatively frequent. We were impressed with the spindle cell carcinoma element in most of our cases but opted for the term giant cell carcinoma because of the prominence of giant cells in all of our cases.

Marked atrophy of parenchyma and fibrosis, in association with duct obstruction, were noted in 12 cases.   The mucicarmine stain was positive in glandular areas in 18 of 20 cases and in the giant cells of 4 of these cases.   Fat necrosis was seen in 3 cases.

Pancreas hemorrhage was prominent in 12 cases and necrosis in 21. There were a few foci of epulis or osteoclast-like cells present, generally near foci of hemorrhage and necrosis, but no osteoid (see below). Cytophagocytosis (mainly erythrocytes) was noted in 9 cases. In situ carcinoma of duct epithelium, atypical duct hyperplasia and papillary hyperplasia were noted in each of 2.

Survival varied from a few weeks (no treatment) to 9 months (chemotherapy and irradiation). The median survival period was 2 months.

GIANT CELL CARCINOMA (EPULIS AND OSTEOID TYPE)

This is a rare tumor (Rosai, 1968). Our patient was a 45-year-old male who presented clinically with jaundice. At exploratory laparotomy at another hospital a frozen section of a mass in the head of the pancreas was diagnosed as giant cell adenocarcinoma of the pancreas and a Whipple procedure was performed. In the resected specimen there was a 7X6 cm. soft yellow-red, well defined mass in the head of the pancreas.

The tumor showed 3 major histologic features: (1) Numerous epulis type giant cells; (2) Bizarre malignant giant cells; and (3) Spindle cells, both benign and malignant. The giant cells were multinucleated and they ranged from benign appearing epulis-like (or osteoclastic) cells to the more bizarre irregular cells seen in the giant cell carcinoma described above. The spindle cells varied from uniform, rather benign fibroblast-like cells to irregular, bizarre anaplastic sarcoma-like cells.

Multiple foci of osteoid tissue in close association with stromal cells and epulis cells were present. In most areas this tumor strikingly resembled the giant cell tumor of bone; in a few focal areas it more closely resembled the giant cell carcinoma described above. Hemorrhage was frequent. The patient died 4 years after the partial pancreatectomy with disseminated pulmonary metastases and a massive pleural effusion which contained malignant tumor giant cells.

In 2 cases seen in consultation, there were several foci of adenocarcinoma of the ductal type present. The longer survival period in these cases as well as the presence of the giant cells suggests that this tumor should be classified separately from the more frequent giant cell carcinoma.

ADENOSQUAMOUS CANCER (Adenoacanthoma, mucoepidermoid, squamous cancer)(18 patients)

This type is seen in many organs and has a mixture of glandular and squamous cell cancer components (at least one-third of the tissue manifesting both malignant squamous cancer and malignant adenocarcinoma components).

Fourteen patients were men and 3 were women, the median age was 63 years, the male/female ratio was 5:1, and all patients were white. Six patients were diabetic; 2 patients had irradiation involving the pancreas area for another malignant tumor; and in 6 patients a second primary tumor was present.

The primary site was head of the pancreas in 9 patients, body in 3 and tail in 1. In 1 patient the cancer involved head, body and tail and in another the body and tail were involved. The median size of the tumors was 6 cm. The tumor (in head of pancreas) was a firm, grey fibrotic irregular mass producing obstruction of main pancreatic duct and cancer bile duct.

In 7 cases there was about equal distribution of glandular and squamous cancers, squamous cancer predominated over glandular carcinoma in 7 cases and in 4 cases the adenocarcinoma component was somewhat in excess.

The adenocarcinoma varied from well differentiated to poorly differentiated adenocarcinoma to focal areas of anaplastic carcinoma.   Mitosis were prominent.   Squamous areas had abundant cytoplastic keratin and "pearls" and intracellular bridges were present in most squamous cancer areas.   In 11 of 12 cases the mucin stain was positive. Desmoplastic response secondary to ductal obstruction was prominent but tumor necrosis was not common.   Perineural invasion was present in 9 of 12 primary tumors.

Metastases were primarily to liver, lymph nodes and peritoneum and were present in 13 cases at time of diagnosis.   The median survival period was 6 months.

MICROADENOCARCINOMA (15 patients)

This is an uncommon type resembling, somewhat, carcinoid tumor (Cubilla and Fitzgerald, 1975).   Nine patients were males and 6 were female.   The median age was 61 years.   Jaundice and distant metastasis to various organs were common.

In 5 patients the tumor was located in the head of the pancreas, in 3 patients it was in the body and in 3 it was body and tail, in 2 it involved head, body and tail, and in 2 patients the site was unknown.   The tumors had a median largest diameter   of 10 cm.; they were gray, firm, but with areas of necrosis.   An adenocarcinoma composed of small glands - smaller than those in the usual duct carcinoma - were present.   Cells were present in sheets or solid foci of cells and the small glands often occurred in the center of a large sea of small cells resembling carcinoid cells.   Nuclei were round to oval and of intermediate size.   The cytoplasm was scant except where glands were formed and then it was moderate in amount and eosinophilic.   There was prominent necrosis.   Mucin was noted in the malignant cells and lumens of glands.   Stains for islet cell or carcinoid granules were negative and in the tumors of 2 patients no cytoplasmic granules were seen by electron microscopy.

Most patients received only palliative treatment.   All but 1 patient died of the disease within days to a few months; the median survival period was 1.5 months.

MUCINOUS ("COLLOID") ("GELATINOUS") ADENOCARCINOMA (9 patients)

This tumor is a well-recognized, although uncommon type.   There were 9 patients, all male, with a median age of 62 years.   Three patients had a long standing history of chronic pancreatitis (one of these had pancreaticolithiasis and another was called an "alcoholic").   Diabetes was present in an additional patient.

Seven tumors occurred in the head of the pancreas and 2 in the body and tail.   The tumors were large (median largest diameter was 7 cm) soft and described as having a "gelatinous" appearance.   They showed large cystic spaces filled with mucin and lined by tall columnar non-papillary, malignant glandular epithelium; another pattern was that of mucinous lakes with floating nests of adenocarcinoma cells; and a third feature (uncommon) was the presence of "signet ring" cancer cells floating in mucinous pools.

The median survival period for all cases was 9 months.   In one patient a "curative" surgical resection (total pancreatectomy) was performed and the patient lived for 15 months.   Four of the cases were diagnosed at autopsy.

CYSTADENOCARCINOMA (MUCINOUS) (3 patients)

This is a well known pancreas tumor, recently clearly separated from serous cyst-adenoma (Compagna and Oertel, 1978). All patients were women and the median age was 54 years. Two patients presented with a large abdominal mass and one with a metastasis to lymph nodes of the left groin. Diabetes, cholelithiasis and the removal of a pancreatic cyst were each present in different patients.

All tumors were located in the tail of the pancreas. They were large (median largest diameter of 18 cm.), gray, multiloculated cysts containing mucinous fluid. Focal solid areas were noted in two cases.

Cysts of varying size from very small to very large, filled with mucin, were pre-sent. The cyst wall was lined by tall columnar cells with basal nuclei and abun-dant clear cytoplasm filled with mucigen granules. In all cases, prominent intra-cystic papillary projections of cells were noted, some with, and some without, fibrovascular stroma. In most histologic sections areas of benign neoplastic epithelium, atypical epithelium, and foci of adenocarcinoma were present, both in the epithelium of the cyst wall and in the fibrous stroma. In a few areas the stroma beneath the epithelium resembled ovarian stroma.

The metastatic tumor varied from an orderly low-grade cystic adenocarcinoma in two cases to a poorly differentiated duct adenocarcinoma in the third patient.

All patients underwent partial pancreatectomy. Two patients died of metastatic disease 17 and 60 months after the pancreatectomy, and the third was lost to follow-up a few months after surgery.

ACINAR CELL CARCINOMA (6 patients)

Acinar cell carcinoma has long been recognized as a distinctive type. There were 4 men and 2 women, with a mean age of 54 years. Four patients presented with a distant metastasis from an occult primary cancer. None of our patients had fat necrosis of subcutaneous tissue or of bone.

The tail or body of the pancreas was involved in 3 cases and the head in 3. Tu-mors were large, had a median diameter of 5 cm., and were grey to tan, firm with minimal amounts of stromal fibrosis. Necrosis was prominent.

Characteristic acinar formation by malignant acinar cells with a small central lu-men was present in many areas. The acinar cells were large and polyhedral with a basal round nucleus and abundant granular cytoplasm containing coarse cytoplasmic granules. In some areas poorly formed acini were present and in other areas ana-plastic foci composed of polyhedral to round cells with considerable eosinophilic coarse cytoplasm were noted. In some fields there were small round cells resem-bling lymphoma cells. Focal glandular features, with cells resembling pancreatic duct cells containing mucin in the apical border of the cells, were identified in some cases. Electron microscopy showed zymogen granules in the 1 case examined by this technique.

At the autopsies of four patients widespread dissemination of the cancer was noted. No tumor was resected. Palliative therapy was given to 5 patients. Medi-an survival period was 9 months.

PANCREATICOBLASTOMA

Our case of this rare lesion (Taxy, 1976) was a 3 year old Peruvian boy with an abdominal mass; at exploratory laparotomy a tissue biopsy was diagnosed as neuroblastoma. At Memorial Hospital he was re-explored and a tumor, 4X3X2 cm, in the head of the pancreas was resected.

The predominant pattern was that of small cells with clear, or amphophilic, scanty cytoplasm forming solid sheets. Focally, glandular arrangement of the small cells was noted. The lumens of gland stained for mucin. Mixed with the small cells there were slightly larger, deeply eosinophilic isolated cells. The eosinophilic cell cytoplasm revealed coarse granules resembling zymogenic granules. Irregular nests of well differentiated epidermoid cells without keratinization were noted. Stains for beta and non-beta islet granules were negative. Electron microscopic examination showed dense large granules (zymogen) and abundant rough endoplasmic reticulum in a few cells.

In most tissues spindle cells, chondroid, osteoid and/or bone tissue were prominent.

The patient died with pulmonary metastasis one year after surgery.

PAPILLARY CYSTIC CARCINOMA

Our case of this rare tumor (Oertel, 1975; Hamoudi and colleagues, 1970; Franz, 1959) was that of a 12-year-old girl in whom at exploratory laparotomy an 8 cm. well circumscribed mass involving the body and tail of the pancreas was resected. The cut surface showed a cystic and hemorrhagic tan grey encapsulated tumor.

The predominant histologic pattern was that of sheets of cells surrounding thin-walled vessels containing erythrocytes. In addition, other areas give a distinctive papillary appearance with the spaces between the papillae filled with intact red blood cells. The nuclei of the cells were round or slightly oval and had an inconspicuous nucleolus and a rather finely dispersed chromatin. Mitoses were very rare. The cytoplasmic cell borders were poorly defined.

Focal areas of myxoid degeneration of the stroma were noted and these appeared somewhat similar to myxopapillary ependymomas, or to some mixed tumors of the salivary gland. In some areas the tumor was rather solid with little hemorrhage but the periangiomatous arrangement was always present. Focally there were areas of fibrosis and hemorrhage with fat necrosis and cholesterol clefts. Special stains for beta and non-beta cells, zymogen granules and mucin stains were all negative in the tumor cells. Mucin was noted in myxoid stromal areas.

Oertel (1978) from the Armed Forces Institute of Pathology, Washington, D.C., has accumulated 52 cases (mostly females, many black) and he found metastases in only 2 patients.

ANAPLASTIC CARCINOMA

This group of tumors did not exhibit in most of the tissue the features of the types described above. Many were diagnosed at autopsy and showed diffuse involvement of the pancreas. There was a variety of types: One contained a large cell which resembled anaplastic carcinoma; a second type with small uniform cells was similar to malignant lymphoma; a rare type had moderate-sized cells containing well-outlined, abundant, clear cytoplasm and an eccentric relatively small, poorly defined, irregular nucleus similar to the renal cell carcinoma, except that the cytoplasm contained mucin; and other morphologic patterns were also present.

COMMENT

Whether the delineation of these histological types will lead to the association of one or more with an epidemiological factor, or to a clinical response to a specific chemotherapeutic regimen, is not known, but malignant morphologic patterns   must be the result of an underlying transformation event at the molecular level which in itself is of great biological interest and, probably, importance.

REFERENCES

Alguacil-Garcia, A. and L.H. Weiland (1977). The Histological Spectrum, Prognosis, and Histogenesis of the Sarcomatoid Cancer of the Pancreas. Cancer, 39, 1181-1189.

Biometry Branch National Cancer Institute (1972). Axtell, L.M., S.J. Cutler and M.S. Myers (Eds.), End Results in Cancer, Report No. 4. DHEW Pub. No. 73 End Results Section, 81-84.

Biometry Branch National Cancer Institute (1974). Axtell, L.M. and M.H. Myers (Eds.), Recent Trends in Survival of Cancer Patients, 1960-1971. DHEW Pub. No. 75-767. End Results Section, 30.

Compagna and J. Oertel (1978). Mucinous Cystic Neoplasms of the Pancreas with Overt and Latent Malignancy (Cystadenocarcinoma and Cystadenoma). Am J Clin Path, 69, 573-580.

Cubilla, A.L. and P.J. Fitzgerald (1975). Morphological Patterns of Non-Endocrine Human Pancreas Carcinoma. Cancer Res, 35, 2234-2246.

Cubilla, A.L. and P.J. Fitzgerald (1976). Morphological Lesions Associated With Human Primary Invasive Non-Endocrine Pancreas Cancer. Cancer Res, 36, 2690-2698.

Cubilla, A.L. and P.J. Fitzgerald (1977). Metastasis. Pancreatic Duct Adenocarcinoma. In S. Day, L. Myers, P. Stansly and M. Lewis (Eds.), Cancer Invasion and Metastasis, Raven Press, New York. pp. 81-94.

Cubilla, A.L. and P.J. Fitzgerald (1978). Pancreas Cancer. 1. Duct Cell Adenocarcinoma. In Pathology Annual, Part 1. Appleton-Century-Crofts, New York. pp. 241-287.

Cubilla, A.L., J. Fortner and P.J. Fitzgerald (1978). Lymph Node Involvement in Carcinoma of the Head of the Pancreas Area. Cancer, 41, 880-887.

Franz, V.K. (1959). Tumors of the Pancreas. Armed Forces Inst of Path, Sect 7, Fasc 27 and 28, 27-73.

Guillan, R.A. (1968). Pleomorphic Adenocarcinoma of the Pancreas. An Analysis of Five Cases. Cancer, 21, 1072-1079.

Hamoudi, A.B., K. Misugi, J.L. Gorsfeld and C.B. Reiner (1970). Papillary Epithelial Neoplasm of Pancreas in a Child: Report of a Case with Electron Microscopy. Cancer, 26, 1126-1134.

Krain, L.S. (1975). The Rising Incidence of Cancer of the Pancreas - Further Epidemiologic Studies. J Chronic Dis, 23, 685-690.

Miller, J.R., A.H. Baggenstoss, and M.W. Comfort (1951). Carcinoma of the Pancreas. Effect of Histological Type and Grade of Malignancy on its Behavior. Cancer, 4, 233-241.

Oertel, J.E. (1978). (Personal communication to Dr. Antonio L. Cubilla).

Rosai, J. (1968). Carcinoma of Pancreas Simulating Giant Cell Tumor of Bone. (Electron Microscopic Evidence of its Acinar Cell Origin. Cancer, 22, 333-344.

Silverberg, E. (1978). Cancer Statistics, 1978. CA, 28, 17-32.

Sommers, S.C. and W.A. Meissner (1954). Unusual Carcinomas of the Pancreas. Arch Pathol, 58, 101-111.

Taxy, J.B. (1976). Adenocarcinoma of the Pancreas in Childhood. Report of a Case and a Review of the English Language Literautre. Cancer, 37, 1508-1518.

Biochemistry of Human Liver Cell Carcinoma—Special Reference to Novel γ-GTP Isoenzyme Specific to Hepatocellular Carcinoma

N. Hattori*, N. Sawabu*, M. Nakagen*, K. Ozaki*
T. Wakabayashi*, M. Yoneda* and M. Ishii**

*First Department of Internal Medicine, School of Medicine
Kanazawa University, Japan
**Division of Serology, Saitama Cancer Center, Japan

ABSTRACT

In view of experimental liver cancer studies indicating that hepatoma tissue acquires carcinoembryonic properties with special respect to γ-glutamyl trans-peptidase (γ-GTP), γ-GTP was examined to see whether or not hepatoma-specific γ-GTP isoenzyme was observed in the sera of patients with hepatocellular carcinoma (HCC). Novel γ-GTP isoenzymes were found to be specific for patients with HCC and detectable in 43% of sera from 100 patients with HCC. It can be useful as one of diagnostic indices for HCC to examine γ-GTP isoenzyme patterns. Novel γ-GTP isoenzyme was finally purified from ascites of patients with HCC by procedures including five steps. It was relatively heat-stable and was immunologically indistinguishable from that of HCC and fetal liver. It is highly probable from these results that this specific band is derived from HCC cells and this protein represents one of carcinofetal proteins.

KEYWORDS : Novel γ-GTP Isoenzyme, Hepatocellular Carcinoma, α-Fetoprotein, Carcinofetal Protein, Polyacrylamide Electrophoresis

INTRODUCTION

It is evident that in conventional laboratory tests, biochemical changes in HCC are not so much different from those in hepatic cirrhosis or chronic hepatitis. On the other hand, numerous studies indicate that many hepatic cancers reveal biochemical changes which fall into the following three major categories: 1. Appearance of some carcinofetal antigens such as α-fetoprotein (AFP) and fetal type of isoenzyme. 2. excessive synthesis of hormones and hormone like substances such as PTH and erythropoietin. 3. metabolic abnormalities such as occurrence of unusual fatty acid (eicosatrienoic acid) and hypercholesterolemia. Some of these products have already been used as biochemical marker for the detection of HCC. Among them, AFP is now considered a sensitive test for the diagnosis of HCC, though the prevalences of other products are too low to be of any diagnostic aid. However, 20 to 30% of patients with HCC shows AFP of low concentration less than 200 ng/ml which can be seen commonly in sera of patients with hepatobiliary diseases other than HCC. Additionally, AFP is not always so useful for detecting HCC in an early stage. Therefore, we need a new diagnostic index specific and more sensitive for HCC.

Experimental liver cancer studies (Fiala and colleagues, 1973; Taniguchi and colleagues, 1975; Kalengayi and colleagues, 1975; Tateishi and colleagues, 1976, Cameron and colleagues, 1978) indicated that hepatoma tissue acquired carcino-fetal properties with special respect to γ-GTP activity. Similar to AFP, γ-GTP activity is quite low in the adult liver whereas the activity is extremely high in the fetal liver and in the HCC, and its activity has been found to become higher in some of patients with HCC. These observations strongly suggest that activation of γ-GTP might occur during hepatocarcinogenesis, by acquisition of fetal properties of HCC, and its activity has been found to become higher in some of patients with HCC. These observations strongly suggest that activation of γ-GTP might occur during hepatocarcinogenesis, by acquisition of fetal properties of HCC, and that this fetal isoenzyme would be detectable in patients with HCC. In this regard, we attempted to examine the γ-GTP isoenzyme clinically by using polyacrylamide gradient gel electrophoresis, and discovered the novel γ-GTP isoenzyme which was considered specific to patients with HCC. This work deals with the clinical significance and some of enzymological and immunological properties of this novel γ-GTP isoenzyme.

MATERIALS

Materials consisted of sera obtained from 320 patients with various hepatobiliary diseases including 100 patients with HCC. In 59 out of 100 patients of HCC, the diagnosis was confirmed by autopsy or surgery, while in the other 41 it was established by AFP and/or selective celiac angiography, as well as other clinical and laboratory examinations. Ascitic fluids were also obtained from some of Patients with HCC. Tissue materials were also obtained from HCC, adult liver and fetal liver. Other several kinds of autopsy samples were included in this study. The supernatant of 25,000 x g centrifugation which was solublized by adding 1% Triton X or DOC was used as enzyme extract.

METHODS

γ-GTP Isoenzyme

Electrophoresis was carried out with G.E.-4 apparatus (Pharmacia Fine Chemicals) loaded with polyacrylamide gradient (from 4 to 30%) gel plate at a constant voltatage of 350 V for 3.5 hr or 125 V for 15 hr. in 0.05 M Tris-glycine buffer (pH 8.35). The detail of staining procedure is described in the previous report (Sawabu and coworkers, 1978a).

Purification of Novel γ-GTP Isoenzyme

Ascites obtained from patients with HCC positive in novel γ-GTP isoenzyme were used as the starting material. Purification was carried out by means of the following five steps including ammonium sulfate fractionation, Con A affinity chromatography, Ultrogel chromatography, separation by preparative polyacrylamide disc electrophoresis and elimination by a technique of immunoabsorption using sepharose 4B affinity chromatography coupled with antihuman serum protein and antihuman serum albumin. The detail of procedures for preparative polyacrylamide disc electrophoresis and immunoabsorption using sepharose 4B affinity chromato-graphy was reported elsewhere (Sawabu and coworkers, 1978b).

Preparation of Specific Antiserum and Immunological Method

Rabbits were immunized with the partially purified fraction corresponding to band II recovered at the step of preparative polyacrylamide disc electrophoresis. An antibody rich in γ-globulin fraction was separated from antiserum by ammonium sulfate fraction (0-40% saturation). Further, by a technique of immunoabsorption using sera of HCC with AFP and without novel γ-GTP isoenzyme, antiserum against to novel γ-GTP isoenzyme was obtained. Ouchterlony's double diffusion method was performed in 1.5% agar in Laurell's buffer (pH 8.6) with the specific antiserum.

Enzyme Assay

γ-GTP activity was assayed by the method using γ-glutamyl-p-nitroanilide as a substrate and glycylglycine as an acceptor. Physicochemical properties such as heat stability, pH optimum, Km value for substrate and effect of some cations were determined in the same manner. AFP was determined by the radioimmunoassay.

RESULTS AND DISCUSSION

Clinical Studies on Novel γ-GTP Isoenzyme

Figure 1 shows γ-GTP zymograms of sera from hepatobiliary diseases, demonstrating various electrophoretic bands. By this method, γ-GTP isoenzymes in sera were separated into thirteen bands. Summary of isoenzyme patterns in various disease states were reported elsewhere (Sawabu and coworkers, 1978a). The fastest moving band, band I and Band III are observed in concentrated sera from pathological subject. But these bands other than the band II, II' and I' are not characteristic to any groups of patients studied. On the other hand, the band II which is seen in the region near to ceruloplasmin, the band II' which is occupied between band II and III, and band I' which located at anodic side adjacent to band I can be seen only in sera of HCC. The densitometric tracings of γ-GTP zymogram in the cases of HCC are presented in Fig. 2. The peak corresponding to band II is observed, while band II' is not in the upper half of this figure. On the other hand, the peaks corresponding to band II and II' can be clearly observed in addition to other peaks in the lower half of this figure. The peak corresponding band I' can not be detected by densitometric tracing because of overlapping with band I.

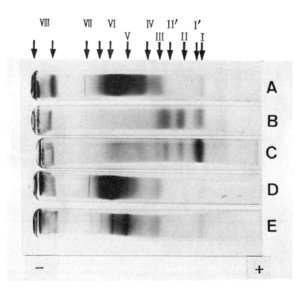

Fig. 1. A: γ-GTP isoenzymogram of serum from alcoholic liver
         injury, B and C: from hepatocellular carcinoma,
         D: from obstructive jaundice due to choledocholithiasis,
         E: from metastatic liver cancer.

Table I. Incidence of Specific γ-GTP Isoenzyme

Diseases	Patients	Patients with specific band		
		II	II'	I'
Hepatocellular carcinoma	100	39	29	36
Cholangioma	5	0	0	0
Metastatic cancer of liver	31	0	0	0
Liver cirrhosis	39	0	0	0
Chronic hepatitis	40	0	0	1
Alcoholic liver injury	23	0	1	1
Subacute hepatitis	6	0	0	0
Acute hepatitis	16	0	0	0
Intrahepatic cholestasis	14	0	0	0
Carcinoma of biliary tract	12	0	0	0
Cholelithiasis	25	0	0	0
Carcinoma of pancreas	9	0	0	0
Total	320	39	30	38

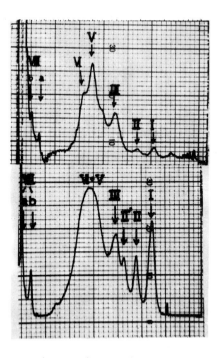

Fig. 2. Densitometric tracing of γ-GTP zymogram from patients of HCC

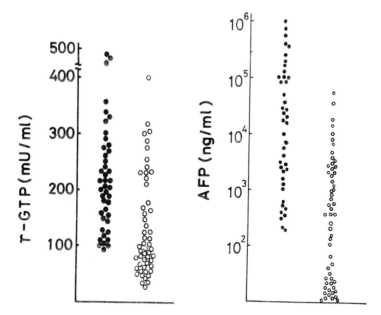

• : with specific band   ○ : without specific band

Fig. 3. Correlation between the appearance of novel γ-GTP
        isoenzyme and serum levels of γ-GTP and AFP in patients
        with HCC.

Table 1 exhibits the results of examination of band II, II' and I' in sera of
patients with various diseases. The band II was detected in 39 out of 100 cases
with HCC, but not in patients with other hepatobiliary diseases. In addition to
band II, band II' and I' were found in 29 and 36 of these 100 cases, respectively.
However, these later two bands were found exceptionally in diseases other than HCC.
That is, out of 220 patients with hepatobiliary diseases other than HCC, only one
patient with alcoholic liver disease exhibited band II', and one each with chronic
active hepatitis and alcoholic liver disease showed band I'. From the results of
isoenzyme patterns in various hepatobiliary diseases, we presumed that band II, II'
and I' could be specific for HCC. The concomittant appearance of all three bands
was observed in 26 cases. That of band II and I', or band II and II' was in 6 and
3 cases, respectively. The appearance of only band II or I' was in 4 cases,
respectively. At least, one of these bands was found to exist in 43 cases out of
100 with HCC. Consequently, positive rate of specific band was 43%.

Several studies have been published on clinical implication of serum γ-GTP isoenzyme
in neoplasm of the liver, demonstrating that the predominant occurrence of slowly
migrating fractions may be diagnostically helpful (Orlowski and Szczeklik, 1967;
Igartua and colleagues, 1973; Patel and O'Gorman, 1973; Hetland and colleagues,
1975; Staeffen and colleagues, 1975). Nevertheless, there has been no report except
for one by Fujisawa and colleagues (1976) on the existence of specific γ-GTP
isoenzyme. They reported the activity in four fractions including postalbumin,
α-, β-, and γ-globulins, and stated that the fraction which was seen in the region
of α-globulin appeared only in sera of HCC, though the incidence, clinical significance and characterization of this specific fraction were not shown. The isoenzyme
which were found to be located at α-globulin were II, II' and III by our method.
The bands II and II' can be detected only in the sera from HCC patients and not in
sera of patients with diseases other than HCC, but band III can be seen not only in

normal sera but also in pathological sera accompanied with an increase of the
intensity of staining reaction of this band. Thus, it is necessary to distinguish
these three bands by using the polyacrylamide gradient electrophoresis, and our
results indicate electrophoretic heterogeneity of hepatoma specific γ-GTP.

Fig. 3 compares the serum activity of γ-GTP in cases of HCC with and without
specific isoenzyme. The specific band could not be detectable in the cases whose
activity of γ-GTP was less than 100 mU/ml. However, the cases without specific
band were seen in the group of which activity of γ-GTP remarkably increased.
These cases were accompanied with a complication such as obstructive jaundice
which could raise the level of serum γ-GTP activity. The incidence of specific
band was 43% in total cases with HCC, and corresponded to 58% in cases whose
activity of γ-GTP was more than 100 mU/ml. As for α-fetoprotein, the same
comparison is shown in Fig. 3. Serum level of AFP was significantly higher in
the cases with specific band than without specific band, and the specific band
was not found in the cases whose level of AFP was lower than 270 ng/ml. Moreover,
the prevalence of specific band may be raised through developing a specific
radioimmunoassay using specific antiserum.

Properties of Novel γ-GTP Isoenzyme

The polyacrylamide disc electrophoresis of the purified fraction corresponding to
band II obtained at the final step using the immunoabsorption could show a single
band for both γ-GTP activity and protein as presented in Fig. 4. Because of the
difficulties in harvesting a sufficient amount of the purified enzyme at the
final step, we examined enzymatic properties of the partially purified enzyme
obtained at the step of preparative polyacrylamide disc electrophoresis.
Analytical disc gel electrophoresis of the partially purified enzyme obtained
at the step of preparative polyacrylamide disc electrophoresis. Analytical disc
gel electrophoresis of the partially purified fraction could exhibit single band
for γ-GTP activity, but a few bands when stained for protein. The enzymatic

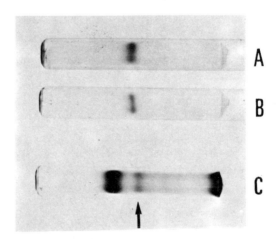

Fig. 4. Analytical disc gel electrophoresis of the purified
fraction obtained at final step. A: stained for
protein, B: stained for γ-GTP activity. C exhibits
γ-GTP isoenzyme pattern of whole serum of HCC patient
for reference. Arrow indicates novel γ-GTP (band II)
isoenzyme.

TABLE 2. Comparison of Physicochemical Properties between Band II and Band I

		band II	band I
Km for γ-glutamyl-p-nitroanilide		1.7 mM	1.8 mM
heat stability		(╫)	(+)
pH optimum		8.0	8.0
effect of cations	(mol)	(%)	(%)
none		100	100
mg^{++}	10^{-2}	115	103
	10^{-1}	140	126
Ca^{++}	10^{-2}	109	119
K^{+}	10^{-1}	97	100
Na^{+}	10^{-1}	96	99
Zn^{++}	10^{-2}	21	22
EDTA	10^{-1}	93	94

properties of purified band II were compared with those of band I, i.e., non-specific band which was prepared from sera of non-malignant patients by using the same steps of purification as shown in Table 2. The value of Km for γ-glutamyl p-nitro-anilide was 1.7mM for the enzyme corresponding to band II. The pH optimum of the enzyme was slightly activated by divalent cations such as Mg^{++} and Ca^{++}. Monovalent cations such as Na^{+} or K^{+} were not activator for this enzyme. Zinc ion was potent inhibitor at a concentration of 10^{-2}M. However, there was no significant difference between band II and band I in Km value for substrate, pH optimum, and effect of cations and EDTA. Heat inactivation of these bands was examined by incubating at 56°C, 58°C and 60°C as illustrated in Fig. 5. Consequently, band II demonstrated stronger heat stability than band I.

The immunological properties of band II were investigated by using antiserum against band II as shown in Fig. 6. Serum with HCC designed to S which was positive in novel γ-GTP isoenzyme was fused against this antiserum by the micro-Ouchterlony procedure, while non-HCC sera designed to D and E with high level of γ-GTP activity were not. In addition, enzyme extracts of HCC and fetal liver reacted with this antiserum to form a continuous line, but adult liver did not. These data indicate that the novel γ-GTP isoenzyme is immunologically indistinguishable from that of HCC and fetal liver, and that this protein is one of the carcinofetal proteins.

Fig. 7 demonstrates γ-GTP isoenzymograms from HCC, fetal liver, adult liver and pathological sera for reference. The specific bands corresponding to band II and II' could be observed in the zymogram from HCC and fetal liver, but not in that from adult liver. It is possible from this result that the specific band is derived from HCC cells and this protein might be responsible for one of carcinofetal proteins.

CONCLUDING REMARKS

We briefly discussed the clinical significance and some of enzymatic and immuno-logical properties of the novel γ-GTP isoenzyme which was discovered by us and was considered specific to HCC. Through further development of radioimmunoassay using the specific antiserum, this novel γ-GTP isoenzyme would be expected to provide a more powerful diagnostic tool in clinical medicine, and also serve as an aid in the field of the research for the hepatocarcinogenesis.

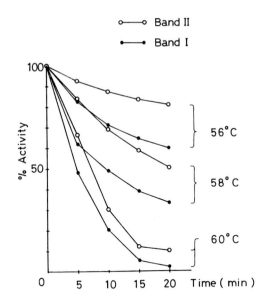

Fig. 5. Comparison of heat stability between band Ⅱ and band Ⅰ

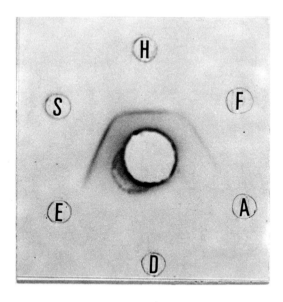

Fig. 6. Ouchterlony test for antiserum against novel γ-GTP
         isoenzyme(central well). H: extract of HCC, S: serum
         of HCC, F: extract of fetal liver, A: extract of
         adult liver, D and E: sera(other than HCC)

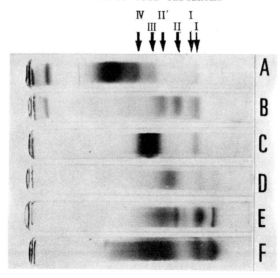

Fig. 7. A and B: γ-GTP zymogram of sera. C: tissue homogenate
      from adult liver, D: from HCC, E: from HCC (after
      autolysis) F: from fetal liver (after autolysis)

ACKNOWLEDGMENT

This work was supported in part by Grants-in-Aid for Cancer Research from the
Ministry of Education, Science and Culture (Dr. Hirai), and from the Ministry
of Health and Welfare (Dr. Suemasu and Hattori)

REFERENCES

Cameron, R., Kellen, J., Kolin, A., Malkin, A. and Farber, E.(1978). γ-GTP in
    putative premalignant liver cell populations during hepatocarcinogenesis.
    Cancer Res., 38, 823-829.
Fiala, S., and Fiala, E.S. (1973). Activation by chemical carcinogens of γ-GTP
    in rat and mouse liver. J. Natl. Cancer Inst., 51, 151-158.
Fujisawa, K., Kurihara, N., Kojima, M., Takahashi, T. and Tanaka, M. (1976).
    Carcinoembryonic character of γ-GTP in primary hepatoma. Leevy, C. M. (Ed.),
    Disease of the liver and biliary tract., S. Karger, Basel. pp. 13-17.
Hetland, Ö., Andersson, T. R. and Gerner, T. (1975). The heterogeneity of the
    serum activity of γ-GTP in hepatobiliary diseases as studied by agarose gel
    electrophoresis. Clin. Chim. Acta, 62, 425-431.
Iguarta, E. B., Domecq, R. and Findor, J. (1973). Isoenzymes of γ-GTP in liver
    diseases. Klin. Wschr., 51, 272-274.
Kalengayi, M. M. R., Ronchi, G. and Desmet, V. J. (1975). Histochemistry of
    γ-GTP in rat liver during aflatoxin B₁-induced carcinogenesis. J. Natl. Cancer
    Inst., 55, 579-582.
Orlowski, M. and Szczeklik, A. (1967). Heterogeneity of serum γ-GTP in hepatobiliary
    diseases. Clin. Clim. Acta, 15, 387-391.
Patel, S. and O'Gorman, R. (1973). Demonstration of serum γ-GTP isoenzyme using
    cellogel electrophoresis. Clin. Chim. Acta, 49, 11-17.
Staeffen, J., Ballen, P., Farrer, J., Beylot, J. Series, C. and Terme, R. (1975).
    Quantitative study of the multimolecular forms of γ-GTP by acrylamide gel
    electrophoresis. Path. Biol., 23, 615-622.
Sawabu, N., Nakagen, M., Yoneda, M., Makino, H., Kameda, S., Kobayashi, K.

Hattori, N. and Ishii, M. (1978a). Novel γ-GTP isoenzyme specifically
     found in sera of patients with hepatocellular carcinoma. Gann, 69, 601-605.
Sawabu, N., Nakagen, M., Senma, T., Hattori, N. and Ishii, M. (1978b).
     Purification and some properties of novel γ-GTP isoenzyme occurred in sera
     of patients with hepatoma. Scand. J. Immunol., 7, Suppl,8, 185-188.
Taniguchi, N., Saito, K. and Takakuwa, E. (1975). γ-GTP from azo dye induced
     hepatoma and fetal rat liver. Biochim. Biophys. Acta, 391, 265-271.
Tateishi, N., Higashi, T., Nomura, T. Naruse, A. Nakashima, K., Shiozaki, H. and
     Sakamoto, Y. (1976), Higher transpeptidation activity and broad acceptor
     specificity of γ-GTPs of tumors. Gann, 67, 215-222.

Combined Nuclear Medicine Procedures for Detection of Hepatocellular Carcinoma

Takeyoshi Imaeda and Hidetaka Doi

*Department of Radiology, Gifu University, School of Medicine,
Gifu City, Japan*

ABSTRACT

For the detection of liver tumors, we have been using combined nuclear medicine procedures comprising radiocolloid liver scintigraphy, radioisotope angiography, ^{67}Ga-tumor scintigraphy, radioimmunoassay of α-fetoprotein (AFP), carcinoembryonic antigen (CEA), HBs-antigen and HBs-antibody, etc. The procedures were evaluated in 158 cases of hepatocellular carcinoma we encountered with during these five years (1973 to 1978). Of the 158 cases, 31 were those that developed hepatocellular carcinoma during the follow-up observation for chronic hepatitis or liver cirrhosis. On the basis of the data obtained from these cases, the possibility of detecting hepatocellular carcinoma earlier in its course was discussed.

High rates of positive diagnosis were seen with radiocolloid liver scintigraphy (96 %), radioimmunoassay of AFP (66%) and a combination of both the procedures (98%). The combined nuclear medicine procedures succeeded in detecting 32 cases of early hepatocellular carcinoma; 15 were detected by a combination of radiocolloid liver scintigraphy and AFP assay, 13 by radiocolloid liver scintigraphy and 4 by the AFP assay. Eight of the 32 cases had their carcinomatous nodules resected. The smallest nodule among those successfully resected was 3.5 x 3.0 x 3.0 cm in dimension. Of the 32 cases, 10 developed hepatocellular carcinoma during the follow-up observation for chronic hepatitis or liver cirrhosis while the remaining 22 had never been subjected to a sustained observation. The prognosis of the patient with hepatocellular carcinoma is generally poor. In fact, death occurred in 70% or more of our cases within six months after detection of carcinoma.

To detect hepatocellular carcinoma in its early stage is an access to favorable prognosis. For this purpose, it seems important to follow the patient with chronic diffuse parenchymal diseases, especially with chronic hepatitis or liver cirrhosis, applying non-invasive procedures including radiocolloid liver scintigraphy, AFP assay, etc.

KEYWORDS

combined nuclear medicine procedures, radiocolloid liver scintigraphy, α-fetoprotein
, detection of early hepatocellular carcinoma, analysis of hepatocellular carcinoma.

METHODS

After the intravenous injection of 10 to 15 mCi of ^{99m}Tc-phytate, radiocolloid liver

scintigraphy was performed under breath-holding by anterior, posterior, right lateral and left lateral projections with a scinticamera (Searle, Pho/Gamma HP).
After the injection of 10 to 15 mCi of ^{99m}Tc-albumin into the right cubital vein, radioisotope angiograms were taken at 2- to 3-second intervals with a multiformat camera to determine dynamics of hepatic blood flow.
The examination by ^{67}Ga-tumor scintigraphy was carried out 24 to 72 hours after the intravenous injection of 2 mCi of ^{67}Ga-citrate.
Serological techniques for AFP, CEA, HBs-antigen and HBs-antibody were performed using a radioimmunoassay kit.

RESULTS

Radiocolloid liver scintigraphy gave the diagnosis of hepatocellular carcinoma in 96% of 158 cases. On the scintigrams, defects were located in the anatomical right lobe of the liver in 58% (33% in the right lateral segment, 24% in the right lateral and left medial segments and 1% in the left medial segment), in the anatomical left lobe in 7% and in both the lobes in 32%. The location of defects was unavailable in 4% of the cases because their carcinomatous nodules were too small, 1 cm or less in diameter (they were detectable by the AFP test or autopsy). The right lobe revealed more defects than the left lobe did. There was little difference in the incidence of solitary defects (50%) and that of multiple defects (46%); remaining 4 % were the cases in which this technique failed to detect defects indicative of hepatocellular carcinoma. There was enlargement of the left lobe by 7 cm or more in the median line in 27 (66%) of 41 cases with a large solitary defect only in the anatomical right lobe. This was prevalent in hepatocellular carcinoma without liver cirrhosis. The enlargement of the left lobe also occurred when the right lobe bore large benign tumors such as cyst, when the right lobe was constricted by massive kidney tumors or when the patient underwent surgical right lobectomy. It may be reasonable to presume that the left lobe was enlarged in compensation for the right lobe attacked with large tumors in our cases and that some of hepatocellular carcinomas were growing slowly. The smallest hepatocellular carcinoma that radiocolloid liver scintigraphy could detect was 3.5 x 3.0 x 3.0 cm in dimension.
When does the radiocolloid scintigram first become suggestive of the presence of hepatocellular carcinoma? We studied it in its retrospective relationship to the diagnosis of carcinoma. Scintigrams were collected from 8 cases that had been subjected to this technique relatively frequently during the one to two years preceding the diagnosis of hepatocellular carcinoma. In 4 of the 8 cases, liver scintigrams taken 6.5 to 9 months before the diagnosis already revealed decreased radioactivity in the liver area that was proved by subsequent diagnosis to almost correspond to the site of carcinoma. In contrast to this, scintigrams from the other four cases were negative 7 to 10 months before the diagnosis of hepatocellular carcinoma; that is, they were free of defects and decrease in radioactivity, and therefore the presence of hepatocellular carcinoma was denied.
So far as half of hepatocellular carcinomas are concerned, it may be that they grow slowly, taking 6.5 months or more, to a noticeable size and that they are finally detected in most cases upon some clinical complaint from the patient.
The AFP test yielding AFP values greater than 400 ng/ml was considered positive. As the result, hepatocellular carcinoma was diagnosed in 66% of cases. The rate means that the AFP test can detect only 2 out of 3 cases of carcinoma.
The AFP value was elevated (above the 400 ng/ml level) in 138 of 1564 cases of liver disease examined by this technique during these five years. These 138 cases included hepatocellular carcinoma (75%), chronic hepatitis (7%), liver cirrhosis (11%), metastatic liver carcinoma (7%) and fulminant hepatitis (1%). The results with this technique were not satisfactory for the detection of carcinoma. As indicated in the above, the 400 ng/ml level was considered to be the lower limit for positive diagnosis. Elevation in AFP values (above 400 ng/ml) accompanying chronic hepatitis and liver cirrhosis was transient in most cases, since AFP as well as transaminase was decreased to normal levels one to four weeks later. However, we experienced a

few cases of liver cirrhosis in which AFP remained elevated for half a year or more. In these cases, we had to carry out radiocolloid liver scintigraphy, X-ray computerized tomography and celiac angiography to know whether or not cirrhosis was complicated by carcinoma. Variation of AFP before and after the diagnosis of hepatocellular carcinoma was studied in 23 cases that had been examined by this technique relatively frequently during the one to two years preceding the diagnosis. We noted there were four patterns of variation:

1) Though tumor masses were small, AFP showed significantly higher levels at the time of diagnosis than the levels obtained one year more earlier. -------- 13 of 23 cases (57%)

2) Though there were clear defects on the radiocolloid liver scintigram, the AFP value was still low. But, after a while when tumors grew to a certain dimension, the AFP test turned into positive. --------- 3 of 23 cases (13%)

A modification of this pattern was recognized in operated cases. In these cases, the preoperative AFP value was not so high, 470 ng/ml. Operation lowered the AFP value to 58 ng/ml, which was re-elevated to a highest value, 199×10^2 ng/ml upon recurrence.

3) The AFP value did not show wide variations but lingered between 20 ng/ml and 400 ng/ml. --------- 4 of 23 cases (17%)

4) AFP remained on the levels less than 20 ng/ml throughout the period under review. --------- 3 of 23 cases (13%)

Another attempt was made to relate AFP values to the growth of hepatocellular carcinoma in 22 cases which had been followed by radiocolloid liver scintigraphy for 4 months or more after diagnosis. The growth of carcinoma was more rapid in 14 cases having AFP values exceeding 10^3ng/ml than in those with AFP values less than 400 ng/ml; the tumor became considerably large in several months and consequently it was only 14% that survived the post-diagnostic one year. The one-year survival rate was 38% in 8 cases having AFP values lower than 400 ng/ml.

Radioisotope angiography was of value in the diagnosis of hepatocellular carcinoma of hypervascular type. The intravenous injection of ^{99m}Tc-albumin promptly produced on the angiogram a region with high radioactivity identified as hepatocellular carcinoma and a region without radioactivity identified as cyst or abscess. In some cases of carcinoma, the region with high radioactivity had a center with low activity, which was found to be caused by central necrosis. The smallest carcinoma that this technique could detect was $4.0 \times 3.5 \times 2.5$ cm in dimension.

Tumor scintigraphy with ^{67}Ga-citrate was useful in determining the extent of hepatocellular carcinoma. It was only in 44% of cases that this technique visualized the cancered area which appeared darker because of its high radioactivity than the normal area on the scintigram. The smallest carcinoma that could be detected by this technique was of a hen's egg size.

If 2.5 ng/ml or more were considered as CEA-positive, the diagnosis of hepatocellular carcinoma was made in 35% of cases. The highest CEA value was 20.0 ng/ml. Nevertheless CEA values were less than 5.0 ng/ml in 88% of all the cases. They were lower in hepatocellular carcinoma than in metastatic liver carcinoma. Though the CEA assay was of less diagnostic value than the AFP test and was deprived of organic specificity, it was most helpful when associated with the AFP test on the same serum sample in discriminating between hepatocellular carcinoma and metastatic liver carcinoma. A relationship of CEA and AFP to diagnosis was studied in 158 cases of hepatocellular carcinoma and 105 cases of metastatic liver carcinoma. Of 116 cases having CEA values less than 9.0 ng/ml and AFP values greater than 20 ng/ml, 112 (97%) were hepatocellular carcinoma and 4 (3%) were metastatic liver carcinoma. On the contrary, all 7 cases having CEA values greater than 10 ng/ml and AFP values greater than 10^3 ng/ml were diagnosed as metastatic liver carcinoma with the primary malignancy in the stomach. HBs-antigens were detected in 42% of 158 cases of hepatocellular carcinoma, the percentage being about twice as high as that in chronic hepatitis (17%) and in liver cirrhosis (26%).

HBs-antibodies were detected in 27% of 158 cases of hepatocellular carcinoma, in 29 % of cases of chronic hepatitis and in 30% of cases of liver cirrhosis. Thus, the

percentage of HBs-antibody positive cases was almost comparable among three diseases. To study variations of HBs-antigen and HBs-antibody titers before and after
the diagnosis of hepatocellular carcinoma were reviewed those cases in which either
HBs-antigen titers or HBs-antibody titers had been determined relatively frequently during the one to two years preceding the diagnosis (4 cases for the HBs-antigen test and 11 cases for the HBs-antibody test). We failed to find a tendency in
the variation of HBs-antigen titers since they were elevated in one case, decreased
in one case but they showed no significant variation in two cases. As to HBs-antibody titers, they were elevated gradually in one case, decreased in five cases but
they showed no significant variation in five cases. Obviously, it is necessary to
try to utilize these parameters with a larger number of cases.
Another investigation was made into a relationship of HBs-antigen to AFP. Of 66
cases in which HBs-antigens were detected, 53 cases (80%) had AFP values greater
than 400 ng/ml. Such high AFP values were noted in only 52 of 92 cases (57%) with
a negative HBs-antigen test. Our 158 cases of hepatocellular carcinoma included
32 cases of early carcinoma. A hepatocellular carcinoma is qualified as early here
if it causes a solitary defect on the radiocolloid liver scintigram and if it involves less than a quarter the right lateral segment only or if its location is limited to the left lateral segment. Of the 32 cases, 15 were detected by a combination of radiocolloid liver scintigraphy and AFP assay, 13 by radiocolloid liver
scintigraphy alone and 4 by the AFP assay alone.
Carcinomatous nodules were surgically resectable in 8 of the 32 cases of early
hepatocellular carcinoma.

CONCLUSION

The best way to improve the cure rates of hepatocellular carcinoma is to detect and
resect carcinomatous nodules earlier in their course. It is recommended to carry
out non-invasive procedures such as radiocolloid liver scintigraphy and AFP test
once or twice every six months on the patient with chronic diffuse parenchymal disease of the liver, especially with chronic hepatitis or liver cirrhosis, for
follow-up purposes.

REFERENCES

Hisada, k. (1977). Systematization of nuclear medicine diagnosis. Nipp. Act.
Radiol., 37, 286-304.
Imaeda, T., Senda, K., Kato, T., Asada, S., Matsuura, S., Yamawaki, Y., Kunieda, T.
and Doi, H. (1976). Clinical evaluation of carcinoembryonic antigen assay in various diseases. Nipp. Act. Radiol., 36, 910-921.
Nishioka, K. (1974). HB antigen and hepatocellular carcinoma. 5th Inuyama Symposium, Tokyo. pp 115-119.
Vogel, C.L., Anthony, P., Mody, N. and Barker, L.F. (1970). Hepatitis-associated
antigen in Ugandan patients with hepatocellular carcinoma. Lancet, II : 621-624.

Clinical Aspects of Hepatocellular Carcinoma

K. Okuda*, N. Suzuki*, Y. Kubo** and H. Obata***

*1st Dept. of Medicine, Chiba Univ. School of Medicine, Chiba, Japan
**2nd Dept. of Medicine, Kurume Univ. School of Medicine, Kurume, Japan
***Institute of Gastroenterology, Tokyo Women's Medical College, Tokyo, Japan

ABSTRACT

The frequency of positive hepatitis B surface antigen (HBsAg) in patients with
hepatocellular carcinoma (HCC) is around 50% in Japan and anti-HB core is more
frequently positive. Patients with chronic hepatitis or cirrhosis positive for
HBsAg tend to develop HCC earlier compared to negative patients. Serum alpha-
fetoprotein (AFP) is most important in early detection of HCC although it
remains low throughout in some cases. In contract to fluctuating AFP levels
below 1000 ng/ml in other liver diseases, AFP remains mildly elevated for some
time with little fluctuation in HCC and at a certain point in the course it begins
to rise continuously at a sharp angle. However, the tumor is already several
centimeters - mostly from 3 to 4 cm - at that time. Other, more sensitive
specific tests are necessary to improve diagnosis further. In Japan, most primary
tumor lesions grow slowly acquiring a capsule, and are hypervascular from the very
beginning. Celiac arteriography is therefore capable of detecting a tumor as
small as 1 cm if it is hypervascular. AFP should be checked periodically in a
patient with chronic liver disease, particularly if he is HBsAg positive, and when
it starts to rise celiac angiography should be done.
There are a number of clinically distinct groups of patients. Besides Berman's
classification of 5 types, we separate those with typical signs of cirrhosis as
the "cirrhotic" type, and those presenting signs of extrahepatic biliary
obstruction "cholestatic" type, etc. The clinical course of patients with an HCC
which has a thick capsule is protracted and may do better without chemotherapy.
The diffuse type of HCC with numerous tumor nodules throughout the liver is
clinically characterized by a rapidly downhill course terminating in hepatic
failure. Celiac angiography not only is useful in assessing the gross anatomical
feature of the tumor, it can also detect tumor growth in the portal and hepatic
veins.

INTRODUCTION

The clinical feature of hepatocellular carcinoma (HCC) is quite variable and it can
also vary with the geographical location, probably because of the different underlying liver diseases. In Africa, especially in Mozambique, HCC occurs in young
ages (Higginson, 1963) often without cirrhosis or chronic liver disease (Steiner,
1960), whereas in Japan and elsewhere it occurs mostly in later ages on the ground
of non-alcoholic cirrhosis (Miyaji, 1976) - after a long course of chronic liver
disease whether the patient was aware of it or not. In the area of low incidence
of asymptomatic carriers of hepatitis B surface antigen (HBsAg), the type of cirrhosis
is predominantly alcoholic, and HCC develops much less frequently in a cirrhotic liver,

but more often after several years of abstinence (Lee, 1966). It is not established
how these epidemiological differences are reflected in the patients with HCC. The
value of serum alpha-fetoprotein (AFP) in early diagnosis is not yet clearly understood, nor are the clinical implications of HBsAg antigenemia in hepatocarcinogenesis established. In this presentation, discussion will limit itself to these clinical problems and recent interests.

HEPATITIS B ANTIGEN AND HEPATOCELLULAR CARCINOMA

In the developing countries in the tropical and subtropical regions, HBsAg carriers
are frequent among general population. The figure stands around 15 % in Taiwan
(Tong and others, 1971) and 2 % in Japan (Nishioka and others, 1973) in contrast to
a few tenths of a percent in European countries. There seems to be a roung correlation between the frequency of carriers and incidence of HCC. The frequency of positive HBsAg among patients with HCC is also high in these areas. In Japan, it is
positive in about half of the patients (Okuda,1976), and anti-HB core (HBc) is more
frequently positive (Kubo and others, 1977). It is not yet clear whether positive
anti-HBc is as closely related to hepatocarcinogenesis as HBsAg is. We studied 124
cases of HCC, 52 of cirrhosis, and 48 of chronic hepatitis in comparison with 299
healthy subjects above age 40. HBsAg was positive in 29.2 % of the patients with
chronic hepatitis, 38.5 % in cirrhosis and 48.9 % in HCC (Fig. 1). If HBsAg positive patients with chronic liver disease were to develop HCC at the same rate, there
should not be any difference in frequency of positive HBsAg among these three groups
of patients. Interpreting it in another way, it seems that HBsAg positive patients
with chronic liver disease develops HCC more frequently or earlier than negative
patients.

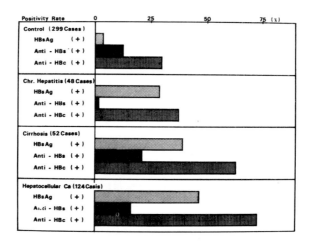

Fig. 1. Frequency of positive tests for HBsAg,
         anti-HBs and anti-HBc in patients with
         HCC, cirrhosis and chronic hepatitis in
         comparison with controls of comparable
         ages.

Liver Cancer Study Group of Japan conducted a survey on a total of 4031 histology
proven cases of primary liver cancer seen during the past 10 years at 153 institutes. They consisted of 2411 cases of HCC, 268 of cholangiocarcinoma, 58 of combined type, 68 of hepatoblastoma and 23 of others. In 25.5 % of the patients with
HCC there was a history of hepatitis or presumable hepatitis whereas 7.5 % of those
with cholangiocarcinoma and none with hepatoblstoma had such history. Our own study

of 258 cases of HCC showed that 34.1 % of the patients had a history of some kind
of surgery, jaundice in 17.1 %, blood trasnfusion in 12.4 % and various liver diseases in 20.4 %. These data strongly suggest that chronic liver diseases related
to viral hepatitis predispose to hepatocarcinogenesis.

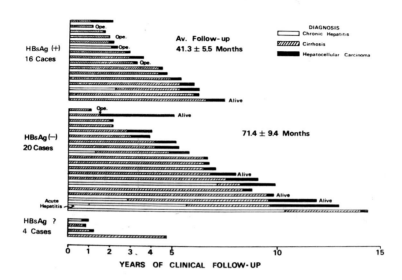

Fig. 2. Clinical follow-up of 40 patients with chronic liver
diseases in whom HCC eventually developed.

We then studied 40 patients who were followed for at least one year and for as long
as 15 years, with an initial diagnosis of cirrhosis, chronic hepatitis or acute
hepatitis and in whom HCC was subsequently detected (Fig. 2). When the follow-up
period before the tumor detection was compared between the patients positive for
HBsAg and negative, there was a significant difference; it was shorter in the former
(41.3+5.5 years) than the latter (71.4+9.4 years). One patient was followed from
post-transfusion acute hepatitis through chronic hepatitis and cirrhosis for 10
years before HCC was detected. One 58 year old man was first treated with corticosteroids for acute hepatitis at another hospital, and then came to us because of
the persistent elevation of transaminases. He was found to be positive for HBsAg
and, due to severe withdrawal reaction, corticosteroids were continued. Fluctuation
of SGOT and SGPT gradually subsided and became nearly normal in 5 years time. One
year or so later, AFP which had been mildly elevated without fluctuation started
to rise, and the diagnosis was unequivacal (Fig. 3). This case gives us a lesson
that corticosteroids may hasten hepatocarcinogenesis. It is also suggested that
when inflammation subsides in the liver after such a course of chronic liver disease, foundation is laid for the development of HCC. It is of interest to postu-
late that cellular immunity has been suppressed by corticosteroids to a point where
damage to the hepatocytes becomes minimal and, at the same time, the immune surveillance against malignant transformation becomes ineffective.

MINUTE HEPATOCELLULAR CARCINOMA AND EARLY DETECTION

In order to obtain information that would aid in the diagnosis of small HCC, minute
HCC's found in the liver at autopsy or surgery were studied. A total of 22 livers,
18 necropsied and 4 resected, bearing one tumor smaller than 4.5 cm in diameter, or
up to 3 tumors smaller than 3.5 cm in the largest diameter, were investigated.

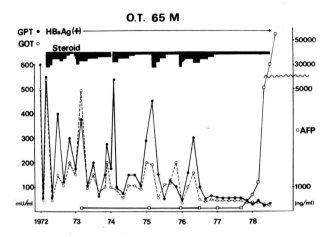

Fig. 3. Clinical course of a 65 year old man, positive for
HBsAg, who was on corticosteroids continuously and
eventually developed HCC. Note that AFP began to
rise after about one year of quiescent SGOT and SGPT.

It was found that most of such minute HCC's were encapsulated suggesting that the
primary or early tumor lesion grows slowly in an expanding fashion (Okuda and
others, 1977). Postmortem angiography also demonstrated that most of such minute
tumor nodules are already hypervascular (Nakashima, 1976). In fact, celiac arteriography demonstrated a small hypervascular lesion or a tumor blush confirming the
suspected diagnosis in many of the cases in which a sharp rise in AFP had suggested
HCC. The smallest HCC ever detected by this procedure has been about 2 cm in our
hands.
Along with development of the technique for the quantification of serum AFP came
varying reports on its positivity rate in patients with HCC (Kew, 1974). Early
reports using the immunodiffusion techniques quoted figures between 45 and 80 % of
positive tests in HCC with suggested geographical differences. For the purpose of
detecting a small HCC and treating surgically, the radioimmunoassay is absolutely
neccessary. It has been shown by others and also by us that the positivity rate
largely depends on at which level one draws a line to separate positive and negative
values. We have measured AFP in 177 cases of HCC, 58 of metastatic liver cancer,
64 of cirrhosis and 69 of chronic hepatitis in comparison with normal controls.
Whereas 94 % of the patients with HCC showed AFP values above 20 ng/ml, the upper
normal level, 38 % of patients with cirrhosis also showed AFP values above it. If
values above 10,000 ng/ml were taken as positive, 64.4 % of HCC patients were positive whereas only 1 out of several hundred other patients showed such a value.
Thus, it is obvious that if an AFP value above 10,000 ng/ml was obtained, the
chances of having an HCC is almost 100 % (Okuda, 1976).
The real problem lies in the differentiation of values below 1000 ng/ml. About 15
% of the patients with HCC show AFP values betwee 20 and 1000 ng/ml, which can not
be distinguished from those in patients with other liver diseases by just one determination. If AFP levels were followed for several months, it would come down to the
normal range in due time if the patient did not have an HCC. By contrast, in HCC
the AFP level is mildly abnormal, say 50 to 200 ng/ml, for a number of months or
even two years and then begins to rise. The rise is sharp with a transitional
period of several months and it continues exponentially. In a typical case, the
rise is so acute and continuous that the diagnosis is unequivocal with no need for

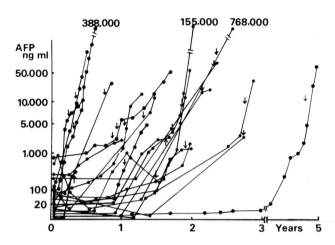

Fig. 4. The serum levels of AFP and the inclinations with
which suspicion of HCC was entertained. The diagnosis
was subsequently confirmed (21 cases).

other tests (Fig. 4). To confirm the diagnosis, celiac arteriography is the most
important.
A second problem is the size of HCC at which AFP starts to rise. Although a number
of reports have been made in Japan in the past several years regarding the size of
HCC detected by sequential determination of AFP, and the smallest one measured less
than 2 cm, our experience has been rather disappointing in that most HCC's detected
by the periodic check of AFP already measured 3 to 5 cm. Apparently, serum AFP
level reflects the capacity of HCC cells to produce AFP. Only a high AFP producing
HCC may be detected while it is still small, and the size of tumor detectable by
the rise of AFP is perhaps inversely correlated with the AFP producing capacity.
The point at which serum AFP starts to rise is an equilibrium breaking point before
which AFP production and its catabolism were in equilibrium. It may also indicate
that tumor growth is slow up to a certain point after which it becomes exponential.
In this respect, it is to be remembered that a considerable proportion of HCC's are
low AFP producers and they can not be detected by AFP (Okuda, 1977a).
Based on these observations, our current policy for the detection of HCC in its
resectable stage is to measure AFP in patients with chronic hepatitis and cirrhosis
at certain regular intervals which are determined according to the degree of hepato-
carcinogenic potential, and whenever AFP levels suggest a possible HCC, liver scan,
ultrasound and, above all, celiac angiography is to be carried out. The potential
is high if the patient is positive for HBsAg and if the AFP level has continuously
been mildly elevated with little fluctuation.

CLINICAL TYPES

Berman (1951) divided his 75 Bantu patients with HCC into 5 distinct clinical types
which he called the "frank," "acute abdominal," "febrile," "occult" and "metastatic"
cancers. However, a considerable proportion of our Japanese counterparts present
sings typical of cirrhosis which we call the "cirrhotic" type. Thus, we have added
a few additional clinical types whose frequencies are given in Table 1.

TABLE 1. Clinical Types of Hepatocellular Carcinoma (376 cases)

Clinical type	No. of cases	Berman's series
Frank	229 (60.9 %)	47 (62.7 %)
Cirrhotic	87 (23.1 %)	
Occult	14 (3.7 %)	12 (16.2 %)
Febrile	8 (2.1 %)	6 (8.0 %)
Acute abdominal	11 (2.9 %)	6 (8.0 %)
Metastatic	11 (2.9 %)	4 (5.3 %)
Cholestatic	7 (1.9 %)	
Hepatitic	3 (0.8 %)	
Unclassified	6 (1.6 %)	
Total	376	75

In the frank type with a large liver and a tumor, cirrhosis is absent or mild as contrasted by the cirrhotic type in which the liver is cirrhotic and the patient expires before the tumor becomes really large. Thus, the frank type is more frequent in South Africa compared to Japan where the cirrhotic type is not uncommon. If the presenting symptoms are high fever with leukocytosis, differntial diagnosis from liver abscess is difficult, and the tumor is usually highly anaplastic. In the metastatic type, HCC is discovered by a lesion outside the liver. In 7 of the 11 cases in our series, a bone lesion was first noted and in the remainder, lung shadows. In the cholestatic type, the patient develops jaundice with upper quadrant pain, and extrahepatic biliary obstruction is suspected. Direct cholangiography will demonstrate an ill-defined filling defect or a tumor growing in a major hepatic duct. We have seen 3 patients who came down with what we thought to be typical of acute hepatitis, and a tumor was subsequently discovered in a cirrhotic liver. Apparently, they had had chronic hepatitis or cirrhosis without notice and and acute excerbation triggered the rapidly progressive course of the chronic liver disease.

Beside these clinical types, several distinct clinical features seem to be closely related to histopathology of HCC. We have seen several patients who lived 5 to 8 years after the discovery of a discrete space occupying lesion on the scan--later confirmed as the tumor. The tumor invariably had a thick fibrous capsule and was a low malignancy histologically. The patient will do better without chemotherapy. If diagnosed early, an encapsulated HCC constitutes a best candidate for resection. Hypercalcemia, or the so-called pseudoparathyroidism is often associated with sclerosing HCC which is not readily distinguished from cholangiocarcinoma (Peters, 1976). A patient with clear cell carcinoma of the liver seems to have a long survival (Edmondson, 1958), although it has been disputed (El-Comeiri and others, 1971).

The diffuse type of HCC (Eggel, 1901) in a strict sense is a vary rare pathological type. We have seen 6 such cases. All had a rapidly downhill course with increasing jaundice and terminating in hepatic failure. The liver had numerous small tumor nodules, apparently intrahepatic metastases from a small primary. Although Peters (1976) described a liver with a diffuse HCC of multicentric development, such HCC seems to be rare in Japan.

In the past, little emphasis was made on the relationship between pathology and clinical findings of HCC. We strongly feel that both are closely related and that more effort be made to correlate the clinical course and prognosis with the pathological findings of the liver and HCC. Such knowledge would assist in predicting prognosis and indirectly improve management of the patient.

DIAGNOSTIC VALUE OF HEPATIC ANGIOGRAPHY

Beside the discussed diagnostic value in the detection of small HCC, selective celiac or, preferably hepatic arteriography provides information on the gross ana-tomy of HCC. For instance, it will give a picture of evenly distributed small tumor stains in the diffuse type of HCC (Okuda and others, 1977c), and will delineate a thin radiolucent rim around the round tumor contour if the tumor is thickly encapsu-lated (Okuda and others, 1977b). With a close study of the relationship between the tumor and arteries, one can dedude whether the tumor is growing in an expanding fashion displacing arteries to the periphery, or it is growing in an infiltraing fashion incasing and embedding arteries in it. It is an important information regarding the benignity and malignity of the tumor.

While invesigating the angiographic feature of HCC by postmortem angiography (Nakashima, 1976), we noted that the tumor thrombus growing in a large portal vein is opacified from the hepatic artery and that the contrast medium runs in thin lon-gitudinal parallel channels along the thrombus. Subsequently, we could demonstrate the same finding antemortem in patients with HCC, and the characteristic angio-graphic sings have been named "thread and streaks" by us (Okuda and others, 1975). Clinical diagnosis of tumor growth in the portal vein precludes the possiblity of surgery and is very important. Similar angiographic finding is also seen in patients with a tumor growing in the large hepatic vein and further into the vena cave (Okuda and others, 1977d). In the presence of such growth, metastases to the lung have already occurred, similarly contraindicating surgery.

We have seen a number of cases inwhich tumor was growing into the inferior vena cava almost occluding it--it never does, however--and further into the right atrium. We have also seen one case in which the tumor bolus was continuous through the tricus-pid valves into the right ventricle with large tumor thrombi in the both pulmonary arteries. Peculiarly and to one's surprise, such a grave clinical condition dose not manifest itself clearly. It is probably because of the severely debilitated general condition of the patient with hypotension, ascites and edema. Hepatic arte-riography often, but not always, demonstrates the tumor growth. For that matter, cavography is more diagnostic. However, one has to take precaution not to send the catheter into the tumor thrombus and should flush with contrast medium in search of tumor growth before entering an hepatic vein.

Hepatic arteriography is also very important when hepatic resection or lobectomy is being contemplated. When a right lobectomy is considered, it is absolutely neces-sary to exclude lesions in the contralateral lobe, and selective left hepatic arte-riography is desired, or at least, special attention is to be paid to the left lobe. If a stereo-angiography apparatus is available, it is to a great advantage to the operator, and Dr. Hasegawa and his associates at National Cancer Center, Tokyo, emphasize its merit in selecting patients and deciding on the proper operative approach.

REFERENCES

Berman, C. (1951). Primary Carcinoma of the Liver. Lewis, London.
Edmondson, H. A. (1958). Tumors of the Diver and Intrahepatic Bile Ducts. Armed
    Forces Inst. Path., Section VII, Fascicle 25, pp. 28-31.
Eggel, H. (1901). Ueber das primäre Carcinoma der Leber. Beitr. Path. Anat. Allg.
    Path. 30, 506-604.
El-Domeiri, A. A., Huvos, A. G., Goldsmith,H. S. and Foote, F. W., Jr. (1971).
    Primary malignant tumors of the liver. Cancer, 27, 7-11.
Higginson, J. (1963). The geographical pathology of primary liver cancer. Cancer
    Res., 23, 1624-1933.
Kew, M. (1974). Alpha-fetoprotein in primary liver cancer and other diseases. Gut,
    15, 814-821.
Kubo, Y., Okuda, K., Hashimoto, M., Nagasaki, Y., Obata,H., Nakajima, Y., Musha, H.,
    H., Sakuma, K. and Ohtake, H. (1977). Antibody to hepatitis B core antigen in

patients with hepatocellular carcinoma. ˋGastroenterology, 72, 1217-1220.

Lee, F. I. (1966). Cirrhosis and hepatoma in alcoholics. Gut, 7, 77-95.

Miyaji, T. (1976). Association of hepatocellular carcinoma with cirrhsis among autopwy cases in Japan durinℌ14 years from 1958 to 1971. Gann, 18, 129-149.

Nakashima, T. (1976). Vascular changes and hemodynamics in hepatocellular carcinoma. In k. Okuda, R. L. Peters (Ed.), Hepatocellular Carcinoma, Wiley, N. Y., pp. 169-204.

Nishioka, K., Hirayama, T., Awkine, T., Okochi, K., Mayumi, M., Sung, J. L., Liu, C. H. and Lin, T. M. (1973). Australia antigen and hepatocellular carcinoma. Gann, 14, 167-175.

Okuda, k., Musha, H., Yoshida, T., Kanda, Y., Yamazaki, T., Jinnouchi, S., Moriyama, M., Kawaguchi, S., Kubo, Y., Shimokawa, Y., Kojiro, M., Kuratomi, S., Sakanoto, K. and Nakashima, T. (1975). Demonstration of growing casts of hepatocellular carcinoma in the portal vein by celiac angiography: the thread and streaks sign. Radiology, 117, 303-309.

Okuda K. (1976). Clinical aspects of hepatocellular carcinoma--Analysis of 134 cases. In K. Okuda, R. L. Peters (Ed.), Hepatocellular Carcinoma, Wiley, N. Y., pp. 387-436.

Okude K., Nakashima, T., Obata, H. and Kubo, Y. (1977a). Clinicopathological studies of minute hepatocellular carcinoma. Anlysis of 20 cases, including 4 with hepatic resection. Gastroenterology, 73, 109-115.

Okuda K., Musha, H., Nakajima, Y., Kubo, Y., Shimokawa, Y., Nagasaki, Y., Okazaki, N., Kojiro, M., Sakamoto, K. and Nakashima, T. (1977b). Clinicopathological features of encapsulated hepatocellular carcinoma. Cancer, 40, 1240-1245.

Okuda, K., Obata, H., Jinnouchi. S., Kubo, Y., Nagasaki, Y., Shimokawa, Y., Motoike, Y., Muto, H., Nakajima, Y., Musha, H., Yamazaki, T., Sakamoto, K., Kojiro, M. and Nakashima, T. (1977c). Angiographic assessment of gross anatomy of hepato-cellular carcinoma: comparison of celiac angiograms and liver pathology in 100 cases. Radiology, 123, 21-29.

Okuda, K., Jinnouchi, S., Nagasaki, Y., Kuwahara, S., Kaneko, T., Kubo, Y., Shimokawa, Y., Nakajima, Y., Takashi, M., Musha, H., Kudo, T., Sakamoto, K., Kojiro, M. and Nakashima, T. (1977d). Angiographic demonstration of growing hepatocellular carcinoma in the hepatic vein and inferior vena cave. Radiology, 124, 33-36.

Peters, R. L. (1976). Pathology of hepatocellular carcinoma. In K.Okuda and R. L. Peters (Ed.), Hepatocellular Carcinoma, Wiley, N. Y., pp. 107-168.

Steiner, P. E. (1960). Cancer of the liver and cirrhosis in trans-Saharan Africa and the United States of America. Cancer,13, 1085-1166.

Tong, M. J., Sun, S. S., Schaeffer, B. T., Chang, N. K., Lo, K. J. and Peters, R. L. (1971). Hepatitis-associated antigen and hepatocellular carcinoma in Taiwan. Ann. Int. Med., 75, 687-691.

Cancer of the Pancreas, Current Diagnostic Approaches

G. Arbeiter

Med. Klinik und Poliklinik, Department of Gastroenterology, Klinikum Steglitz der Freien Universität Berlin, Hindenburgdamm 30, 1000 Berlin 45, Fed. Republic of Germany

ABSTRACT

Four branches of pancreas-diagnostic procedures are currently available: 1. Clinical practice; 2. Laboratory, i.e. functional tests; 3. Physical examinations (nuclear-medical examination, angiography, computerized axial tomography, ultrasonic diagnosis); 4. Endoscopic methods (ERCP, laparoscopy). The diagnostic values of the individual techniques applied to disclose pancreatic cancer are compared with the more recent literature. The results indicate a high sensitivity and specificity for the ERCP, computerized axial tomography and somography. Peritoneoscopic examination of the pancreas including biopsy also is a highly valuable method, without imposing a great degree of stress.

INTRODUCTION

As in all industrialized countries, the morbidity rate of pancreatic carcinoma has increased in the Federal Republic of Germany about 3/4-fold from 1952 to 1972 (Report of the Federal Bureau of Statistics, Wiesbaden). Thus it follows that more attention must be given to pancreatic carcinoma. From the low 5-year survival rate of 0.2% in Japan (Report of the Ministry of Public Welfare in Japan) up to 1.4 to 4.8% in Denmark (according to the Danish Cancer Registry), it is evident that an early and thus timely diagnosis is still very difficult.

CLINICAL ASSESSMENT

There are no pancreas-specific symptoms; the history of the patient with pancreas carcinoma is non-characteristic. The most frequent symptoms according to the literature and our own investigations are: weight loss, anorexia, apigastric pains, nausea, vomiting, increasing icterus, irregular stools. The time that elapsed between the onset of the first symptoms to be attributed to the carcinoma and the first hospitalisation was 8 months and 2 weeks on the average in our group of patients. This long period of time,

in which the symptoms insidiously begin, can well be regarded as a
contributing factor to our inability to make an early diagnosis.

LABORATORY FINDINGS

Routine laboratory diagnostics does not lead us in a direct way to
a diagnosis; at best, it can yield indications for the presence
of an epigastric process. I shall not go into any detail at this
time on the immunological blood tests: the detection of tumor-asso-
ciated antigens: carcinoembryonal antigen, α-feto-protein, pancreatic oncofetal antigen; its value, especially that of the pancreatic
oncofetal antigen, was recently made apparent in a prospective
study by Wood and Moossa (1977). High accuracy for the discovery
of a pancreas carcinoma is quoted in the literature for the secre-
tin-pancreocymin test (Di Magno and others, 1977; Dreiling, 1951,
1975).
In the following, I should like to present a tabulated synopsis
of the accuracy quota of modern physical examination procedures
in cases of pancreatic carcinoma, which shows a selection from
the more recent literature. For a better comparison, the results
of the authors, as far as it was possible on the basis of the literature, are reported in sensitivity and specificity. "No. of
cases" means the number of patients examined in each respective
study and not the number of carcinoma patients. Always Only the
first author of the group will be mentioned. The absolute values
after the percentages of sensitivity indicate, in each respective
case, the right positive examination results in relation to the
number of examined patients with proven pancreas carcinoma.
The absolute values after the percentages of specificity signify
the number of right negative examination results in relation to
the number of patients without carcinoma.

PANCREATIC SCANNING

The evaluation of pancreatic scanning by different authors ranges
from "method of choice in the beginning of pancreas diagnostics"
(Schmidt, 1975) to "grave doubts on the justification of the method" (Bachrach and others, 1972). Pancreatic scanning shows a
high sensitivity, but the difficulties arise from the low organ
specificity of 75-Se-methionine. Corresponding to the protein synthesis rate, the radioactively labelled amino acid is accumulated
in various organs such as the liver and gastrointestinal tract
and results in overshadowing effects. All attempts to increase
the percentage uptake amount of the 75-Se-methionine in the pancreas or to find more specific radiopharmaceuticals have remained
unsuccessful up to the present time. For this reason, developments
in scanning systems including computer evaluation cannot lead
to any significant improvement of pancreas diagnostics in the field
of nuclear medicine. Our experiences show, that space-occupying
lesions are only recognizable in a size of over 4 to 5 cm in diameter. With satisfactory practicability of the examination, the
diagnostic evidence is questionable because of the low specificity
(table 1). In addition, there is a high risk involved in the radiation exposure to 75-Se-methionine with the physical half-life
of 121 days and an effective half-life of 50 to 90 days. For this
reason, we are of the opinion that pancreatic scanning should be
avoided if possible, and it is no longer performed at our institute.

TABLE   1   Value of Pancreatic Scanning in Pancreatic Cancer

Author	No. of Cases	Pancreatic Scan. Sensitivity %		Specificity %	
Barkin (1977)	46	96	27/28	25	3/12
Di Magno (1977)	70	92	30/33	33	10/29
Eaton (1968)	45	89	8/9	70	7/10
Fitzgerald (1978)	184	75	27/36	69	20/29
Mac Carthy (1972)	393	94	47/50	91	77/85
Wood (1976)	89	56	10/18	--	

ENDOSCOPIC RETROGRADE CHOLANGIO-PANCREATOGRAPHY

The undoubtedly great significance of the ERCP or ERP is illustrated by table 2 which makes evident the high sensitivity and,
above all, the specificity of the method. Pancreas diagnostics is
unthinkable without this combined gastroenterological and radiological technique.

TABLE   2   Value of ERCP in Pancreatic Carcinoma

Author	No. of Cases	E R C P Sensitivity %		Specificity %	
Ariyama (1977)	32	90	29/32	--	
Di Magno (1977)	70	95	20/21	90	28/31
Fitzgerald (1978)	184	73	8/11	79	15/18
Freeny (1978)	118	95	20/21	--	
Hatfield (1976)	61	90	18/20	100	
Rohrmann (1974)	300	74	17/23	--	
Satake (1975)	133	94	15/16	--	
Stadelmann (1974)	54	100	42/42	--	
Wood (1976)	89	88	51/58	--	

Mr. Pollard will be discussing this diagnostic method in detail.
The disadvantage of this technique is, however, that the cannulisation of the papilla and, after successful cannulisation, the
achievement of a positive pancreatogram as well as, not least
of all, the subjective tolerance by the patient are decidedly dependent upon the skill of the examining physician; this makes it
an extremely demanding method. In addition, it has also been established that not every pancreas carcinoma originates in the pancreatic duct; thus a small percentage of pancreas carcinomas will
always evade ERP-diagnostics.
With the development of the new fiber endoscopes (as, for example,
the instrument GIF P$_2$ by Olympus) the still existing technical
difficulties - also in connection with the operated stomach - will
certainly be reduced in the future.

ULTRASONIC DIAGNOSTICS

Sonography is a further extremely valuable method which has the advantage of being both: non invasive and non ionizing. There are many reports which show that there is high sensitivity and speci- ficity (table 3). According to the general opinion of the

TABLE   3   Value of Sonography in Pancreatic Carcinoma

Author	No. of Cases	Sonography Sensitivity %		Specificity %	
Barkin (1978)	46	91	30/33	68	9/13
Di Magno (1977)	70	73	25/34	82	25/31
Engelhardt (1970)	12	100	11/11	--	
Filly (1970)	37	80		--	
Fitzgerald (1978)	184	67	18/27	72	13/18
Kremer (1977)	481	77	57/61	95	321/338
Mac Cormack (1977)	28	86	24/28	--	
Rettenmaier (1975)	3982	88	38/43	90	
Seat (1976)	1900	73	19/26	100	
Stuber (1972)	250	88	7/8	--	
Weill (1973)	163	88		--	
Wood (1976)	89	76	19/25	--	

authors, the tumor must have a diameter of at least 2 cm in order to be detected by sonography. According to Rettenmaier (1976), who has performed sonographies in almost 4.000 patients, the dif- ferential diagnosis between chronic pancreatitis and pancreas carcinoma is one of the most difficult sonographic diagnoses, among other things, because pancreas carcinoma areas can be sur- rounded by a focal pancreatitis. In addition, it is often diffi- cult to distinguish pancreas tissue from enlarged retroperito- neally located lymph nodes. Metastases in the pancreas cannot be differentiated from the primary pancreas carcinoma.

ANGIOGRAPHY

The special problems of pancreatic angiography are caused by the blood vessel supply of the organ. Selective injections of contrast medium into the celiac trunc and the superior mesenteric artery result in a sufficient visualisation only of the large pancreatic arteries and veins. With this method of selective angiography only 70 - 80 % of the pancreatic carcinomas can be detected. With the superselective injection technique (gastroduodenal arte- ry for the head, splenic artery for the tail, dorsal pancreatic artery for the body) and pharmaco-angiography (vasoconstrictor Angiotensin, vasodilators Bradykinin, Tolazolin) for better re- sults can be achieved. In table 4 the results of angiography of some authors are listed, most of them performed the selective and superselective method.

TABLE   4   Value of Arteriography in Pancreatic Carcinoma

Author	No. of Cases	Arteriography Sensitivity %		Specificity %		Technique
Ariyama (1977)	32	96				selective, partly supersel.
Di Magno (1977)	70	69	18/26	95	36/38	selective, partly supersel.
Eaton (1968)	45	80	4/5	100	3/3	selective
Fitzgerald (1978)	184	83	78/94	68	25/37	selective
Freeny (1978)	118	86	6/7	--		selective, partly supersel.
Mac Gregor (1973)	100	93	42/45	93	28/30	pharmaco-angiography
Weill (1973)	163	80		--		
Wood (1976)	89	67	12/18	--		selective, partly supersel.

Tumor vascularity in pancreatic carcinomas is usually sparse.
Therefore, tumors are often charcaterized by focal areas of
absent vascularity or indirectly by blood vessel compression,
displacement or occlusion (Goldstein, 1974).
One of the major advantages of angiography in pancreatic carcinoma is its ability to predict resectability. The required standards for the prediction of resectability are as follows (Ary-
yama and others, 1977):
   1. Encasement should be confined to intrapancreatic arteries.
   2. No invasion of portal or superior mesenteric veins should
       be present.
   3. There should be no metastases.
80 % of pancreatic carcinomas diagnosed angiographically show:
no resectability.
Of the 20 % who are operated after angiography show no resectability   in 50 % of the cases during the operation.

COMPUTERISED AXIAL TOMOGRAPHY

Computerised axial tomography is another non invasive diagnostic
technique which is new, but promising. The literature up to now -
as far as pancreatic carcinoma is concerned - is still very
limited.

TABLE   5   Value of Computerised Axial Tomography in Pancreatic
              Carcinoma

Author	No. of Cases	C T Sensitivity %		Specificity %	
Barkin (1977)	46	82	27/33	92	12/13
Fitzgerald (1978)	184	94	31/33	60	12/20

The 2 literature examples in table 5 show a high sensitivity. At
our institute Dr. Wegener and Dr. Souchon examined 2343 patients
by computerised axial tomography. 9 patients were suffering from

pancreatic carcinoma proven by operation or autopsy. In all 9 cases CT showed a pancreatic mass.
The specificity of this procedure varies in the literature. At
this time our radiologists are busy with the evaluation of their
cases. Difficulties in this very expensive method lie within the
fact that pancreatic tumor masses can not exactly be differentiated from normal pancreatic parenchyma.
All examination procedures metioned up to now, which - when used
in combination - yield an even greater accuracy, have one thing in
common: none of them have been able to decisively improve the
resectability of the pancreas carcinoma and the 3-year or 5-year
survival rate of the patients. As I have already mentioned, the
history of our patients with proven pancreas carcinoma extented
over 8 months, on the average. By the time patients first come
to the clinic for a clarification of their complaints, they usually already have an advanced carcinoma. In connection with this,
I should like to discuss the signisficance of laparoscopy in cases
of pancreas carcinoma.

LAPAROSCOPY

Up to now, little investigation has been done on the value of laparoscopy in the diagnostics of the pancreas carcinoma. In 1973,
Meyer-Burg presented the results of laparoscopy in cases of pancreas carcinoma including laparoscopic fine-needle aspiration
cytology or puncture with a Vim-Silverman needle.

Technique

The technique of inspection, palpation and biopsy of the pancreas
is done according to the method described by Meyer-Burg (1972)
as well as Look, Henning and Lüders (1972) in order to inspect
the body of the pancreas, the liver is elevated with the rear
part of the laparoscope optic. Thus the body tissue, visible
through the lesser omentum, can be observed. The head of the
pancreas lies within the duodenal curve where it is seen through
the tissue layer of the greater omentum.

Laparoscopic criteria for a head carcinoma

Compact protrusion in the area of the duodenal curve, very often
the sign of the extrahepatic cholestasis with a smooth liver surface and a distended elastic gallbladder with a blue-green shining
wall (Courvoisier syndrome).

Laparoscopic criteria for a corpus carcinoma

Compact protrusion in the corpus area with irregular surface, lesser omentum immovable or only movable to a small degree. Isolated
tail tumors cannot be detected by laparoscopy, but fortunately
they are relatively rare.

Results

Since 1974 we have performed 2215 laparoscopies and we have examined by laparoscopy 35 patients with pancreas carcinomas that
had been proven by autopsy (n = 13) or operation (n = 22) (table 6)
The correct diagnosis was made 19 times in the group of operated
patients and 7 times in the cases proven by autopsy. (9 x head
carcinoma, 8 x body carcinoma, 2 x head and body carcinoma, 1 x
total carcinoma). In 8 cases, a peritoneal carcinosis and/or

metastatic liver was detected and, in one case, the examination
was unsuccessful because of extended adhesions in the condition
following an epigastric operation. 7 of 13 pancreas carcinomas
proven by autopsy were described by laparoscopy (4 x head carcinoma, 3 x body carcinoma). In the remaining 6 patients, a peritoneal carcinosis and/or metastatic liver was found, but a primary tumor could not be detected.

TABLE   6   Results of Laparoscopy in 35 Cases with Proven
                 Cancer of the Pancreas

Pancreatic carcinoma	n	LAPAROSCOPY				Carcinomatosis of the peritoneum and/or the liver
Operation	22	9	7	2	1	2
Autopsy	13	4	3			6
	$\sum$ 35			$\sum$ 26		$\sum$ 8

A laparoscopy was performed in most patients with several tentative diagnosis or clinical problems.
43 patients were presented for laparoscopy for the sole purpose
of excluding a pancreas carcinoma (table 7). A carcinoma was

TABLE   7   Results of Laparoscopy in 43 Cases with Clinically
                 Suspected Pancreatic Carcinoma

	n	Laparoscopy of the pancreas		
		normal	suspected carcinoma	cytol.
Pancreatic carcinoma suspected clinically	43	29	14	9 normal

correctly ruled out in 29 times, which was proven by the course
of the disease or the operation (mostly cholecystectomy). In 14
cases, the suspicion was raised of a pancreas carcinoma or the
diagnosis was made: "carcinoma not to be excluded". The operation
revealed a metastasising tumor (colon carcinoma, prostate carcinoma) in 2 of these cases and a hemorrhagic pancreatic necrosis
in one of them; cytological material was taken 9 times in these
14 cases, each time without pathological findings. This corre-
sponds to a specificity of about 70 %.

          Cytology

We consider the removal of cytological or histological material
to be necessary only in macroscopically unclear cases. If there
is an invasive growth in neighboring organs or even a peritoneal
or liver carcinosis, we consider the pancreas biopsy to be su-
perfluous. In the 35 patients with proven carcinoma, a fine-
needle aspiration was performed 7 times, 5 times with positive

indication of a carcinoma. In table 8 you find a compilation of
authors with different approaches to pancreatic cytology. Of those
operated patients in whom a pancreas carcinoma had been discovered
by laparoscopy, none achieved the 5-year survival time. In the
literature, 0.1 to 2 % is reported for the 5-year healing period.
Thus laparoscopy does not contribute towards improving the resectability of a carcinoma; it's value lies rather in the fact that,
with the aid of an inexpensive method which puts the patient under
little stress, a diagnosis can often be rapidly obtained which
can save the patient an operation, depending on the extend of the
disease.

TABLE   8   Value of Cytology in Pancreatic Carcinoma

Author	No. of Cases	Cytology Sensitivity %	Specificity %	Technique
Di Magno (1977)	70	22 7/26	88 33/37	duodenal aspiration
Fitzgerald (1978)	184	14 4/29	100	duodenal aspiration
Forsgren (1973)	40	97 28/29	91 10/11	laparotomy, percutaneously
Hancke (1975)	25	81 17/21	100 4/4	sonography guided aspirat.
Hatfield (1976)	61	54 14/26	100	pure pancreatic juice
Oscarson (1972)	20	100 2/2	100 5/5	angiography guided aspirat.
Smith (1975)	7	68	62	sonography guided aspirat.

REFERENCES

1. ARIYAMA, J., SHIRAKABE, H., IKENOBE, H., KUROSAMA, A., OWMAN,T.
   (1977): The diagnosis of the small resectable pancreatic carcinoma. Clin. Radiol. 28, 437-444.
2. BACHRACH, W.H., BIRSNER, J.W., IZENSTARK, J.L., SMITH, V.L.
   (1972): Pancreatic scanning: A review. Gastroenterology 63,
   890-910.
3. BARKIN, J., VIMING, D., MIALE, A., GOTTLIEB, S., REDLHAMMER,
   D.E., KALSER, M.A.(1977): Computerized tomography, diagnostic
   ultrasound and radionuclide scanning. Comparison of efficacy in
   diagnosis of pancreatic carcinoma. J. Amer. Med. Ass. 238,
   2040-2042.
3. DiMAGNO, E.P., MALADELADA, J.R., TAYLOR, W.₤., GO, V.L. (1977):
   A prospective comparison of current diagnostic tests for pancreatic cancer. New Engl. J. Med. 297, 737-742.
4. DREILING, D.A. (1951): Studies in pancreatic function. IV. The
   use of the secretin test in the diagnosis of tumors in and
   about the pancreas. Gastroenterology 18, 184-196.
5. DREILING, D.A. (1975): Secretion analysis: Secretin testing
   in pancreatic cancer. J. Surg. Oncol. 7, 101-105.
6. EATON, S.B., FLEISCHLI, D.J., POLLAND, J.J., NEBESAR, R.A.,
   POTSAID, M. (1968): Comparison of current radiologic approaches
   to the diagnosis of pancreatic disease. New Engl. J. Med. 279,
   389-396.
7. ENGELHART, G., BLAUENSTEIN, U.W. (1970): Ultrasound in the

diagnosis of malignant pancreatic tumors. GUT 11, 443-449.

9. FILLY, R.A., FREIMANIS, A.K. (1970): Echographic diagnosis of pancreatic lesions. Ultrasound scanning techniques and diagnostic findings. Radiology 96, 575-582.

10. FITZGERALD, P.J., FORTNER, J.G., WATSON, R.C., SCHWARTZ, M.K., SHERLOCK, P., BENUA, R.S., CUBILLA, A.L., SCHOTTENFELD, D., MILLER, D., WINAWER, S.J., LIGHTDALE, C.J., LEIDNER, S.D., NISSELBAUM, J.S., MENENDEZ-BOTET, C.J., POLESKI, M.H. (1978): The value of diagnostic aids in detecting pancreas cancer. Cancer 41, 868-879.

11. FORSGREN, L., ORELL, S.(1973): Aspiration cytology in carcinoma of the pancreas. Surgery 73, 38-42.

12. FREENY, P.C., BALL, T.J. (1978): Evaluation of endoscopic retrograde cholangiopancreaticography and angiography in the diagnosis of pancreatic carcinoma. Amer. J. Roentgenol. 130, 683-691.

13. GOLDSTEIN, H.M., NEIMAN, H.L., BOOKSTEIN, J.J. (1974): Angiographic evaluation of pancreatic disease. Radiology 112, 275-282.

14. HANCKE, S., HOLM, H.H., KOCH, F. (1975): Ultrasonically guided percutaneous fine needle biopsy of the pancreas. Surg. Gynec. Obstet. 140, 361-364.

15. HATFIELD, A.R.W., SMITHIES, A., WILKINS, R., LEVI, A.J. (1976): Assessment of endoscopic retrograde cholangiopancreatography (ERCP) and pure pancreatic juice cytology in patients with pancreatic disease. GUT 17, 14-21.

16. KREMER, H., KELLNER, E., SCHIERL, W., SCHUMM, C., WEIDENHILLER, S., ZÖLLNER, N. (1977): Sonographische Pankreasdiagnostik. Münch. med. Wschr. 119, 1449-1452.

17. LOOK, D., HENNING, H., LÜDERS, C.J. (1972): Darstellung und Biopsie des Pankreaskopfes bei der Laparoskopie. Z. Gastroenterol. 10, 109.

18. McCARTHY, D.M., BROWN, P., MELMED, R.N., AGNEW, J.E., BOUCHIER, I.A.D.(1972): ^{75}Se-selenomethionine scanning in the diagnosis of tumours of the pancreas and adjacent viscera: The use of test and its impacton survival. GUT 13, 75-87.

19. McCORMACK, L.R., SEAT, St.G., STRUM, W.B. (1977): Pancreatic carcinoma. J. Amer. Med. Ass. 238, 240.

20. McGREGOR, A.M.C., HAWKINS, J.F. (1973): Selective pharmacodynamic angiography in the diagnosis of carcinoma of the pancreas. Surg. G nec. Obstet. 137, 917-921.

21. MEYER-BURG, J. (1972): The inspection, palpation and biopsy of the pancreas by peritoneoscopy. Endoscopy 4, 99-101.

22. MEYER-BURG, J., ZIEGLER, U., PALME, G., KIRSTAEDTER, H.J. (1973): Peritoneoscopy in carcinoma of the pancreas. Endoscopy 5, 86-90.

23. OSCARSON, J., STORMBY, N., SUNDGREN, R.(1972): Selective angiography in fine-needle aspiration cytodiagnosis of gastric and pancreatic tumours. Acta Radiologic. Diagn. 12, 737-749.

24. RETTENMAIER, G. (1976): Leistungsfähigkeit der Sonographie bei Erkrankungen der Bauchspeicheldrüse. In: Die Untersuchung der Bauchspeicheldrüse. Bartelheimer, Classen, Ossenberg, Hrsg., Thieme, Stuttgart, p. 83-97.

25. ROHRMANN, C.A., SILVIS, St.E., VENNES, J.A. (1974): Evaluation of the endoscopic pancreatogramm. Radiology 113, 297-304.

150   G. Arbeiter

26. SATAKE, K., UMEYAMA, K., KOBAYASHI, K., MITANI, E., TATSUMI, S., YAMAMOTO, S., HOWARD, J.M. (1975): An evaluation of endoscopic pancreatocholangiography in surgical patients. Surg. Gynec. Obstet. 140, 349-354.
27. SCHIRMEISTER, J., KRAUTH, G. (1975): Klinik und internistische Diagnostik des Pankreas-Carcinoms. Langenbecks Arch. klin. Chir. 339, 259-266.
28. SCHMIDT, H.A.E. (1975): Nuclearmedizinische Diagnostik des Pankreas-Carcinoms. Langenbecks Arch. klin. Chir. 339, 247-251.
29. SCHULTZ, N.J., SANDERS, R.J. (1963): Evaluation of pancreatic biopsy. Ann. Surg. 158, 1053-1057.
30. SEAT, S.G., McCORMACK, L.R., STRUM, W.B. (1976): Ultrasonic scanning in diagnosis of pancreatic malignancy. Gastroenterology 70, 2.
31. SMITH, E.H., BARTRUM, R.J., CHANG, Y.C., D'ORSI, L.J., LOKICH, J., ABBRUZZESE, A., DANTONO, J. (1975): Percutaneous aspiration biopsy of the pancreas under ultra sonic guidance. New Engl. J. Med. 292, 825-832.
32. STADELMANN, O., SAFRANY, L., LÖFFLER, A., BERNA, L., MIEDERER, E., PAPP, J., KÄUFER, C., SOBBE, A. (1974): ERCP in the diagnosis of pancreatic cancer. Experiences with 54 cases. Endoscopy 6, 84.
33. STUBER, J.L., TEMPLETON, A.W., BISHOP, K. (1972): Sonographic diagnosis of pancreatic lesions. Amer. J. Roentgenol. 116, 406-412.
34. WEILL, F., BECKER, J.C., KRAEHENBUHL, J.R., HERIOT, G., WALTER, J.P. (1973): Atlas clinique de radiographie ultrasonore. Masson & Cie., Eds., Paris, p. 132.
35. WOOD, R.A.B., MOOSSA, A.R., BLACKSTONE, M.O., BOWIE, J., COLLINS, P., LU, C.T. (1976): Comparative value of four methods of investigating the pancreas. Surgery 80, 518-522.
36. WOOD, R.A.B., MOOSSA, A.R. (1977): The prospective evaluation of tumour - associated antigens for the early diagnosis of pancreatic cancer. Brit. J. Surg. 64, 718-720.

The Radiological Diagnosis of Carcinoma
of the Pancreas

O. Pascal* and E. C. Jennings**

*Assoc. Chief, Dept. of Diag. Radiol., Roswell Park Memorial Institute,
Buffalo, New York
**Chief, Dept. of Diag. Radiol., Roswell Park Memorial Institute,
Buffalo, New York

ABSTRACT

With the alarming increase in the rate of Carcinoma of the pancreas, new dimensions
in earlier radiological work up for a definitive diagnosis become imperative if we
hope to alter for the better the present grim mortality figures. Routine upper
gastro-intestinal barium examinations including hypotonic duodenography are frequently inconclusive and when deformity is portrayed the disease is usually far advanced.
Also celiac arteriography when positive often indicates an unresectable tumor. With
the advent of gray scale ultrasound early direct visualization of the head and body
of the pancreas becomes possible in addition to the biliary tract and adjacent vascular structures. Percutaneous ultrasonically guided needle biopsies can accelerate
the diagnosis of a suspected pancreatic mass and could obviate the need of an
exploratory laparotomy. Computerized axial tomography where available also has a
high diagnostic accuracy rate. Of the non-invasive studies, ultrasound has a higher
accuracy rate than barium studies or radioiostope scans. Of the invasive studies,
it has a comparable accuracy to angiography except in islet cell tumors. A new
attitude to earlier diagnosis should therefore be fostered to combat the current
widespread sense of defeatism in dealing with this disease.

KEY WORDS

Early pancreatic tumor visualization, routine radiology, angiography, ultra-sound,
C.A.T.

INTRODUCTION

Carcinoma of the pancreas has been increasing at an alarming rate in the population
of the United States and Canada over the past 20 years with the male incidence
slightly higher than the female. Coincidental with this, there has been a non-
commensurate fall in the rate of gastric cancer. The American Cancer Society esti-
mates approximately 25,000 new cases in the United States for 1978 with more than
24,000 deaths.

Until an accurate laboratory test is found, new dimensions in early diagnostic radiological work up becomes mandatory if we hope to combat the widespread pervasive sense
of defeatism current in dealing with this disease. The laboratory findings to date
are mostly inconclusive, with the most widely used routine upper gastro-intestinal
barium examination found to be most often normal or equivocal; and yet, if there is

to be more than an isolated salvage case, early diagnosis becomes imperative without resorting in every case of low suspicion to a diagnostic laparatory as recommended by Haubruch and Berk.(1976).

From an anatomical consideration the problem we faced in the past for early diagnosis is the organ's lack of visibility by most of the previously known procedures. Radiologically we have been exploiting each organ that is immediately related to the pancreas for the indirect signs on that organ, and when a deformity is portrayed, it is usually an indication of far advanced disease within the pancreas, or complications as a result of the disease spread.

In an upper intestinal barium G.I. series, we look for indentation of the greater curvature of the antral areas of the stomach, double densities, or invagination on the mesial side of the second and third portions of the duodenum. If there is any suspicion, we follow this up with hypotonic duodenography following injection with glucogon and paying particular attention to the mucosal pattern.

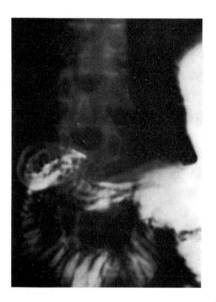

Fig. 1. Hypotonic duodenography showing a double density in second portion of duodenum from an adenocarcinoma of head of pancreas.

If the above examinations are inconclusive or even if they are positive, further study frequently involves an angiographic examination by means of a Seldinger technique via a femoral approach with the use of various shaped catheters. Contrast agents such as Urographin is injected into the celiac and superior mesenteric arteries.

Celiac arteriography when positive often indicates an unresectable tumor. (Douglas, 1978). The poor vascularity of pancreatic carcinoma makes early diagnosis difficult

since it rarely portrays a tumor stain with celiac injection only as do islet cell
or carcinoid tumors.   In advanced cases, displacement of vessels, stenosis and encasement is seen.   Use of adrenalin to reduce the blood flow in normal vessels can
be helpful.   (Herlinger, 1978).   Our aim is to fill the gastroduodenal, dorsal
pancreatico-duodenal branches.   A significant number of early cases could be diagnosed with super selective injection since it provides a high level of accuracy,
(Herlinger, 1978).   but it is time consuming and takes skilled hands.

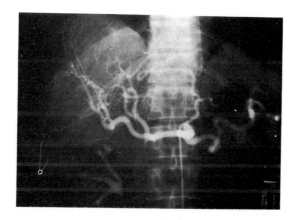

Fig. 2.   A celiac axis angiogram showing pointed stenosis of the gastroduodenal
artery from an adenocarcinoma in the head of the pancreas.

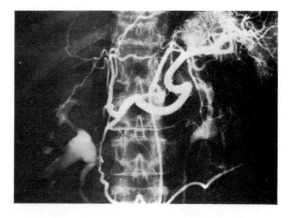

Fig. 3.   Celiac angiography with stretching of the proximal part of the gastroduodenal artery and the superior pancreaticoduodenal artery by a large mass in the head

of the pancreas.

While radionuclide scanning of the pancreas is theoretically an ideal approach, it
has a number of deficiencies, with more than 15% of normals not visualized plus
inability to separate a number of cases from an enlarged liver. In addition there
are 12% false negatives and 9% false positives. (Douglass, 1978). Gallium scans
may permit visualization in 40% or more of pancreatic malignancies but inflammatory
processes can give confusing similar appearance. (Langhammer, 1972).

Percutaneous transhepatic cholangiography, spleno-portography, endoscopic retrograd
cholangiopancreatography (E.R.C.P.), all of these examinations demonstrate the
effects of contrast in the lumina of vascular or organ structures. The effects of
tumor invasion may show on the biliary tree in those with obstructive jaundice with
dilatation of the biliary radicles or common bile duct or a courvoisier gall bladde
or in filling defects in the splenic, superior mesenteric and portal veins in the
venous phase of angiography.

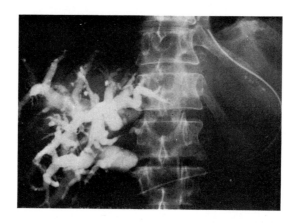

Fig. 4. Transhepatic cholangiogram with obstruction and dilatation of the common
hepatic duct in the porta hepatis.

With the advent of gray scale ultrasound, direct visualization of the head and body
of the pancreas became possible in most cases, besides the visualization and assess
ment of biliary tract and the adjacent vascular structures. We feel a new attitude
to earlier diagnosis should therefore be fostered.

The average patient has a time lapse from the first vague symptoms of three or more
months before a definitive diagnosis is made. (Douglass, 1978). It is our impress
ion that the size of the head and the body of the pancreas can now be evaluated
earlier. And, provided the pancreas is not hidden by stomach or bowel gas or the
patient is not excessively obese, the pancreas can be visualized in 85% of cases.
In addition, an early dilated pancreatic or biliary duct can be looked for and
tumors of the pancreas can be suspected even if not demonstrable; and not left unti
there is a contour deforming abnormality on adjacent structures.

Real time, refinement in transducers and improved electronics, all spell for better resolution with more detail. Where there is still some doubt and where computerized axial tomography C.A.T. is available, problems of assessing the size of the pancreas for a possible lesion becomes relatively simple in most cases. C.A.T. has a high accuracy rate (86%) (Haaga, 1977) and its most potential advantage would be in patients where there is a high suspicion. Transverse cuts in serial sections can give the total extent of tumor and in addition, gas in the stomach and bowel does not obstruct the organs as in ultrasound. The C.A.T. in many cases would preclude the exploratory laporatomy as a diagnostic technique. Its disadvantages are few: financial, X radiation and thin patients with little peri-pancreatic fat. Where ultrasound is concerned, the thinner the patient and less fat the better.

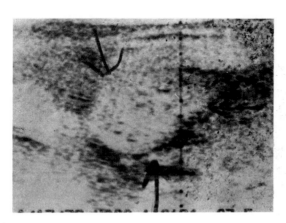

Fig. 5. Ultrasound. Transverse cut showing a large mass in the head of the pancreas squeezing down on the aorta and I.V.C. and a dilated gall bladder.

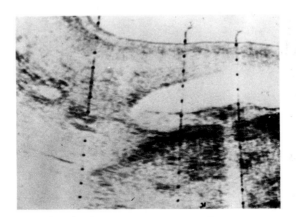

Fig. 6. A case of non functioning gall bladder on two consecutive examinations. The ultrasound shows a longitudinal cut with an enormously elongated gall bladder at lower border of liver.

It is our feeling notwithstanding the reservation shown by a number of clinicians and surgeons that percutaneous ultrasonically guided needle biopsies for pancreatic tumors is a simple, safe technique which can accelerate the diagnosis of a suspected pancreatic mass. We also feel that the procedure is relatively atraumatic or not more so than that of a thoracentesis. It is not to be compared with a debilitating and expensive laparatomy. It also could eliminate uninformative time delay testing.

The accurate placement of a 21 gauge biopsy needle under B mode ultrasound should
be performed early.

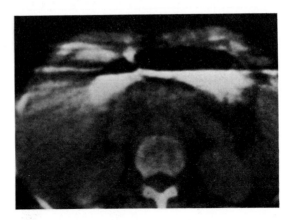

Fig. 7. A C.A.T. scan with contrast in the stomach and the pancreatic mass filling
the lesser sac. Calcifications are present in the pancreas.

Since we now have a multiplicity of diagnostic procedures for imaging, we are faced
with choices. Of the non-invasive studies, ultrasound has a higher accuracy rate
than barium studies or radioisotope scans. (Perlmutler, 1977). Of the invasive
studies, ultrasound has a comparable accuracy to angiography except in islet cell
tumors.

In conclusion, one notes a steady rise in the incidence of cancer of the pancreas
with as yet no improvement of the grim mortality figures. We must stress the need
for increased early suspicion on the part of the clinicians to the patients with
low suspicion index. Immediate consultation with the radiologist for the sequence
of simple x-ray diagnostic procedures followed by ultrasound of the liver and pancr
as where suspicion is low is mandatory and if possible, C.A.T. where it is high.
The early use of ultrasound and ultrasound guided needle biopsies just might alter
for the better the present mortality figures.

REFERENCES

Bartrom, R.J., Jr. and Crow, H.C.: (1977) Gray Scale Ultrasound. Saunders, Phila
    London, Toronto, pp. 191-202.

Douglass, H.O., Karakousis, C.P. and Nava, H.: (1978) Guide to the Diagnosis of
    Pancreatic Cancer, Part 11. Hospital Medicine, pp. 40-55.
Haaga, J.R. and Alfidi, R.J.: (1977) Computed Tomographic Scanning of the Pancreas
    Radiologic Clinics of North America. Vol. XV., No. 3, pp. 367-376.

Haubruch, W.S. and Berk, J.S.: (1976) Tumors of the Pancreas. Medical Aspects of
    Exocrine Tumors. Gastroenterology, 3rd Edition, Ed. Bockus, J.L. Vol. 111,
    pp. 1102-1121. W.B. Saunders Cc. Phila, London, Toronto.

Herlinger, H. and Finlay, D.B.L.: (1978) Evaluation and Follow Up of Pancreatic
    Arteriograms. A New Role for Angiography in the Diagnosis of Carcinoma of the
    Pancreas. Clin. Radiol. 29, pp. 277-284.

Langhammer, H. 'and colleagues': (1972) 67 Ga for Tumor Scanning. J. Nucl. Med.
    13:25.

Perlmutler, G.S.:   (1977)   Abdominal Gray Scale Ultrasonography.   John Wiley and Sons,
    pp. 167-213.

Liver Tumors—Surgical Treatment

Martin A. Adson

Professor of Surgery, Mayo Medical School, Rochester, Minnesota, USA

ABSTRACT

Personal experience with resection of 46 primary solid tumors of the liver is reported. There was but one operative or postoperative hospital death. Survival rates following resection of 34 primary hepatic malignancies are ten-year, 22 per cent; five-year, 36 per cent; three-year, 60 per cent. All patients with benign solid tumors are living without recurrent tumor.

Past experience with removal of small hepatic metastases revealed that of 20 patients having multiple metastases resected, there were no five-year survivors. In contrast, resection of apparent solitary metastases in 40 patients resulted in 42 per cent and 28 per cent five- and ten-year survival rates respectively.

Encouraged by this experience, we have taken a more aggressive approach in the management of liver metastases from colorectal cancer. This ongoing study involves 20 who have had major hepatic resections for lesions generally much larger than those removed in the earlier series. Operative risk is acceptable and results encourage continuing aggressiveness. However, analysis of this group reveals a point of diminishing returns in dealing with larger lesions and continuing experience will be useful in defining more specifically the possible limitations of resective surgery for metastatic hepatic tumors.

INTRODUCTION

My discussion of surgical treatment of hepatic tumors will be limited to the two most common lesions for which surgery is considered in our Clinic and in my country. These are: Primary Solid Tumors and Metastatic Colo-Rectal Cancers.

Before I relate my personal experience with resection of 46 Primary Solid Tumors, let me emphasize four characteristics of this group of patients: 1 - All were adults; 2 - Most had relatively differentiated malignancies; 3 - No patient had cirrhosis of the liver; and 4 - Some patients had used oral contraceptives. This characterization is important because different epidemiologic factors appear to have influence in different countries; therefore, the tumors that I resect may be different from the tumors that some of you must deal with.

This is not a truly large experience, for such tumors are not really common. However, I think it is large enough to justify some conclusions about the risks and benefits of resection of such tumors as they are seen in my country.

Although surgical treatment of the 46 Primary Solid Tumors involved an equal number of men and women, the incidence of malignant tumors occurring in the two sexes is strikingly different. Benign tumors in men were uncommon, whereas benign and malignant tumors were encountered with nearly equal frequency in women. (Fig. 1)

46 SOLID HEPATIC TUMORS

Fig. 1.

	MALIGNANT	BENIGN
23	13 (3 - oral cont.)	10 (7 - oral cont.)
23	21	2

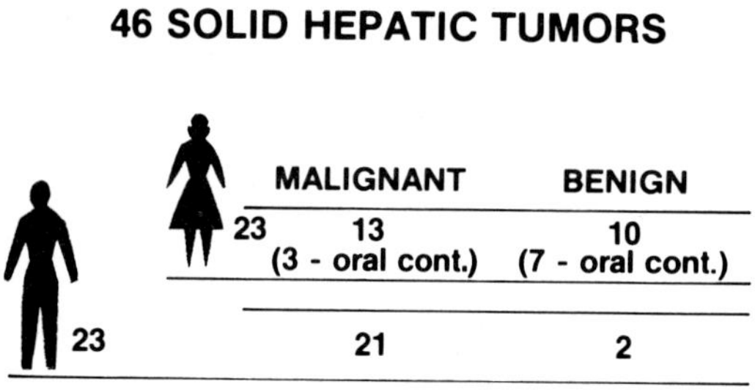

Also shown on Figure 1 is the association of the use of oral contraceptives with some solid tumors. Although there is not time to analyze the uncertain and some-what controversial aspects of this relationship, several observations deserve mention: 1) benign hepatocytic adenomas have occurred much more frequently in women since oral contraceptives have been widely used, 2) the Center of Disease Control in our country in its study of 79 patients with hepatocytic adenomas and an equal number of matched controls found a 500 times increased risk of develop-ing such tumors for patients who had taken oral contraceptives for 7 or more years, and 3) we and others have observed co-existence of hepatocytic adenoma and malignant hepatoma in the same tumor in women who have used oral contracep-tives -- an apparent transition from benign to malignant tumor tissue.

Let us return to more factual observations concerning the surgically treated series. All but three of the malignant tumors were hepatocellular carcinomas (there being two cholangiocarcinomas and one angiosarcoma) -- and all benign tumors were hepatocytic adenomas.

The occurrence of tumors with respect to the age of patients is seen on Fig. 2. Benign tumors were seen most often in women of childbearing age, and two-thirds of malignant tumors in men were seen at the two extremes of adult life.

PRIMARY SOLID HEPATIC TUMORS
•AGE DISTRIBUTION•

Fig. 2.

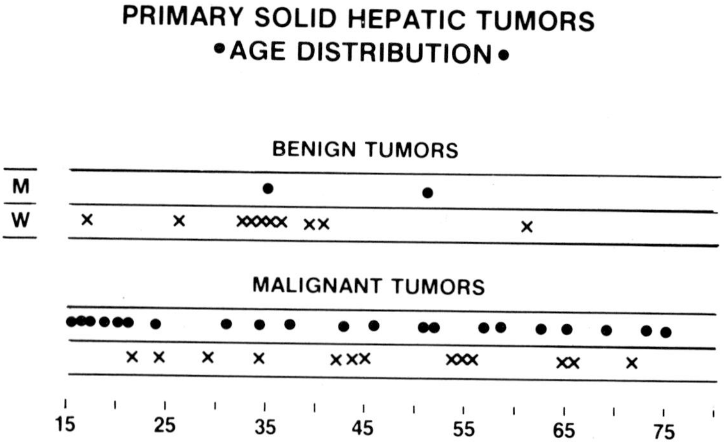

The size of tumors varied considerably. (Fig. 3). Four lesions were less than 9 cm. in size, and the dimensions of the rest varied from 9 to 29 cm. -- with an average diameter of 14 cm. These variations in size are reflected in the varying extent of resection required for treatment.

46 SOLID HEPATIC TUMORS
EXTENT OF RESECTION

Fig. 3.

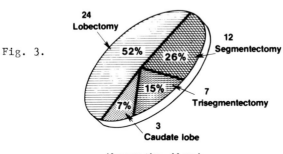

24 Lobectomy — 52%

12 Segmentectomy — 26%

7 Trisegmentectomy — 15%

3 Caudate lobe — 7%

(Average size - 14 cm.)

Our resectability rates were high ∼∼ approximately 80 per cent of those patients seen in surgical consultation. This fact is probably related to pre-operative selection -- some of this by medical colleagues who did not seek surgical consultation for obviously unresectable lesions, and also some selection resulting from the reliability of angiographic techniques for assessment of resectability.

The risk and results of resection can be summarized briefly. (Fig. 4) There was but one operative death in the series (the result of uncontrollable hemorrhage from the vena cava during removal of a large hepatocytic adenoma of the caudate lobe) -- and there were no deaths during postoperative hospital convalescence and no deaths related to postoperative complications.

46 PRIMARY SOLID HEPATIC
TUMORS

Fig. 4

	(34) Malignant	(12) Benign
	13	10
	21	2
HOSPITAL †	0	1
% SURVIVAL:		
10 YR	22	100
5 YR	36	100
3 YR	60	100

Observations relating to survival of patients treated by hepatic resection are encouraging. Eleven patients who survived resection of benign tumors all are living and well from one to 16 years after operation. The 3, 5 and 10-year survival rates of patients having malignant tumors resected are 60 per cent, 36 per cent and 22 per cent respectively.

This experience has led me to conclude that an aggressive surgical approach in the management of primary hepatic malignancy is justified by acceptable low operative risk and by encouraging survival rates.

Decisions about surgical treatment of benign tumors are only occasionally difficult. Solid benign tumors reported in this series were resected when they were large and symptomatic, when differentiation between benign and malignant tumor could not be made (a common occurrence in our early experience), and when discontinuance of oral contraceptives was not followed by prompt regression of tumors.

It is likely that these results of surgical treatment are, in large part a function of the natural history of the types of tumors seen in my country. Again, I emphasize the fact that none were associated with cirrhosis, most were relatively differentiated malignancies, and multicentric tumors involving both lobes were uncommon.

Now, let me consider the role of surgery in the management of metastatic colorectal cancers. Although many types of cancers may spread to the liver, the results of resection of metastatic colo-rectal malignancies have been studied most extensively. This is because these tumors are so common, tend to be relatively differentiated slowly growing lesions, and the control of the primary tumors is more often possible than for other visceral cancers.

However, despite these favorable features, the number of patients that may be benefitted by hepatic resection is disappointingly few. It is important to place this basic truth in perspective. Clinical and autopsy studies show that at least 20 per cent of patients with colo-rectal cancer have hepatic metastases. However, only one-fourth of these lesions are solitary or unilobar. Therefore, only 5 per cent of patients have theoretically resectable hepatic lesions -- and more than half of these patients harbor other undetectable foci of disseminated cancer.

Despite this frustrating and humbling statistic, we do see patients with apparently resectable hepatic metastases, and we must try to make decisions in their favor.

My interest in this subject was kindled by the progress of a friend's wife whose liver metastasis I resected in 1969. Although this lesion was so large as to require trisegmentectomy, she is still living 9 years after that operation. In 1974, as she lived on, her remarkable progress stimulated Dr. Stephen Wilson and I to review our institutional experience with resection of colo-rectal metastases. That study has been published and can be summarized briefly at this time.

Between 1950 and 1973, 60 of our Clinic patients had hepatic metastases from colo-rectal cancer resected. (Fig. 5) Forty lesions appeared to be solitary and 20

HEPATIC METASTASES FROM
COLORECTAL CANCERS

Fig 5.

Resection for 60 Patients, 1950-1973

Lesions, No. : 40 solitary, 20 multiple

Primary tumor: 80% Broders' grade 1 or 2

Lesion size: 75% 5 cm or smaller

50% Duke's C

were multiple. Three-fourths of the lesions were 5 cm. or less in size. Approximately 80 per cent of the cancers were well differentiated, and slightly more than half of the primary tumors had involved the regional lymphatic nodes. There was but one operative death following the 60 operations.

The results of resection as seen in analysis of survival data were unexpectedly favorable. (Fig. 6) Although no patient who had multiple metastasis resected lived for 5 years; 15 or 36 (42 per cent) of patients with apparently solitary lesions lived for 5 years after removal of the metastatic lesion. Ten-year survival analysis (Fig. 7) was similarly surprising in that 8 or 28 (or 28 per cent) of patients who had apparent solitary lesions removed lived for 10 years.

RESECTION OF HEPATIC METASTASES — RESULTS
5-Year Survival Analysis

Lesions	No.	Patients Surviving 5 years
Solitary	36	15
Multiple	18	0
Total	54	15

Fig. 6

RESECTION OF HEPATIC METASTASES — RESULTS
10-Year Survival Analysis

Lesions	No.	Patients Surviving 10 Years
Solitary	28	8
Multiple	14	0
Total	42	8

Fig. 7

Being surprised by these results, and having concern about some unapparent selective bias in surgical treatment, we found in our Clinic files 60 other patients who had similar hepatic lesions that had been examined by biopsy but not resected at the time of colonic resection.

This group was matched by age and sex with the study group. Differences with respect to the grade and incidence of nodal involvement of the primary lesion, and the size and number of metastases are not statistically significant. Thus, these patients constitute the best "control" group that we could find for comparison of survival data. (Fig. 8) These comparative survival curves show clearly the favorable effect of resection of solitary metastases upon survival.

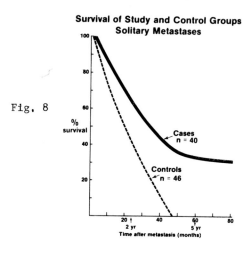

Fig. 8

Efforts to evaluate prognostic factors other than the number of metastatic lesions by statistical analysis were invalidated by the small size of patient samples in various categories. However, some interesting observations concerning those patients who did survive for from 5 to 23 years after resection of hepatic metastases are noteworthy. Of these 15 patients, all had apparent solitary lesions, 6 had primary tumors that involved regional lymphatics, 3 had undifferentiated cancers. Interestingly, all patients who survived 10 years or more were women. These observations suggest that only the presence of multiple metastases, anatomic or technical factors, or an obviously uncontrolled primary lesion can be considered as absolute contraindications to hepatic resection of metastases from colo-rectal cancer.

We can conclude from this study that small, solitary hepatic metastases found at the time of operation for the primary tumor should be removed -- for removal of such lesions involves little surgical risk and a surprising proportion of patients are benefitted.

However, this study provides us with a less definite guide to the management of some of the hepatic metastases that we have seen more often in recent years. With widespread use of nuclear scanning, computerized tomography, and biologic indicators such as CEA assy, we now see more liver metastases that are detected some time after the colonic resection, are larger, or are symptomatic. Unfortunately, analysis of our earlier series does not provide a definite guide to management of such lesions -- for the great majority of tumors resected in the earlier series were small, asymptomatic, or found incidentally during colonic resection.

The first consideration in the surgical management of larger metastatic tumors is the question of operative risk. That question we have answered. Since 1974, my colleague, Dr. J. A. van Heerden, and I have performed 20 major hepatic resections for colo-rectal cancer. There have been no operative deaths.

The next question in whether or not a significant number of patients will be benefitted by such aggressive surgical treatment. Our conclusions concerning results of treatment are preliminary -- for longer observation of treated patients who are still living is required. However, results are somewhat encouraging.

Sixteen of the 20 patients just mentioned had large metastases resected more than one year ago, and thus, are suitable for preliminary survival analysis. To these 16, I have added 4 major resections from the earlier series that I personally performed.

The extent of resection and the average size of these lesions is shown on Fig. 9. Also noted here is the fact that 6 of these lesions proved to be multiple despite our efforts to define solitariness angiographically or by computerized tomography.

Also, 7 of the 14 solitary lesions had associated extrahepatic foci of tumor. These unfavorable features make it clear that we are reaching a point of diminishing returns as we resect larger metastatic lesions. Nevertheless, survival analysis is somewhat encouraging. Of these 20 patients, 80 per cent lived for one year, 75 per cent lived for 18 months, and nearly 50 per cent lived for 2 or more years after resection. Nine patients are still living (6 without evidence of recurrent tumor) 18 or more months after resection.

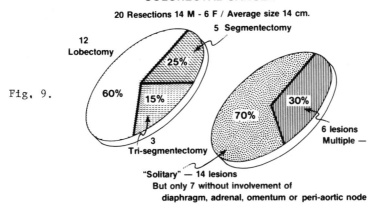

HEPATIC METASTASES —
COLORECTAL CANCER

20 Resections 14 M - 6 F / Average size 14 cm.

Fig. 9.

Only with longer observation of these living patients will definite conclusion about results of resection of these larger lesions be justified. However, the survival curve for these patients is remarkably similar to the curve derived from our earlier study (Fig. 10) -- and a classification of results taking into account both length of survival and palliation of symptoms is somewhat encouraging (Fig. 11). Thus, we are persisting in our aggressive surgical treatment of hepatic metastases from colo-rectal cancer. At the same time, however, we are trying to be more discriminating in our use of angiographic and computerized tomographic studies in the pre-operative selection of such patients. In addition, we are now combining surgical treatment with the use of adjuvant chemotherapeutic agents.

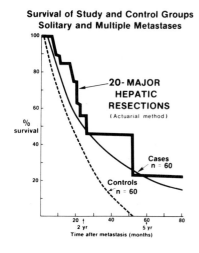

Survival of Study and Control Groups
Solitary and Multiple Metastases

Fig. 10

METASTATIC COLORECTAL CANCER —
26 MAJOR HEPATIC RESECTIONS

SUMMARY (26 Pts)

RESECTION CLEARLY BENEFICIAL   5
DEFINITE SURGICAL FAILURE   5
PROBABLE SURGICAL FAILURE   3
RESULT DEBATABLE   5
ULTIMATE RESULT UNKNOWN   8

Living without & with rec-12 , D-14

Fig. 11

Surgery of the Pancreatic Cancer

José María Mainetti

Escuela de Oncología Provincia de Buenos Aires, 8-706 La Plata 1900
Argentina

ABSTRACT

The "duodenopancreatic complex" is the visceral content of a mediastinal region, which we have called the supramesocolonic abdominal mediastinum. This complex lies astride the portomesenteric axis and makes up an anterior visceral mediastinum that covers Luchka's region or posterior abdominal mediastinum. Therefore, every cancer of the pancreas is a mediastinal one and carries by its location, size, lack of a capsule or microscopic degree of differentiation, a bad prognosis. Cephalic duodenopancreatectomy might be sufficient only in favourable lesions placed in the periampullary region, less than 2 cm. in diameter and surrounded by normal pancreatic tissues or reactive pancreatitis, which keeps the tumor separated from the portomesenteric trunk or other vital structures. In the experience of the author, from 1946 to 1974, 65 out of 130 duodenopancreatectomies were performed for cancer at the head of the pancreas; tumors ranged from 3 to 9 cm. in diameter and the three-year survival rate was 6%. Better surgery and a more aggressive approach is needed now, and the answer could be regional pancreatectomy under axiological values.

Key words: Cancer of the pancreas; cephalic duodenopancreatectomy; oncological duodenopancreatectomy.

INTRODUCTION

At present, any treatment for cancer of the pancreas offers a dismal outlook, and its surgery is regarded with skepticism.Surgical confer - mism and looking upon the pancreas as an "untouchable" have turned it into a taboo.
We shall try to show some negative aspects in this field of modern surgery, which are chiefly due to histological malignancy and topogra - phic situation of the "duodenopancreatic complex".

CANCER OF THE PANCREAS
PERIOD 1946-1974

TUMORS AT THE HEAD		110 cases
Duodenopancreatectomy	65	
By-pass procedures	45	
TUMOR AT THE BODY AND TAIL		60
Corporocaudal resections	20	
Exploratory laparatomy		
and other procedures	40	
TOTAL (personal serie)	170	170

Fig. 1

CANCER OF THE HEAD
SO-CALLED RADICAL SURGERY

CEPHALIC D-P	65
Total D-P	4
Resection porto mesenteric	4

Fig. 2

PANCREATIC CARCINOMA
MORTALITY - SURVIVAL

CEPHALIC D-P

Mortality	22 %
3 year survival rate	6 %
5 year survival rate	0 %

BY-PASS

2 year survival only in 2 cases

CORPORO-CAUDAL RESECTIONS

18 months survival in one case

Fig. 3

MATERIAL - METHODS

The author has delved into his own surgical material dating from 1946
to 1974.During that period (Fig.1) 170 operations were performed;110
for tumors at the head and 60 for tumors at the body and tail of the
pancreas.In 65 out of 110 tumors of the head, a duodenopancreatectomy was performed, implying a high operative rate and aggressive appre -
ach on tumors ranging from 3 to 9 cms.in diameter.Total duodenopancrea -
tectomy was done in four cases, and resection of the portomesenteric
vein, also in four cases (Fig.2).Mortality was accordingly high (22%).
Three-year survival rate was 6%. There was no five-year survival(Fig.
3).In 45 by-pass operations two cases lived for nearly two years.In
the group of 60 cases of cancer at the body and tail of the pancreas,
there were 20 corporocaudal resections, some of them with visceral
extension (stomach,colon,suprarenal,left kidney).Denervation opera-
tions(splanicectomy plus vagotomy,bilateral thoracolumbar sympathec-
tomy)gave very transient results.In this group of cancer at the body there was only one case which survived for 18 months (Mainetti,
1976).
Microscopic findings(Fig.4) in the 170 operations submitted,were carcinoma in 157,lymphosarcoma in 4,cystoadenocarcinoma in 4 and nesidio-
blastoma in 5.
Oncological duodenopancreatectomy in the same period(Fig.5) was performed by the author in 130 cases:65 for cancer at the head of the
pancreas,25 at the ampulla of Vater,10 for cancer of the biliary tract,
5 for cancer of the duodenum and duodenojejunal junction,15 for cancer
of the anthropyloric region and 6 for preduodenal colon cancer (Maine -
tti,1974).
By oncological duodenopancreatectomy we understand the removal of the
"duodenopancreatic complex" for tactical purposes in surgery of the
upper digestive tract.This denomination surpasses the limits of the
pathology encompassing the periampullary region and head of the pancreas, which obviously requires that strategy and involves besides,
all tumors from the fore or middle gut,which for anatomoembryologi-
cal reasons have their lymph drainage in this crossroad.In most of
these cases duodenopancreatectomy is a true oncological operation,it
might be a radical one, a safer procedure than in cases of cancer of
the pancreas.
Cancer of the head of the pancreas stands for 50% of our cephalic duo-
denopancreatectomies.We rely upon gross findings,preoperative (cholangiography, selective arteriography) and peroperative(choledocus or
Wirsung distention,regional nodes)in making a diagnosis and adopting
a decision,without resorting to a biopsy of the pancreas itself,which
involves in many ways an unreliable or risky manoeuver.Biliary decompression is considered an essential previous manoeuver in patients
with severe jaundice.
After Whipple,there was a sound revision,embryoanatomical,physiologi-
cal,clinical and therapeutical of the duodenopancreatic complex as a

CANCER OF THE PANCREAS
MICROSCOPIC FINDINGS
(Period 1946-1974)

Operations	170
Carcinoma	157
Lymphosarcoma	4
Cystoadenocarc.	4
Nesidio blastoma	5

Fig. 4

ONCOLOGICAL DUODENOPANCREATECTOMY
PERIOD 1946-1974

Cancer of the pancreas	69
Ampulla Vater	25
Biliary tract	10
Duodenum	5
C.antropyloric region	15
Pre-duodenal colon cancer	6
	130

Fig. 5

PANCREATIC MALIGNACIES

1- SITE (abdominal mediastinum)
2- SIZE (capsule)
3- DIFFERENTIATION
4- TYPE OF SURGERY

Fig. 6

"pattern unit" of resection (Mainetti,1969)and we have prefered
Child's way of reconstruction and lately adopted some modifications
for preventing postoperative acute pancreatitis or leakage at the pan-
creato-jejunal anastomosis.We have found safer the isolated jejunal
loops (Valdoni,1974),or two separate intestinal loops for biliary and
pancreatic anastomosis (Machado,1976).

DISCUSSION

Bearing in mind the "untouchability" and "failure" on the surgical
treatment of pancreatic malignancies,we must therefore consider some
very important factors (Fig. 6), namely,site,size and capsulation of
the tumor,histological differentiation and type of surgery.
The duodenopancreatic complex is placed over the celiac region or posterior abdominal mediastinum,which contains the aorta,inferior vena
cava,solar plexus and chyle cistern,where lymphatic intestinal trunks
arrive.It represents the visceral content of this region,lying astride the portomesenteric axis and covering the posterior mediastinum,
making up by itself an anterior mediastinum. This anatomical situation explains the inadequacy of the simple partial or total duodenopancreatectomy for cancer.Corporocaudal resections or Whipple operation are generally palliative procedures,tumors are in size from 3 to
10 cm.in diameter, even small tumors may not be capsulated,pancreatic
capsule is broken and extension to the vascular structures of the mediastinum is easily accomplished.Extension to portal vein,to the superior mesenteric artery,to the aorta and solar plexus are outstanding
features, even in very small tumors according to their location (Fig.
7).Site, size of the tumor,lack of a capsule,operative manouvers(biopsy) give reason for the short-term postoperative survivals(Fig. 8).
It is known that there are only a few cases of favorable lesions,which
are those placed at the periampullary region,less than 2 cm.in diameter and surrounded by enough normal pancreatic tissues or reactive
pancreatitis,which keep the tumors separated from the portomesenteric
trunk.
Grade of microscopic differentiation is important.Tumor registries
showed that only 1% of the undifferentiated carcinomas have lived for
5 years.(Baylor S.,Berg J.,1973).Cystoadenocarcinomas and nesidioblas-
tomas have a better prognosis.Five-year survival rate after duodenopancreatectomy ranges from 0 to 15%,average 4%(Shapiro,1975).It has
been emphasized that a more careful pathological investigatión is needed (Baylor,1973)
Type of surgery.Some surgeons think that in the present state of detection and treatment of cancer of the head of the pancreas,only palliative by-pass surgery is worth while, and the future may be expected to become somewhat brighter with an aggressive multidisciplinary
medical approach (Crile,1970).Other surgeons think,even though the
number of long-term survials is small, the only cure for carcinoma of
the pancreas remains resection,and one is left with the important con-

CARC. AT THE UNCINATE PROCESS AND ITS EXTENSION.

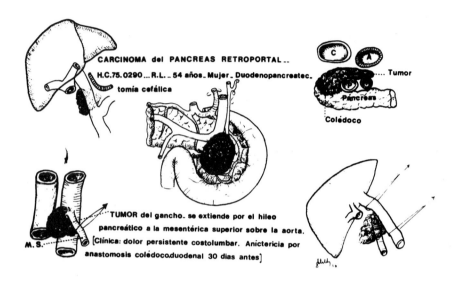

CARCINOMA del PANCREAS RETROPORTAL...
H.C.75.0290...R.L._54 años_Mujer_Duodenopancreatec._tomía cefálica

Tumor
Páncreas
Colédoco

TUMOR del gancho_ se extiende por el hileo pancreático a la mesentérica superior sobre la aorta. [Clínica: dolor persistente costolumbar. Anictericia por anastomosis colédoco.duodenal 30 dias antes]

M.S.

Fig. 7

This figure shows cancer at the uncinate process extending over the posterior surface of the portal vein and involving the superior mesenteric artery up to the aorta.
Pain and jaundice are outstanding signs at this location. Even in very small tumors the extension accounts for a bad prognosis.

22740_INFILTRATING TUMOR 3 cm diameter.
      CEPHALIC D-P.
      LONG-TERM SURVIVAL 3 YEARS
Demise: PERITONEAL SEEDING.

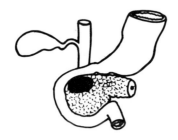

24 248_NODULAR INFILTRATING TUMOR ENCLOSED
      BY REACTIONAL PANCREATITIS.

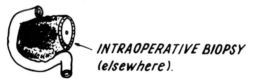

INTRAOPERATIVE BIOPSY (elsewhere).

Demise: 14 MONTHS LATER
          WOUND SEEDING.

Fig. 8

These figures have been sketched from small tumors of our operative records to show the usefulness of pathomorphologic criterium and to avoid,
if possible, any operative biopsy.

ONCOLOGICAL CRITERIA

I-BIOLOGICAL

      Classification (oncotaxonomy)

      Staging

      Prognosis

II-TACTICAL

      Anatomo-embry."Surgical units"

      Technique:"Oncological asepsis"

      Phisiopathology

III-ANTHROPOLOGICAL

      The four dimensions of a man

      Selective Surgery

      Wisdom

Fig. 9

sideration of reducing the operative mortality to levels that appro-
ximate those to by-pass procedures (Shatney,1975).
The choice of by-pass depends on the local conditions and general state of the patient;it ranges from a cholecistogastrostomy to a triple
diversion, according to the surgeon's experience.
The so-called cephalic duodenopancreatectomy will do only for a few
favorable periampullary lesions.In agreement with Dr.Joseph Fortner
this operation is called number O.On the basis of disatisfaction
with the results of duodenopancreatectomy, some surgeons,in the last
decade,have renewed interest in total duodenopancreatectomy(Moroni
1968,Plian 1975,Shatney 1975).
In our opinion, total duodenopancreatectomy is not the answer to the
problem of a tridimensional exceresis in the supramesocolonic mediastinum. A new answer seems to have been given by Joseph Fortner in
1973 with the introduction of regional pancreatectomy (Fortner 1973,
74,77).Regional pancreatectomy faces the vascular structures,as much
important as a cause of inoperability and failure.We knew long time
ago (Evans,1954)that resection of the portomesenteric axis should be
mandatory for cancer at the pancreas,and now,we have learnt how to
improve technique and fill the venous gap without resorting to a
graft,and be aquainted with further possibilities of regional pancreatectomy.
Fortner has devised two types of regional pancreatectomy.The operation is an en-block resection of the pancreas with adjacent soft tissues and transverse mesocolom,regional lymph nodes and pertinent vascular structures.Type 1 operation is an in-block resection of the pancreas with the portal vein,which is repaired by direct anastomosis,
without a graft.Additional removal of the hepatic and/or superior mesenteric arteries for more extensive cancers is Type II operation.
Using regional pancreatectomy Fortner has doubled resectability from
18% to 40%; one-year survival has increased from 36 to 62%,and his
operative mortality has been the same as in Type O procedure,16,6%.
We are in favor of an aggressive surgical approach in this condition
in which we have seen the inefficency of other therapeutical procedures,where the surgeon ought to do his best for forwarding a workable
patient to the therapist and break the psychological barrier of surgical conformism.
Aggressive oncological surgery is based on values or axiological criteria which we have evolved in three items (Fig. 9).
Oncological criterium is related to the natural history of the disease, its classification (Oncotaxonomy)staging and prognosis.
Oncotactical criteria have a great bearing on operability, on anato-
moembryological ground with the knowledge of "Zygotic planes", science of cleavage, and the establishment of surgical units.Physiopatho-
logy applied before,during and after the operation is able to revert
inoperability and provide safer results.From an anthropological point
of view,man is more important than mass.Mind or spirit than matter,
other dimensions play a role, and the surgeon is compelled to choose

between palliative or aggressive surgery according to his wisdom.

CONCLUSION

Oncological criteria support a more aggressive approach in the supra-mesocolonic mediastinum for cancer at the pancreas, than the conventional cephalic duodenopancreatectomy. Regional pancreatectomy seems to be a true oncological operation.

REFERENCES

BAYLOR, S. and BERG, J, (1973) Cross classification and survival characteristics of 5000 cases of cancer of the pancreas. Jour. of. Surg. Oncology, V, 335-358.

CRILE, G. (1970) The advantages of bypass operations over radical pancreatic duodenectomy in the treatment of pancreatic carcinoma, S.G.O., 150, 1049

EVANS, B.P. and Ochsner, A, (1954) The gross anatomy of the lymphatics of the human pancreas. Surgery, 36, 177-90.

FORTNER, J.G (1973) Resection of cancer of the pancreas: a new surgical approach. Surgery, 73, 307-320.

FORTNER, J.G. (1974) Recent Advances in pancreatic surgery. The Surg. Clin of N.A., 54, 859-863.

FORTNER, J.G. (1977) Regional Pancreatectomy. Annals of Surgery, 186, 42-50

MAINETTI, J.M (1969) Duodenopancreatectomía oncológica. Arq. de Gastr. (Brasil), VI, 133.

MAINETTI, J.M (1974) Oncological duodenopancreatectomy. N.Y. Acad. of Med. November 14.

MAINETTI, J.M. (1976) Cancer de Pancreas. Quirón VII, 29

MORONI, J. (1968) Tumores pancreáticos. XXXIX Congreso Argentino de Cirugía.

MACHADO, M. and coworkers (1976) A modified technique for reconstruction of the alimentary tract after pancreaticoduodenoctomy. S.G.O. 143, 27.

PLIAN, M.B. and W.A. Remine (1975) Furfther evaluation of the total pancreatectomy. Arch. Surg. 110, 506.

SHATNEY, Cl and. J. Castellano (1975) Total pancreatectomy. Liver pancreas. Ed. Najarian J.

SHAPIRO, Th.M. (1975) Adenocarc. of the pancreas. Statistical analysis of biliary bypass Vs Whipple's Resection in good risk patients. Ann. of Surg. 182, 715

VALDONI, P. (1974) pancreatodigiunostomiaisolata. Chirurgia abdominale. Vallerdi. Milan.

Cancer of the Pancreas — Radiation Therapy*

R. R. Dobelbower, Jr.

The Department of Radiation Therapy and Nuclear Medicine,
Thomas Jefferson University Hospital, Philadelphia, Pa. 19107, U.S.A.

ABSTRACT

Thirty-six patients with locally extensive, unresectable adenocarcinoma of the pancreas received precision high dose (PHD) radiation therapy with a 45 million volt (MV) betatron. A histologic diagnosis of cancer was established at laparotomy in every case. The gross margins of the tumor were outlined with radio-opaque clips in all but one case. The clipped tumor volume plus a 1-to 3-cm margin was irradiated to a minimum dose of 5900 to 7000 rad in 180 rad fractions over 7 to 9 weeks. For slender patients, a "mixed beam" technique was employed: opposed lateral 45-MV photon beams mated to an anterior "mixed beam" consisting of 50% 45-MV photons and 50% 15-35 million electron volt (MeV) electrons. The choice of electron energy depended upon the depth of the posterior margin of the target volume. For non-slender patients, a "box" technique consisting of 3 or 4 fields of 45-MV photons was used. Where indicated, fields were shaped to conform the isodose distribution to the shape of the target volume. PHD radiotherapy was generally well tolerated. During treatment, only 7 patients experienced significant nausea, vomiting, diarrhea or anorexia. Late gastrointestinal radiation reactions were observed in 7 patients (severe in 3 patients). Relief of pain occurred in 20/29 patients and anorexia improved in 6/12 patients following PHD radiotherapy. The projected survival of patients with unresectable pancreatic cancer treated with PHD radio-therapy seems comparable to that of patients with resectable disease operated for cure.

Key Words: Pancreas, Cancer, Precision Radiation Therapy, High Energy Electrons

INTRODUCTION

Until recently, the role of external beam radiation therapy has been largely palliative as regards cancer of the pancreas (Dobelbower and co-authors, 1978). In the orthovoltage era, definitive doses were not delivered because of the inherent limitations of the relatively low energy beams then in use and because of 2 major anatomic factors: the deep location of the pancreas in the upper abdomen and its relative proximity to various radioresponsive structures such as the spinal cord, kidneys, stomach, small bowel and liver. Perhaps as a consequence of these circumstances, cancer of the pancreas acquired a reputation of "radio-resistance" (Borgelt, Dobelbower and Strubler, 1978). It appears that this notion has largely persisted, even well into the megavoltage era, in spite of the fact that occasional long term survival has been observed after high dose radiotherapy for pancreatic cancer in the form of local application of various radioisotopes (Handley, 1934; Henschke, 1956; Hilaris and Roussis, 1975; Pack and McNeer, 1938). Haslam, Cavanaugh and Stroup (1973) reported improved survival in a group of 23 patients with locally unresectable pancreatic cancer treated to a dose of 6000 rad

---

*Supported, in part, by U.S. Public Health Service grants CA-09137 and CA-11602 from the National Cancer Institute, U.S. Department of Health, Education and Welfare and by a grant (JCFC 26313) from the American Cancer Society.

in 10 weeks in double split-course fashion with opposed fields of external beam
Cobalt-60 (^{60}Co) teletherapy. Acute morbidity necessitated cancellation or
interruption of therapy in 10% of their patients. Dobelbower, Strubler and
Suntharalingam (1976) postulated that even higher doses of external beam
irradiation were necessary to control pancreatic cancer. They described techniques
employing high energy photons and electrons to deliver high doses of radiation to
pancreatic tumors, while largely sparing the spinal cord, kidneys, liver and gut.
Preliminary reports based on observations of 18 patients indicated that precision
high dose (PHD) radiotherapy with high energy electrons and photons was well
tolerated, and that survival of patients so treated compared favorably to that
reported by Haslam, Cavanaugh and Stroup (Dobelbower and co-authors, 1978).
Thirty-six pancreatic cancer patients have now been treated with PHD techniques,
and observations from this group form the basis for this report.

MATERIALS AND METHODS

Patient Characteristics
Thirty-six patients with adenocarcinoma of the pancreas were treated. Patient age
ranged from 35 to 83 years with a median age of 65 years. Twenty-five patients
were male; eleven, female. Thirty-two were white; four, black. Eighteen were
smokers; eighteen, non-smokers. The most common symptoms at the time of diagnosis
were jaundice, pain and weight loss (Table 1).

TABLE 1   Symptoms of Pancreatic Cancer Patients

Symptom	Number of Patients	Symptom	Number of Patients
Jaundice	30	Vomiting	11
Pain	29	Pruritis	9
Weight Loss	25	Steatorrhea	6
Dark Urine	18	Diarrhea	6
Light Stool	18	Constipation	6
Nausea	14	Abdominal Distention	2
Anorexia	12	Fever	2

Pre-treatment baseline studies included complete blood count, serum bilirubin
and other standard liver function studies, chest radiography, upper gastrointestinal radiography, intravenous pyelography with a cross-table lateral
view to define the antero-posterior location of the kidneys, and isotope scans
of liver, spleen, bone and brain. Recently abdominal ultrasound and computerized
transaxial tomography were routinely used in treatment planning.

Each patient underwent at least one abdominal laparotomy at which time biopsies
were obtained, radio-opaque clips were placed (in all but one patient) to define
the gross extent of tumor, and bypass surgery was performed on the biliary tract
and/or the gastrointestinal tract. One patient was treated for massive local
recurrence following a Whipple procedure (Table 2).

TABLE 2   Extent of Surgery

Procedure	Number of Patients
Laparotomy, Biopsy	36
Clip Tumor Margins	35
Biliary Bypass	28
Gastrointestinal Bypass	18
No Bypass (only clips)	4
Whipple Procedure	1

The diagnosis was confirmed histologically before treatment in every case, usually by direct pancreatic biopsy (Table 3).

TABLE 3   Sites of Positive Biopsy

Site	Number of Patients
Pancreas	20
Lymph Node	10
Peripancreatic Tissue	10
Other (Stomach, Mesentery, etc.)	8

No patient with distant metastasis or hematogenous spread to the liver was included in this study, but no patient with resectable disease was included either. In general, the pancreatic cancers were rather extensive (Table 4).

TABLE 4   Extent of Pancreatic Cancer

Structure	Number of Patients	Structure	Number of Patients
Pancreas		Lymph Nodes	
Ampulla	3	Peripancreatic	9
Head	32	Peribiliary	3
Neck	12	Portahepatic	2
Uncinate Process	4	Preaortic	1
Body	13	Other	3
Tail	4	Other Local Structures	
Whole Pancreas	3	Common Bile Duct	13
Blood Vessels		Retroperitoneal Tissues	13
Superior Mesenteric	7	Mesentery	8
Vena Cava	4	Peripancreatic Fat	4
Portal Vein	3	Ligament of Treitz	2
Aorta	1	Peritoneum	2
Gut		Mesocolon	1
Duodenum	8	Spleen	1
Stomach	2		
Small Bowel	2		

Treatment Techniques.

External beam irradiation was delivered from a 45-MV betatron to a target volume encompassing the clipped tumor volume plus a 1-to 3-cm margin. If the posterior margin of the target volume was 12 cm or less from the anterior surface of the abdomen (19 patients), patients were treated with a "mixed beam" technique (Fig. 1) with opposed, lateral 45-MV photon fields and an anterior "mixed beam" (50% 45-MV photons and 50% 15-to 35-MeV electrons). The choice of electron energy was based upon the posterior extent of the target volume. (Dobelbower, Strubler and Suntharalingam, 1976). If the posterior margin of the target volume was more than 12 cm from the anterior surface of the abdomen, patients were treated by a four-field photon technique (10 patients, Fig. 2) or a three-field photon technique (7 patients, Fig. 3).

Where indicated, fields were shaped with blocks or castings to conform the isodose distribution to the shape of the target volume. The target volume, usually encompassed by the 90-95% isodose curve, was irradiated in daily 180 rad fractions, 5 days per week, to a minimum dose of 5900 to 7000 rad over a 7 to 9 week period. With the "mixed beam" and three-field photon techniques, all fields were treated daily; with the four-field photon technique, two fields were treated daily.

R. R. Dobelbower

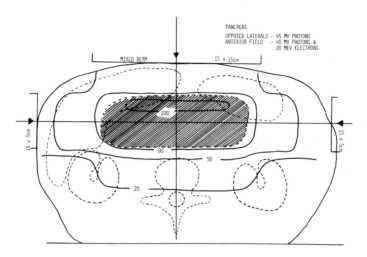

Fig. 1.   "Mixed beam" technique for
treating locally extensive pancreatic cancer

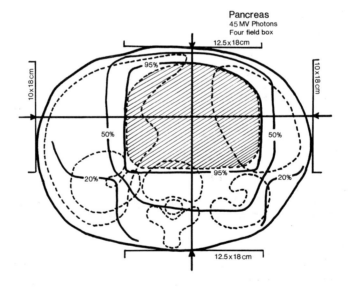

Fig. 2.   Four-field 45-MV
photon technique for treating
locally extensive pancreatic cancer

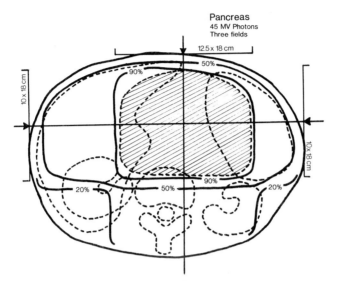

Fig. 3.   Three-field 45-MV
photon technique for treating
locally extensive pancreatic cancer

The average target volume was 1000 cm^3 or less. The dose to the spinal cord was
always less than 3500 rad. A portion (1/8 to 1/2) of the total renal parenchyma
was within a relatively high dose volume.

No patient has been lost to follow-up, which ranges from 2-1/2 to 67 months post
diagnosis. Twelve patients received adjuvant chemotherapy at the discretion of
their referring physicians. Six of these 12 patients received only 5-Fluorouracil
(5-FU); 2 received 5-FU and Thioquanine; 2 received 5-FU and a Nitrosourea, and
2 received 5-FU as part of a multi-drug adjuvant regimen.

Actuarial survival data were determined by the Berkson-Gage method (Berkson and
Gage, 1950).

RESULTS

Acute Morbidity.
Of 36 patients entered into the study, four failed to complete treatment as
planned: two because of rapid progression of local disease and rapid deterioration
of general condition, one because of the appearance of osseous metastasis near the
end of the proposed course of treatment, and one because of psychiatric/social
factors. These patients received minimum tumor doses of 3600, 4800, 6100 and 1300
rad, respectively, but were not excluded from calculations for survival data. The
proposed course of treatment was significantly interrupted in two additional
patients: one for persistent post-operative fever and hepatic abscess, and another
because of E. coli-caused sepsis. Treatment was rather well tolerated by the
remaining patients. Of the 36 patients, only six reported significant nausea. One
of these was the patient with sepsis and one was a patient with rapid local
progression of disease. Four of these six patients experienced episodes of
vomiting during the course of radiation therapy. Three patients experienced
significant diarrhea during the course of radiation therapy: the patient with

sepsis, the patient with hepatic abscess and the single patient treated for recurrence after a Whipple procedure. All three of these patients had diarrhea prior
to commencement of irradiation. One patient reported profound anorexia (in
addition to significant nausea and vomiting) during irradiation, but this was
present prior to treatment.

Late Morbidity.
In 27 patients at risk for six months or more, we have observed seven patients with
clinically significant long term radiation reactions. Five patients developed
gastrointestinal bleeding and six developed symptoms of gastritis (Table 5).

TABLE 5   Gastrointestinal Reactions Following PHD
          Radiotherapy for Pancreatic Cancer

Patient Reaction	Severity*	Time of Onset (Months Post Treatment)	Minimum Tumor Dose (rad)	Treatment Technique
DD Gastritis	1	9 Mo.	6840	4-Field
FD Bleeding	1	6 Mo.	6480	4-Field
TD Gastritis	3	11 Mo.	6480	4-Field
Bleeding	3	13 Mo.		
NF Gastritis	1	12 Mo.	6300	Mixed
RH Gastritis	1	6 Mo.	6120	Mixed
Bleeding	1	2 Mo.		
RR Gastritis	2	7 Mo.	6300	Mixed
Bleeding	2	5 Mo.		
SS Gastritis	1	7 Mo.	6840	4-Field
Bleeding	2	7 Mo.		

*Severity 1- Mild/Moderate   2- Severe   3- Life Threatening

In all but two instances, the reactions listed in Table 5 coincided temporally
with local recurrence of cancer and, hence, might actually represent manifestations
of local tumor activity rather than radiation complication.

Seven patients developed mild pancreatic insufficiency two to ten months after
beginning PHD radiation therapy. Three of these seven were also patients who
experienced gastrointestinal bleeding. In every case the symptoms of pancreatic
insufficiency were controlled by oral enzyme replacement. Two patients developed
elevated fasting blood sugar levels subsequent to PHD radiotherapy.

No patient died of radiation complications, and there have been no cases of
radiation myelitis or clinically significant hepatic or renal damage. In the post-
treatment isotope liver scans of nine patients, we observed areas of decreased
uptake of isotope corresponding to that portion of the hepatic parenchyma
included in the high dose treatment volume. This defect was usually observed
within two months of treatment and was associated with abnormalities of liver
function tests in four patients. The defect usually resolved spontaneously
between 12 and 24 months after PHD radiotherapy.

Palliation of Symptoms.
Appetite improved in six of twelve anorexic patients, and relief of pain occurred
in 20 of 29 patients. Fifteen patients lost five pounds or more during therapy
while the weight of the remaining 21 patients either remained stable or increased.

Survival.
Six of 36 patients are alive as of October 1, 1978. Five of these are clinically
free of disease 5 to 38 months after diagnosis. The sixth patient has locally
recurrent cancer 16 months after diagnosis. He has been receiving adjuvant 5-FU

since completion of PHD radiotherapy. The remaining five living patients have received no adjuvant chemotherapy. The actuarial survival rate in this series for 12 months post-diagnosis is 49% (Fig. 4).

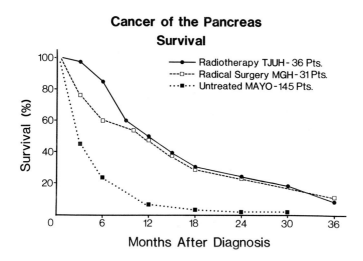

Fig. 4.   Comparison of survival rates of
36 patients treated with PHD radiotherapy
(Thomas Jefferson University Hospital),
31 patients treated with radical surgery
(Massachusetts General Hospital) and
145 patients receiving no treatment
(Mayo Clinic).

Of the 30 patients that have died, two died of causes other than cancer. One patient, clinically free of cancer, died of a myocardial infarction five months after diagnosis. Post mortem examination revealed microscopic evidence of residual disease. Another patient was clinically free of cancer when he died of a fecal impaction three months after diagnosis. Only nine of 36 patients showed evidence of metastatic disease at any time. Of the 28 patients who died of cancer, only five died primarily because of metastatic disease.

DISCUSSION

The relatively low doses of external beam irradiation (4000-5000 rad) that may be safely delivered to the pancreas by opposed fields may afford some degree of palliation (20-40%) but fail to affect survival (Billingsley, Bartholomew and Childs, 1958; Miller and Fuller, 1958). Higher doses (e.g. 6000 rad) given by opposed fields of ^{60}Co in double split course fashion provide enhanced survival, but at the cost of increased frequency and severity of radiotherapy complications (Haslam, Cavanaugh and Stroup, 1973). The thesis of the present pilot study is that by tailoring the dose profile to the tumor profile, even higher local tumor doses can be achieved without greatly adding to morbidity. In order to tailor the dose profile to the disease profile, yet largely spare the surrounding normal tissues, it is necessary to determine with some degree of certainty not only the location of the tumor, but also that of surrounding normal tissues. Recent advances in computerized tomography and ultrasonagraphy notwithstanding, we have

yet to find a better method of tumor localization than the marking of the
gross margins of disease with radio-opaque clips at the time of laparotomy.
The morbidity of this procedure is very small. The single patient for whom
the tumor was <u>not</u> outlined at surgery (RH, Table 5) promptly developed
evidence of local recurrence of cancer in addition to hemorrhagic gastritis
at a dose somewhat lower than the other patients in this study who developed
delayed gastrointestinal reactions. This suggests a geometric miss and
underscores the necessity to accurately define the tumor volume.

Surgeons are generally reluctant to biopsy the pancreas, especially if it
appears that a resection would not be feasible. This is primarily due to
the fear of leakage of pancreatic fluid with subsequent fistula and/or
peritonitis. In 20 patients with positive biopsy specimens obtained
directly from the pancreas, we have observed neither pancreatic fistula
nor peritonitis as a complication in spite of subsequent high doses of
external beam radiation. Surgeons should be encouraged to histologically
confirm a clinical diagnosis of pancreatic cancer, even if the lesion
appears unresectable, and especially if there is no evidence of
dissemination of the disease.

Acute morbidity was observed in seven patients, and in at least three of
these, other factors (sepsis, hepatic abscess, rapidly progressive disease)
may have contributed to the morbidity. Severe or life-threatening delayed
morbidity was limited to the gastrointestinal tract and was observed in
only three patients. The numbers of patients are too small to lend any
meaning to a dose-response analysis at this point. In view of the survival
benefit obtained (Fig. 4), the morbidity of PHD radiotherapy for unresectable pancreatic cancer seems justified. It is important to note that Fig. 4
compares survival of patients with <u>resectable</u> disease treated surgically
to projected survival of patients with <u>unresectable</u> disease treated with
PHD radiotherapy. The two seem quite comparable to the three year point.
The apparent initial advantage of radiotherapy over surgery may reflect
acute surgical mortality. The projected median survival for this group
of patients with unresectable regional disease is 12 months. The median
survival for untreated patients with regional disease is six months
(Moertel and Reitermeier, 1969).

One-third of the patients in the present study received adjuvant chemotherapy, mostly 5-FU. This was not a random allocation, hence a
statistical analysis of differences in survival between the adjuvant
chemotherapy group and the PHD radiation only group would not be valid.
However, the average survival time of those patients that received
adjuvant chemotherapy is presently 15-3/4 months as compared to 12
months for the radiotherapy only group. Although conclusive data are not
yet available, it seems that there is a suggestion of a survival
advantage for patients with locally unresectable pancreatic cancer who
receive chemotherapy in addition to radiotherapy (Dobelbower and co-
authors, 1978). Only nine of thirty-six patients in this study developed
metastatic disease, and of twenty-eight patients who died of cancer,
metastasis was the cause of death in only five. This suggests that
pancreatic cancer often kills by local growth without widespread dissemination and illustrates the need for development of effective local
therapeutic measures.

SUMMARY

PHD radiotherapy with high energy photons and electrons is well tolerated
by patients with locally unresectable adenocarcinoma of the pancreas. The
survival pattern of patients so treated seems comparable to that of
patients with resectable disease treated surgically.

REFERENCES

Berkson, J. and R.P. Gage (1950). Calculation of survival rates for cancer.
  Proc. Mayo Clin., 25, 270-86.
Billingsley, J.S., L.G. Bartholomew and D.S. Childs (1958).
  A study of radiation therapy in carcinoma of the pancreas. Proc. Mayo
  Clin., 33, 426-430.
Borgelt, B.B., R.R. Dobelbower, Jr. and K.A. Strubler (1978).
  Betatron therapy for unresectable pancreatic cancer: A preliminary report.
  Am. J. Surg., 135, 76-80.
Dobelbower, R.R., Jr., B.B. Borgelt, N. Suntharalingam and K.A. Strubler
  (1978). Pancreatic carcinoma treated with high-dose, small-volume
  irradiation. Cancer, 41, 1087-1092.
Dobelbower, R.R., Jr., K.A. Strubler and N. Suntharalingam (1976). Treat-
  ment of cancer of the pancreas with high-energy photons and electrons.
  Int. J. Radiat. Oncol., 1, 141-146.
Handley, W.S. (1934). Pancreatic cancer and its treatment by implanted
  radium. Ann. Surg., 100, 215-233.
Haslam, J.B., P.J. Cavanaugh and S.L. Stroup (1973). Radiation therapy in
  the treatment of irresectable adenocarcinoma of the pancreas. Cancer, 32
  1341-1345.
Henschke, U.K. (1956). Interstitial implantation with radioisotopes. In
  P.F. Hahn (Ed.), Therapeutic Use of Artificial Radioisotopes, John Wiley
  & Sons, New York.
Hilaris, B.S. and K. Roussis (1975). Cancer of the pancreas. In B.S. Hilaris
  (Ed.), Handbook of Interstitial Brachytherapy. Publishing Sciences Group,
  Inc., Acton, Mass.
Miller, T.R. and L.M. Fuller (1958). Radiation therapy of carcinoma of the
  pancreas. Am. J. Roentgenol., 80, 787-792.
Moertel, C.G. and R.J. Reitermeier (1969). Advanced Gastrointestinal Cancer -
  Clinical Management and Chemotherapy. Harper and Row, New York.
Pack, G.T. and G. McNeer (1938). Radium treatment of pancreatic cancer. Am.
  J. Roentgenol., 40, 708-714.

Chemotherapy of Pancreatic Cancer

P. S. Schein, F. Smith, P. V. Woolley, D. F. Hoth and J. S. Macdonald

Vincent T. Lombardi Cancer Research Center, Georgetown University Medical Center, Washington D.C. 20007, U.S.A.

Cancer of the pancreas is the fourth leading cause of cancer-related mortality in the United States. Despite its overall importance in the field of oncology, there has been remarkably little systematic investigation of nonsurgical therapies for this disease.

During the past three years there has been a resurgence of interest in pancreatic cancer. I will briefly review the rationale and design of some of the more recently developed therapeutic programs, and where possible give direction for future therapeutic investigation.

Between 40 to 70 percent of patients with pancreatic cancer will present with locally unresectable disease; tumor that has spread into the regional lymph nodes, has invaded into the adjacent viscera lymph nodes, has invaded into the adjacent viscera, or has surrounded essential blood vessels. Childs (Moertel, 1969a) has examined the efficacy of external radiation therapy of 3,500 to 4,000 r, to the region of the pancreas and compared the survival with that of a comparable group of patients who were untreated. Radiation therapy made no impact on the survival of these patients, nor was there any evidence of symptomatic palliation.

A control trial was subsequently conducted at the Mayo Clinic (Moertel, 1969b), comparing a combined modality approach of radiation therapy, 4000 rads of split-course irradiation, with 5-fluorouracil (5-FU) on the first three days of each radiation course. The survival results were compared with that achieved by patients receiving radiation alone. There was some improvement of survival in patients receiving the combined modality approach; the mean survival for 5-FU plus radiation was 10.4 months versus 6.3 months for radiation alone.

Investigators at Duke University (Haslam, 1973) reported that higher doses of radiation therapy may be more efficacious. Six-thousand rads of split-course radiation therapy was delivered to the pancreas of patients with locally unresectable disease. A 24 percent two-year survival was reported which compared favorably with the historical control group of patients at the Mayo Clinic who were not treated. One problem with the analysis was that many patients had received concomitant chemotherapy with the radiation.

In 1974 Gastrointestinal Tumor Study Group designed the following treatment program: The basic treatment arm from the previous Mayo Clinic study of 5-FU combined

with 4000 rads of split-course radiation therapy was chosen as the control. This
was compared with 6,000 rads of radiation therapy, again with 5-FU being administered on the first three days of each course, and 6000 rads of radiation therapy
alone, as proposed by the Duke investigators.

The overall median survival for radiation alone was   5   months, which was dis-
tinctly inferior to both the combined modality approaches. In contrast, median
survival for 6,000 rads of radiation therapy plus 5-FU was 10.5 months and for
4,000 rads plus 5-FU 8.5 months (Moertel, 1976c). There is no statistical difference between the survivals in the two combined modality arms. 5-FU appears to
make an important additive impact when combined with radiation therapy, perhaps as
a radiation sensitizer and in part through its intrinsic cytotoxic action.

What is the status of chemotherapy for cancer of the pancreas? Chemotherapy has
been traditionally withheld until the patient has reached an advanced stage of
disease. There are surprisingly few clinical trials that have examined the activity of individual single agents for this specific tumor. At the time an analysis of existing data was compiled three years ago, there were only four drugs for
which adequate clinical information were available.

5-FU has been shown to produce objective responses in 20 percent of patients with
this disease. Mitomycin-C and streptozotocin, a drug we have used for islet cell
carcinoma, also appear to have activity for pancreatic adenocarcinoma (Schein,
1977). The nitrosourea BCNU, which has been employed in many combination chemotherapy programs, has not been demonstrated to have single agent activity; in contrast, this drug is known to be effective for gastric cancer. Methyl CCNU has
produced a 10 percent response rate when used as a single agent (Moertel, 1976d).
Chlorozotocin, a new non-myelosuppressive nitrosourea, is now undergoing clinical
trial in the Gastrointestinal Tumor Study Group.

One of the important aspects of any systematic approach to developing a therapy
for pancreatic cancer is, therefore, an attempt to define the activity of the individual single agents in this disease. We must obtain this background information if effective drug combinations are to be designed in the future. In a study
recently completed by the Gastrointestinal Tumor Study Group (Schein, 1978b) three
agents, which represented important drugs in the field of medical oncology, were
specifically tested for efficacy in pancreatic cancer. The patient population
consisted of cases of advanced measurable disease, which allowed for an objective
assessment of the effectiveness of the individual agent. Two of fifteen patients
(13 percent) responded to adriamycin. No activity could be demonstrated for methotrexate, and only one of thirteen patients treated with actinomycin-D responded.
Although the activity of adriamycin is not all that we might hope for, this drug
may be more effectively used in combination therapy in patients with less advanced
disease, as in the FAM regimen.

It had been claimed that spiranolactone and testalolactone had a synergistic effect when combined with 5-FU for the treatment of pancreatic cancer. A controlled
randomized trial using lactone with chemotherapy has recently been completed,
and lactone therapy was shown to have no activity (Moertel, 1977e).

There have been several attempts to design effective combination chemotherapy regimens using the limited number of agents available for this purpose. Kovach and
coworkers at the Mayo Clinic (1974) have conducted a randomized controlled trial
of 5-FU and BCNU as a single agent, and the combination of 5-FU plus BCNU. Surprisingly, the combination resulted in a 33 percent rate of response compared
with 16 percent for single agent 5-FU and no activity for BCNU. The final end
point for any clinical trial is the impact on survival. The 5-FU plus BCNU combination, despite its somewhat enhanced remission rate, did not increase survival

when compared with single agent therapy.

At the Vincent T. Lombardi Cancer Research Center at Georgetown University Medical Center (Wiggans, 1978) we have recently completed a Phase II clinical trial of a new combination that incorporated the three agents which we believed had demonstrated activity in this tumor - 5-FU, mitomycin-C, and streptozotocin (SMF). Mitomycin-C is administered as a single dose every nine weeks. In the past this drug was commonly given in a loading schedule. We now recognize this is an inappropriate method, since mitomycin-C has delayed hematologic toxicity that appears some four weeks after single dose administration. The SMF regimen produced a 43 percent objective response rate in patients with measurable disease. The median duration of response is in excess of 8 months, and four patients remain in remission. Importantly, there was evidence of survival benefit in patients who did respond. The three-month survival of nonresponders is quite typical of what has been previously reported for patients with advanced measurable disease, and this compares with a median survival of 8 months in the responding group with patients alive and in continued remission as long as three years despite their initial presentation with advanced metastatic disease.

Following the demonstration that adriamycin has activity as a single agent, a Phase II trial was initiated at the Lombardi Center using the FAM regimen. This program had previously been demonstrated to produce a 50% objective response in patients with advanced gastric cancer. The FAM regimen is administered in eight-week cycles. 5-FU is injected intravenously at a dose of 600 mg/m^2 on days 1 & 8, 29 & 36. Adriamycin is administered at a dose of 30 mg/m^2 on day 1 and 29. Mitomycin, 10 mg/m^2, is injected on day 1 only. The cycle is repeated on day 58. Over the past 15 months that this study has been active, twenty-five patients with advanced measurable disease have been treated and ten (40 percent) have achieved a partial response. In addition, two cases evidenced stabilization of their disease. The median duration of response is 8 months, with a range of 3+ to 13+ months. The median survival of the responding patients is in excess of 9 months, range 3+ to 14+, in contrast to a three-month median for nonresponders.

What can we look for in the future? Progress in chemotherapy for pancreatic cancer will require the identification of more effective chemotherapeutic agents. This will allow for the design and development of effective drug combinations, an approach that has resulted in substantial improvement in survival for other tumors. The radiation therapists have a number of leads they are currently pursuing. The implantation of ^{125}I has attracted interest, and there are data in the literature to support further exploration of this approach. An alternative involves the use of intraoperative external radiation beam, in which patients are opened and the pancreatic and adjacent regions are subjected to electron beam irradiation, with single doses in excess of 1,000 rads. This approach has been piloted in Japan and is currently undergoing clinical investigation at Howard University in Washington, D.C.

The use of fast neutrons has some interest because of the reduced requirement for oxygen for cytotoxicity when compared with photons. A preliminary trial of neutron therapy plus 5-FU is currently undergoing evaluation at the Lombardi Center (Macdonald, 1978) in collaboration with the Manta Project. Thirteen patients with locally advanced pancreatic cancer have been treated. Forty-five percent have demonstrated a partial response, with a median survival of responding cases of 8+ months (range 5-18 months). One patient was re-explored at six months, with no evidence of tumor. This trial is still in progress and, importantly, the 2000 rad neutron dose appears to be adequately tolerated. For those who do not have access to a cyclotron there is hope that in the future we will develop radiation sensitizers that will achieve the same result: a selective increase in the sensitivity of anoxic cells to conventional photon therapy.

Haslam, J. B., Cavanaugh, P. J., and Stroup, S. L. (1973). Radiation therapy in the treatment of unresectable adenocarcinoma of the pancreas. Cancer, 32, 1341-1345.

Kovach, J. S., Moertel, C. G., Schutt, A. J., Hahn, R. G., and Reitemeier, R. J. (1974). A controlled study of combined 1, 3-bis-(2-chloroethyl)-1-nitrosourea and 5-fluorouracil therapy for advanced gastric and pancreatic cancer. Cancer, 33, 563-567.

Macdonald, J., Smith, F., Ornitz, R., Rogers, C., Woolley, P., and Schein, P. (1978). Phase I-II trial of fast neutron radiation with and without 5-fluorouracil for locally advanced psncreatic and gastric adenocarcinoma. Proc. Am. Soc. Clin. Oncology, 19, 377.

Moertel, C. G., Childs, D. S., Reitemeier, R., Colby, M. Y., and Holbrook, M. A. (1969a). Combined 5-fluorouracil and supervoltage radiation therapy of locally unresectable gastrointestinal cancer. Lancet, 2, 865-867.

Moertel, C. G., and Reitemeier, R. J. (1969b). Advanced Gastrointestinal Cancer. Clinical Management and Chemotherapy. Harber and Row, New York.

Moertel, C. G., Lokich, J. J., Childs, D. S., Schein, P. S., and Lavin, P. T. (1976). An evaluation of high dose radiation and combined radiation and 5-fluorouracil (5-FU) therapy for locally unresectable pancreatic carcinoma. Proc. Am. Assoc. Clin. Oncology, 17, 244.

Moertel, C. G., Douglass, H. O., Hanley, J., and Cqrbone, P.P. (1976). Phase II study of methyl-CCNU in the treatment of advanced pancreatic carcinoma. Cancer Treat. Rep., 60, 1659-1661.

Moertel, C. G., and Lavin, P.T. (1977). An evaluation of 5-FU, nitrosourea, and "Lactone" combinations in the therapy of gastrointestinal cancer. Proc. Am. Soc. Clin. Oncology, 18, 344.

Schein, P. S, Macdonald, J. S., and Widerlite, L. (1977a). Biology, diagnosis and chemotherapy management of pancreatic malignancy. In, Advances in Pharmacology, Academic Press, New York. pp. 107-142.

Schein, P. S., and Gastrointestinal Tumor Study Group (1978b). Randomized Phase II clinical trial of adriamycin, methotrexate, and actinomycin-D in advanced measurable pancreatic carcinoma. Cancer, 42, 19-22.

Wiggans, R. G., Woolley, P. V., Macdonald, J. S., Smythe, T., Ueno, W., and Schein, P. S. (1978). Phase II trial of streptozotocin, mitomycin-C and 5-fluorouracil (SMF) in the treatment of advanced pancreatic cancer. Cancer, 41, 387-391.

Gastric Cancer

Early Gastric Cancer—Clinical and Morphological Aspects

H. Sugano*, K. Nakamura*, Y. Kato* and K. Takagi**

*Dept. Path. Cancer Inst., Tosima, Tokyo 170, Japan
**Dept. Surg. Cancer Inst., Hosp., Japan

ABSTRACT

Early gastric cancer is described in various aspects. Data were based on some 5,000 gastric cancer cases resected during the past 30 years. Prognosis of early cancer is good, with around 90% of 5-year survival rate. Among early cancer, prognosis of the elevated type consisting of differentiated carcinoma was less favorable than that of depressed type consisting mainly of undifferentiated carcinoma. The frequency of elevated type is less common than that of depressed type. The elevated type was often found in older people and in male, while the depressed one in younger people and in female. The analysis of early cancer and microcarcinoma indicated that differentiated carcinoma mainly arises from the metaplastic mucosa and undifferentiated carcinoma, from the non-metaplastic mucosa. The frequency of early cancer reaches around 30% in major cancer hospitals in Japan, and the rate for curative operation has increased, as a result of prognosis of gastric cancer gradually becoming favorable. Several evidences of early gastric cancer may reveal that early cancer stays as early cancer for a long period. These findings clearly indicate that stomach cancer is curable when it is treated within the period of early gastric cancer.

INTRODUCTION

In the history of the study on gastric cancer during the past 50 years, there were several epoch-making advancements in its carcinogenesis, pathology, diagnosis, and treatment areas. Among them, one of the most striking achievements was establishment of the concept of early gastric cancer and its diagnosis and treatment. It is being postulated that the technical improvement of surgery has brought an improvement in prognosis of stomach cancer by about 20%: Early cancer, however, has brought an enormous improvement, seemingly by 60-80%. Therefore, it is emphasized that detection and treatment of early gastric cancer is extremely important, and early detection is now technically possible. For example, at the major cancer hospitals in

Japan, one-third of gastric cancer cases at the present time belong to early cancer.

In this paper, early gastric cancer will be discussed in various aspects. Data were based on some 5,000 gastric cancer cases operated at the Cancer Institute Hospital, Tokyo during the past 30 years from 1946 to 1972.

1. Definition of Early Gastric Cancer and Its Frequency

It is generally accepted that early cancer is a mostly curable cancer at the time of treatment, and a stage I cancer is appropriate as the early cancer.

In the case of gastric cancer, there is some discrepancy about definition of early gastric cancer. According to the General Rules of the Japanese Research Society for Gastric Cancer (1965,1974), early cancer is defined as the same as superficial cancer which involves the mucosa and submucosa of the gastric wall indifferent to lymph node involvement. There is an objection to this definition, however, because it is not adequate to use early cancer in the case of superficial cancer with lymph node involvement. In fact there are several percentage of lymph node metastasis among superficial cancer cases. Another opinion is that stage I cancer should correspond to early cancer. Table 1 shows the crude 5-year survival rate for gastric

TABLE 1   5-year Observed Survival Rate by Prognostic Factors[*]

Stage		Depth of Invasion		Lymph Node Metastasis	
I	87 (%)	m	95 (%)	n_0	77 (%)
II	52	sm	87	n_1	51
III	23	pm	69	n_2	26
IV	6	ss	48	n_3	9
		s_1	43	n_4	5
		s_2	22		
		s_3	5		

[*] Curative operation for solitary tumor at
    Cancer Institute Hospital (1947-65)

cancer by three prognostic factors; clinical stage, depth of tumor invasion of the gastric wall, and grade of lymph node metastasis (Takagi and co-workers, 1978). In this paper, the crude survival rate will be used. It is noted that, among these three, the rate by depth is most accurately reflected in the prognosis of gastric cancer The 5-year rate is 95 and 87% for mucosal (m) and submucosal (sm) cancer, respectively, and 90% for superficial (m plus sm cancer), whereas the rate is 87% for stage I cancer and 77% for all cancer without lymph node metastasis. From these results, it is reasonable to define early gastric cancer as either superficial cancer including both m and sm cancer or stage I cancer. It seems to be practical and convenient to use superficial cancer as early cancer, and it will be adopted in this paper.

The frequency of early gastric cancer is not high, 469 cases (14.9%) among 3,145 cases among curative operation cases in our Hospital. From the viewpoint of time trend, early cancer was below 10% before 1960. By the active introduction of double contrast method of x-ray examination added with endoscopy and biopsy for the detection of gastric cancer, the rate of early cases increased gradually and it reached about 30%. As a result of the increase of early cancer and curative operation cases, as well as the improvement in the treatment, prognosis of overall resected gastric cancer cases has gradually increased from about 40% to about 60% during the past 30 years.

2. Morphology of Early Gastric Cancer

According to Japan Gastroenterological Endoscopy Society (1962), early cancer is classified by macroscopical features into several types; protruded (Type I), elevated (IIa), flat (IIb), depressed (IIc) and excavated (III). Some cases showed combined form of these types, such as elevated and depressed (IIa+IIc).

Practically it is useful to divide early gastric cancer into two types, elevated and depressed, by the level of the surrounding normal gastric epithelium. The elevated type consists of both protruded and elevated types and the depressed one, of both depressed and excavated ones. Case distribution showed 18.2 and 81.8% for elevated and de- pressed type, respectively, among 269 cases of early cancer (Sugano and Nakamura, 1972). It is noted that depressed type is common in Japan and this type often shows ulceration or ulcer scar resembling chronic peptic ulcer. Therefore, it was formerly thought that chronic ulcer became malignant and stomach cancer in Japan was char- acterized with such a type of ulcer cancer. It is clear by now that, such a cancer is not an ulcer cancer but cancer with ulceration (Sugano and Nakamura, 1967).

Early gastric cancer is histologically divided into two categories; differentiated (papillary, papillotubular or tubular cancer) and undifferentiated (poorly differentiated tubular, trabecular or signet ring cell cancer). The former is gland-forming and the latter non- gland-forming, and 39.0 and 61.0%, respectively, in case distribution. Elevated type is mostly identified as differentiated carcinoma (94%), and depressed one as both differentiated (26.8%) and undifferentiated carcinoma (73.2%). Among 95 cases of signet ring cell carcinoma, 98% of them belonged to depressed type and only 2% to elevated one.

The size of early cancer at the surface of the mucosa ranges from 5 to over 41 mm. It was noted that the frequency of elevated type de- creased with size, while that of depressed increased. Therefore, we can understand that the depressed type often infiltrates widely into the superficial layer of the stomach. In fact, there were a consid- erable number of superficial spreading cancer. Among 269 cases of early cancer, 100 cases (37.1%) was over 41 mm in diameter and most cases belonged to undifferentiated carcinoma.

The age distribution of early cancer is interesting. Depressed type was common among younger patients, while elevated type was more fre- quent in the older; the peak age of the former was in the 40s, mainly consisting of femeles and that of the latter is in the 60s, mainly consisting of males.

3.   Survival Rate and Lymph Node Metastasis in Early Cancer

As mentioned above, prognosis of early cancer is excellent.   The
5-year survival rate for m and sm cancer is 95 and 87%, respectively.
The survival rate and rate of lymph node metastasis of early cancer
is different in m cancer and sm cancer, and it is also different in
elevated and depressed type, as well as the histological type.

According to the analysis of 184 cases of early gastric cancer
resected during 1950 to 1963 (Nishi and Seki, 1970), elevated type
mainly consisted of sm cancer '(83.3%), and depressed one, of m cancer
(33.0%) and sm cancer (67.0%).   The 5-year survival rate in the above
early cancer cases was 78.4% in elevated type and 93.8% in depressed
one.   In the elevated type, none of m cancer showed lymph node metastasis, but sm cancer showed 38%, while the rate for positive node was
11% in m cancer and 20% in sm cancer in depressed type.

As to histological difference, the 5-year survival rate for papillotubular and tubular carcinoma was 75% and 83%, respectively, in
elevated type, and that for tubular and undifferentiated carcinoma
was 94% and 83%, respectively, in depressed type.

Thus the prognosis of elevated type was less favorable than the depressed type, and that of differentiated carcinoma less favorable
than undifferentiated one in early cancer.   The difference in prognosis between elevated and depressed type, and in that between differentiated and undifferentiated carcinoma was resulted from the
difference in the frequency of submucosal involvement and hematogenous and lymphatic metastasis (Nishi and Seki, 1970; Sugano, 1971,
Sugano and Nakamura, 1972).   Namely, elevated type or differentiated
carcinoma easily involved the submucosa and often showed hematogenous
metastasis to the liver and multiple lymph node metastases.   It is
interesting that prognosis of early cancer was not so different
according to tumor size in either elevated or depressed type, age or
sex of the patients.

Furthermore, it may be pointed out that the prognosis of sm cancer
depends on the degree of involvement of the submucosal layer.   Cancer
with slight to moderate involvement tends to show much favorable
prognosis than that of sm cancer with deep or massive involvement
(Kato and co-workers, 1978).

In conclusion, prognosis of early cancer is not related to tumor size,
or age and sex of the patients, but is related to macroscopic and
histological type, depth of tumor invasion, and lymph node metastasis.
These factors closely correlate with each other as described above.
Among these factors, macroscopic type, elevated or depressed, is the
most important feature for the prognosis of early cancer.

4.   Morphogenesis of Gastric Cancer on the Basis of Analysis of Early Cancer, especially of Microcarcinoma

Early gastric cancer cases provide a very good tool for the analysis
of development of gastric cancer, because early cancer and its surrounding mucosa may preserve their original features more accurately
than in advanced cancer.   Probably, a smaller cancer is a better
example for this purpose.   Among the early cancer, microcarcinoma

(Nakamura and co-workers, 1969; Nakamura, Sugano and Kato, 1978) is the most profitable lesion for the analysis of development of gastric cancer.

The relationship between cancerous lesion and its surrounding mucosa was examined in m cancer of 6-40 mm in diameter (Nakamura and co-workers, 1969). In differentiated carcinoma cases, the surrounding mucosa showed 92.7% of moderate to marked intestinal metaplasia and 7.3% of none to mild degree. On the contrary, in undifferentiated cancer cases, the mucosa showed 60.5% of moderate to marked degree of metaplasia and 39.5% of none to mild degree. These data indicated that differentiated carcinoma was closely related to the intestinally metaplastic mucosa and that undifferentiated one to both the metaplastic and non-metaplastic mucosa. Probably metaplasia of the gastric mucosa would occur and its intensity would increased during the period in which cancer became larger.

We obtained 130 foci of microcarcinoma less than 5 mm in diameter, which were mainly histologically found by thorough serial cutting of the whole stomach (Nakamura, Sugano and Kato, 1978). Among 130 foci, 112 were differentiated and 18 undifferentiated carcinoma. In differentiated carcinoma cases, the surrounding mucosa of the micro-cancer showed 68.5% of marked intestinal metaplastic, 16.9% of slight to moderate intestinal metaplastic, and 0.77% of non-metaplastic original epithelium, while the surrounding tissue of undifferentiated carcinoma showed 77.8% of non-metaplastic and 22.2% of slight intestinal metaplastic epithelium. Therefore, it is strongly suggested that undifferentiated carcinoma arises from the non-metaplastic gastric epithelium, and differentiated one from both the metaplastic and ron-metaplastic, mostly from the metaplastic, epithelium.

Histochemical and electron microscopic findings of tumor cells in microcarcinoma were compared with those of the non-metaplastic and the metaplastic gastric epithelium (Nakamura and co-workers, 1969). The findings of undifferentiated cancer resembled that of the non-metaplastic foveolar epithelium and those of differentiated cancer, resembled that of the intestinal metaplastic epithelium.

Furthermore, in overall gastric cancer cases, the ratio of differentiated/undifferentiated cancer (DUR) increased with age (Nakamura and co-workers, 1969; Sugano, 1971). The ratio of intestinal metaplastic to non-metaplastic epithelium (MNR) of the stomach also increased with age in the analysis of the stomach resected for chronic gastric ulcer. Comparison of these two figures showed a parallel increase with age, but the MNR preceded the DUR. It is interesting that the DUR is over 1 at the age of 50s and older, while MNR is over 1 at 40s and older. There is a 10-year difference between the appearance of intestinal metaplasia and that of gastric cancer.

From these data it may be concluded that differentiated carcinoma mainly arises from the metaplastic gastric mucosa and undifferentiated carcinoma from the non-metaplastic gastric mucosa.

5. Natural History of Early Gastric Cancer - Early Cancer as a Latent Cancer of the Stomach

It has been postulated that early cancer, especially mucosal cancer, mostly stays as early cancer for a long time. This assumption has arisen from the following evidences.

a) Out of 125 foci of microcarcinoma as mentioned above, only 10 foci were clinically detected, and others were histologically found by thorough cutting of the resected stomachs, which were mainly operated for early gastric cancer. The frequency of microcarcinoma was around 7%. This indicates that there is a possibility of a considerable number of latent microcarcinoma in the gastric mucosa, and microcarcinoma may gradually develop into usual early cancer.

b) It is surprising that the frequency of stomach cancer among aged people (78 year-old in average) was very high, and it was 13.3% among autopsy cases at the Yoikuin Hospital (the Tokyo Metropolitan Almshouse) (Yamashiro and co-workers, 1978). Among these gastric cancer cases, 34.4% were early cancer.

C) According to the data of mass survey screening for gastric cancer (Fujii, Fuchigami and Osaki, 1978), the frequency of gastric cancer is 0.15% and the one-half of these cancers were early cancer.

d) According to retrospective clinical follow up study on gastric cancer (Nakamura and co-workers, 1976; Nakamura and co-workers, 1978), some early cancer showed no change in the size for several years.

e) In the case of recurrence of gastric cancer in the remnant stomach at the surgical stump (Sugano, 1971), mucosal cancer took sometimes a few to several years to become clinically detectable cancer.

The former three items show that many latent early cancers may be present in the gastric mucosa without any clinical signs, and latter two indicate that early cancer, especially mucosal cancer, sometimes takes long time to become larger. These findings may partly support a postulation that early cancer mostly stays as early cancer for a considerable period. Therefore, it is anticipated that gastric cancer is curable by treatment while it is in the stage of early cancer.

REFERENCES

Fujii, A., Fuchigami, A. and Ohashi, Y. (1978). Report on Gastric Cancer found by mass survey. Proc. 31th Meeting of Jap. Res. Soci. Gastric Cancer. Sapporo, Aug. 25, p.24.

Japan Gastroenterological Endoscopy Society (1962). Definition of Early Carcinoma of the Stomach. Proc. Jap. Gastroenterol. Endoscopy Soc.

Japanese Research Society for Gastric Cancer (1965, 1974). The General Rules for the Gastric Cancer Study in Surgery and Pathology. Kanehara Publ. Co. Tokyo. 56 pp. and 76 pp.

Kato, Y., Watanabe, I., Sugano, H., and Nakamura, K. (1978). Clinically Favorable and Unfavorable Early Gastric Cancer. Proc. 31th Meeting of Jap. Res. Soci. Gastric Cancer. Sapporo, Aug. 25, p.50.

Nakamura, K., Sugano, H., Takagi, K., and Kumakura, K. (1969). Histogenesis of Carcinoma of the Stomach with Special Reference to 50 Microcarcinoma : Light- and Electron-microscopic, and Statistical Studies (in Japanese). Jap. Jour. Cancer Clinics,

15, 627-647.
Nakamura, K., Sugano, H., Sugiyama, N., Maruyama, M., Baba, Y., and
    Takagi, K. (1976). Clinical and Histological Features of
    Scirrhous Carcinoma (in Japanese with English Summary). Stomach
    and Intestine, 11, 1275-1284.
Nakamura, K., Ashizawa, S., Takada, Y. and others (1978a). The
    Relationship between the Size and Time in Gastric Cancer (in
    Japanese). Stomach and Intestine, 13, 89-93.
Nakamura, K., Sugano, H., and Kato, Y. (1978b). Histogenesis of
    Microcarcinoma of the Stomach mesuring less than 5 mm in the
    largest diameter. XII Cancer Congress, Buenos Aires. Oct.
Nishi, M., and Seki, M. (1970). Prognosis and Depth of Tumor Inva-
    sion in Early Gastric Cancer (in Japanese). Medicine, 26, 102-
    116.
Sugano, H., and Nakamura, K. (1967). Analysis of Ulcer Cancer (in
    Japanese). Jap. Jour. Cancer Clinics, 13, 477-484.
Sugano, H. (1971). Early Gastric Cancer and Its Behavior (in Japa-
    nese) In Symposium-34: Pathology and Problems in Early Gastric
    Cancer. Proc. 18th General Assemble of Japan Medical Association,
    Tokyo, pp.1003-1007.
Sugano, H., and Nakamura, K. (1972). Pathology of the Elevated Type
    of Early Gastric Cancer (in Japanese). In Medicine Series-No.8,
    Early Carcinoma of the Stomach, Nanzando Co., Tokyo, pp.59-70.
Takagi, K., Nakajima, J., Adachi, H., Ohashi, I., and Oota, H. (1978).
    Prognosis of Gastric Cancer (in Japanese). Operation, 32, 161-
    169.
Yamashiro, M., Nakamura, K., Hashimoto, H., Kanazawa, G. and Kubo, T.
    (1977). Gastric Lesions in the Aged-Review of Autopsy Cases
    (in Japanese with English Summary). Stomach and Intestine, 12,
    615-625.

X-ray Examination of the Stomach for Detection of Early Gastric Cancer

M. Kurihara

Department of Internal Medicine, Juntendo University, Tokyo, Japan

ABSTRACT

277 cases with 312 lesions of early gastric cancer have been found in our department in the past 9 years (1968-1977) by the combined use of a barium meal study
with a double contrast method and gastroscopy with biopsy. In this paper, the past
9 years are divided into three periods (1968-1971,1972-1974,1975-1977) and early
gastric cancers detected in each period are clinically, radiologically and pathologically reviewed and compared in order to define the role of a barium meal study
in the diagnosis of early gastric cancer. Of the 312 lesions of early gastric
cancer, 85 were detected in the first period, 101 in the second period and 126 in
the third period. The ratio of early gastric cancers to the total number of gastric
cancers detected in our department is on the rise in each period. The higher
detectability of early gastric cancers on the anterior wall was achieved in the
later period and this seems to be due to the introduction of a barium thin layer
method into the routine barium examination of the stomach. Furthermore, the detected number of minute early gastric cancers less than 10 mm in the largest diameter
increases in each period. It was very difficult to discriminate 42 lesions of
ulcerated gastric cancer from benign ulcer without analyzing fine mucosal abnormalities on the radiographs. Therefore, emphasis should be placed on careful film-
ing of the stomach with a combination of a barium thin layer, barium filling,
double contrast and compression method and on careful analysis of fine mucosal
abnormalities visualized on the radiographs.

The combined use of a barium meal study with a double contrast method and gastroscopy with biopsy has greatly facilitated the detection of early gastric cancer.
A barium meal study plays an important role in the diagnosis of early gastric
cancer, particularly in detecting rather vague mucosal abnormalities of early
gastric cancer and in discriminating them from those of other benign gastric
lesions. In this paper, the methodology of a barium meal study is historically
reviewed and early gastric cancers detected in the past 9 years are clinically,
radiologically and pathologically analyzed for the further improvement of a barium
meal study.

277 cases with 312 lesions of early gastric cancer have been found in our department in the past 9 years (1968-1977). Dividing the past 9 years into three periods
(1968-1971,1972-1974,1975-1977), the detected number of early gastric cancers is 85
(80 cases) in the first period, 101 (93 cases) in the second period and 126 (104

cases) in the third period. The ratio of early gastric cancers to the total number
of gastric cancers detected in our department is 38 % in the first period, 42 % in
the second period and 44 % in the third period. These figures show that improvement of diagnostic methodology has brought successful results in early detection
of gastric cancer year by year. Furthermore, the ratio of early gastric cancers on
the anterior wall to the total number of early gastric cancers is 25 % in the
first period, 31 % in the second period and 33 % in the third period. This fact is
another evidence showing the improvement of diagnostic methodology for early
gastric cancer. Fig. 1 shows 'pick-up' diagnosis of early gastric cancer on the
anterior wall. 34 out of the 93 early gastric cancers (36.6%) on the anterior wall
were picked up by a barium thin layer method, and 53 % of the 34 early gastric
cancers were less than 30 mm in the largest diameter. The prone view of the anterior wall of the stomach by a barium thin layer method is taken in the first place
at a routine barium examination of the stomach. This view can be produced by about
50 ml of 50 w/v% barium suspension and about 350 ml of air. The exposure conditions
for this view are 120 kv, 50 mA and 0.02-0.06 sec. when a 85 cm focus-film distance
equipment with grid (8:1) is used. Fig. 2 shows two prone views of the anterior
wall. On the left side view taken at a routine x-ray examination, an irregular-
shaped depression with converging mucosal folds is suggestive of malignancy. On
the other hand, the right side view taken at a preoperative detailed examination
clearly shows early gastric cancer type IIc. The postoperative diagnosis of the
resected specimen (Fig. 3) was early gastric cancer type IIc on the anterior wall
18 x 17 cm in size and the histological diagnosis was intramucosal carcinoma of
signet ring cell type (Fig. 4).

The ratio of minute early gastric cancers less than 10 mm in the largest diameter
to the total number of early gastric cancers is 4 % in the first period, 7 % in
the second period and 18 % in the third period. More minute early gastric cancers
were detected in the later periods, and this also depends upon the improvement of
diagnostic methodology for early gastric cancer. From the viewpoint of distribution of 33 minute early gastric cancers, they were discovered in the whole area of
the stomach except for the cardiac region and fornix. The commonest part for
minute early gastric cancer in our series is the greater curvature. Table 1 shows
the relationship between the type and size of minute early gastric cancers less
than 10 mm in the largest diameter. Between 5 and 10 mm in the largest diameter, a
depressed type of early gastric cancer is twice number of a protruded type.
52.9 % of the minute early gastric cancers less than 5 mm in the largest diamter
were superficial flat type, type IIb, 35.3 % were depressed type and the remaining
11.8 % were protruded type. As shown in Table 2, out of 16 minute early gastric
cancers between 5 and 10 mm in the largest diameter, 9 were picked up by a barium
meal study and the remaining 7 were by gastroscopy. A preoperative accurate diagnosis was made in 75 % of them by a barium meal study, in 81 % by gastroscopy and
in 100 % by biopsy. On the other hand, none of 17 minute early gastric cancers
less than 5 mm in the largest diameter was diagnosed as carcinoma by a barium meal
study or gastroscopy. Biopsy materials showed positive identification of carcinoma
in 4 of them. The remaining 13 minute early gastric cancers were confirmed at the
postoperative histological examination. Consequently, the results indicate that
the limiting size of minute early gastric cancer for a barium meal study or gastro
-scopy is 5 mm in the largest diameter. Fig. 5 is a supine double contrast view of
the stomach in a patient with a minute early gastric cancer. A small irregular-
shaped depression surrounded by converging mucosal folds, which is highly suggestive of malignancy, is clearly visualized on the posterior wall of the angular
region. A minute early gastric cancer 7 x 5 mm in size is noted in the post-
operative resected specimen (Fig. 6 a,b). The histological diagnosis was intramucosal carcinoma of signet ring cell type (Fig. 7).

The another subject to be discussed in the diagnosis of early gastric cancer is
how to discriminate depressed type early gastric cancers from benign ulcers.

Table 3 shows the diagnostic process of 42 lesions of gastric cancer which were initially diagnosed as benign gastric ulcer at a barium meal study or gastroscopy. 32 out of the 42 gastric cancers (76.2%) were diagnosed as carcinoma at the follow -up barium meal study or gastroscopy, but the remaining 10 (23.8%) were still thought as benign ulcer even at the preoperative detailed barium study or gastro- scopy. They were also considered as benign ulcer by their macroscopic appearances in the resected specimens. Table 4 shows the schematic illustrations of 10 gastric cancers where the preoperative diagnosis was benign ulcer. Retrospectively, in 6 out of the 10 cancers, a cancerous erosion around the ulcer crater can be pointed out on the x-ray views as shown in Table 5. Therefore, a diagnosis of carcinoma may be possible if a careful attention is paid to the cancerous erosion around the ulcer crater. Fig. 8 is the resected specimen of a patient with early gastric cancer type III. A cancerous erosion is hardly recognizable even in the resected specimen. However, the histological examination showed tubular adenocarcinoma invading the submucosal layer (Fig. 9 a,b). When careful analysis of x-ray find- ings on the double contrast view (Fig. 10) is retrospectively made, an irregular- shaped erosion is suggestive of cancerous infiltration.
Thus, in the diagnosis of minute early gastric cancer or benign-looking early gastric cancer of depressed type, emphasis should be placed on careful analysis of the fine mucosal abnormalities visualized on the radiographs in order to decrease false negative or positive diagnoses.

TABLE 1 TYPES OF MINUTE EARLY GASTRIC CANCERS (≤ 1 CM)

	I, IIa	IIb	IIc, III	TOTAL NO. OF LESIONS
> 5 MM	5 (31.3%)	-	1 1 (68.7%)	1 6
≤ 5 MM	2 (11.8%)	9 (52.9%)	6 (35.3%)	1 7

(20 CASES WITH 33 LESIONS)

TABLE 2 DIAGNOSIS OF MINUTE GASTRIC CANCERS (≤ 1 CM)

	NO. OF LESION	DIAGNOSIS	X-RAY	GASTROSCOPY	BIOPSY
> 5 MM	1 6	PICK-UP	9	7	
		PREOPERATIVE	12 (75%) "CANCER"	13 (81%) "CANCER"	16 (100%) "CANCER"
≤ 5 MM	1 7	PREOPERATIVE	4 (23%) "BENIGN"	4 (23%) "BENIGN"	4 (23%) "CANCER"
		OVERLOOKED	13 (77%)	13 (77%)	13 (77%)

TABLE 3 FALSE NEGATIVE CASES AT INITIAL DIAGNOSIS

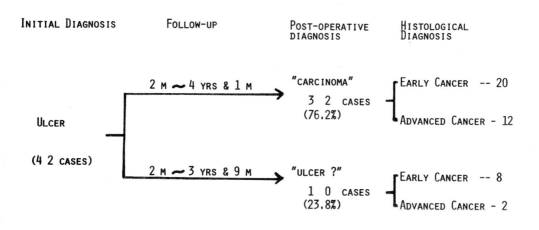

INITIAL DIAGNOSIS	FOLLOW-UP	POST-OPERATIVE DIAGNOSIS	HISTOLOGICAL DIAGNOSIS
ULCER (4 2 CASES)	2 M ∼ 4 YRS & 1 M	"CARCINOMA" 3 2 CASES (76.2%)	EARLY CANCER -- 20 / ADVANCED CANCER - 12
	2 M ∼ 3 YRS & 9 M	"ULCER ?" 1 0 CASES (23.8%)	EARLY CANCER -- 8 / ADVANCED CANCER - 2

TABLE 4 SCHEMATIC ILLUSTRATION OF GASTRIC CANCERS
DIFFICULT TO DISTINGUISH FROM BENIGN ULCER

EARLY CANCER TYPE III			
TYPE III - LIKE ADVANCED CANCER			
EARLY CANCER TYPE III + IIC			
EARLY CANCER TYPE IIC + III			

ULCFR   SCAR

CANCER

Table 5

RETROSPECTIVE ANALYSIS OF X-RAY FINDINGS IN 10 FALSE NEGATIVE CASES

	Histological Diagnosis	Diagnosed as "ca" by X-ray
Type III	2	(1)
Advanced cancer looks like type III	2	(1)
Type III + IIc	3	(3)
Type IIc + III	3	(1)
Total	1 0	(6) (60.0%)

Fig. 1   "PICK-UP" OF EARLY GASTRIC CANCER AT THE ANTERIOR WALL

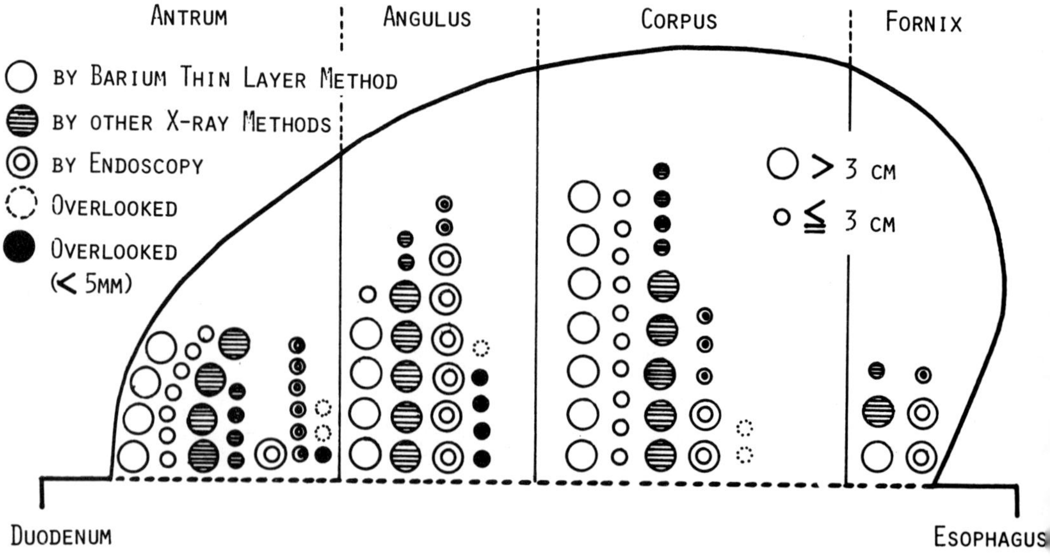

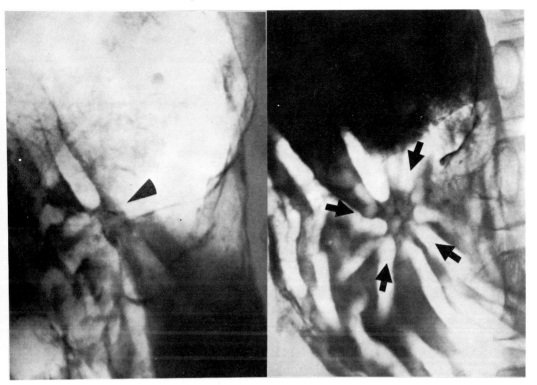

Fig. 2 The prone views of the anterior wall of the stomach by a barium thin layer method in a patient with an early gastric cancer type IIc on the anterior wall. The left side view taken at a routine x-ray examination shows an irregular-shaped depression with converging mucosal folds suggestive of malignancy. The right side view clearly shows an early gastric cancer type IIc.

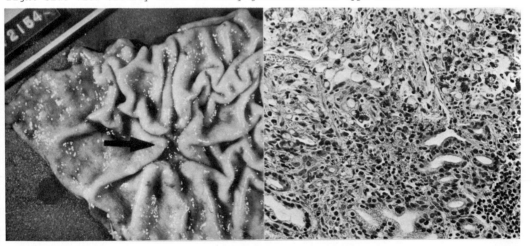

Fig. 3 The resected specimen with an early gastric cancer type IIc 18 x 17 mm in size on the anterior wall of the stomach.

Fig. 4 The histological section showing signet ring cell carcinoma.

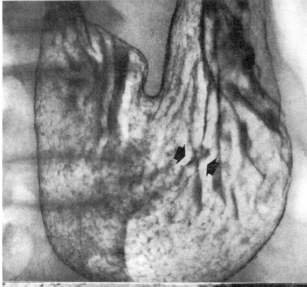

Fig. 5 The supine double contrast view of the stomach in a
patient with a minute early
gastric cancer type IIc.
An irregular-shaped depression
surrounde by converging mucosal
folds is well visualized.

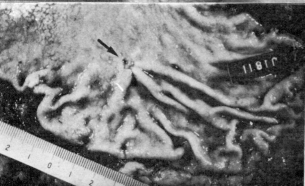

Fig. 6a The resected specimen with a minute
early gastric cancer type IIc 7 x 5 mm in size.

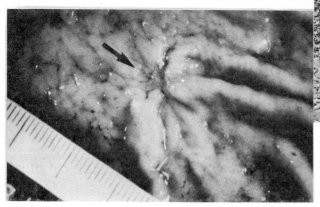

Fig. 6b The close-up view of an minute early
gastric cancer.

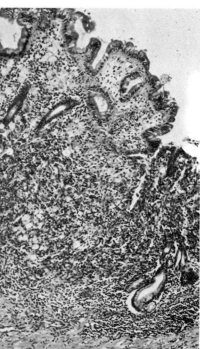

Fig. 7 The histological section
showing signet ring cell carcinoma.

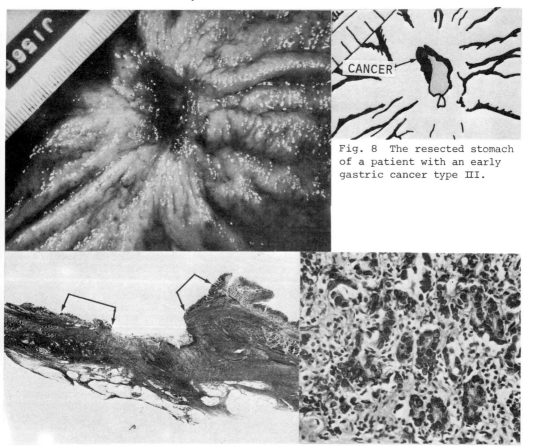

Fig. 8 The resected stomach of a patient with an early gastric cancer type III.

Fig. 9a The low magnification of a histological section. Arrows indicate cancerous infiltration.

Fig. 9b Tubular adenocarcinoma is noted on the moderate magnification of the histological section.

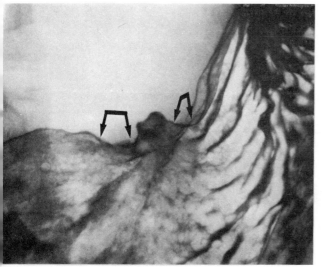

Fig. 10 The supine double contrast view of the stomach. Retrospectively, an irregular-shaped cancerous erosion can be pointed out on the double contrast view. Arrows indicate a cancerous erosion.

Early Diagnosis of Gastric Cancer in Japan

K. Kawai*, Y. Akasaka*, Y. Kohli** and F. Misaki*

*Department of Preventive Medicine,
**The 3rd Department of Internal Medicine, Kyoto Prefectural University of
Medicine, Kyoto, Japan

ABSTRACT

In this paper the present status of endoscopic diagnosis of early gastric cancer
in Japan is reported. Recently in this country the dye spraying method has been
adopted to diagnose early gastric cancer as a subsidiary method in endoscopy,
and it is noticeable that with this method early gastric cancer is more easily
diagnosed by endoscopy. Furthermore, the developing site of early gastric cancer
may be detected with this method not only from the difference of patterns of the
phyloric gland mucosa and the fundic one, but also from the difference in
staining of the gastric mucosa with methylene blue.

INTRODUCTION

Japan's death rate from malignant diseases grows larger every year. In 1976, the
number of deaths from malignancy reached 140,893 and it accounted for 20.0% of all
deaths in Japan. It is exceeded only by cerebrovascular accidents in the morti-
lity statistics. It is a remarkable feature in Japan that gastric cancer is most
common in malignant diseases. In the same year, the number of deaths from gastric
cancer was 50,092 and its rate to all malignant diseases reached 38.2% in male and
32.7% in female. It is a national interest, therefore, to lower the mortality
from this disease.
In this paper, we would like to report the present status of endoscopic diagnosis
of early gastric cancer in Japan and some problems awaiting solution.

Incidence

From 1958 to 1976, 283 cases of early gastric cancer were found in our clinic.
Using these cases, some statistical studies were tried on the incidence of early
gastric cancer, and significance of roentgenography and endoscopy were discussed
for diagnosing early gastric cancer.
Table 1 shows the analysis of 283 cases of early gastric cancer from 1958 to 1976
at three-year intervals. During the first three years, only 3.7% of 83 cases of
resected gastric cancer were of early cancer, while it occupied 42.2% during the
last three years.
Table 2 shows the age and sex distribution of early and advanced gastric cancer
operated. The peak of age distribution was seen from the fourties to the sixties,

211

TABLE 1   Yearly Distribution of Early Gastric Cancer

Diagnosis Period	Stomach Cancer	Early Gastric Cancer (%)
1958-1960	83	3 (3.7)
1961-1963	114	19 (16.7)
1964-1966	122	39 (32.0)
1967-1969	151	50 (33.1)
1970-1972	216	96 (44.4)
1973-1975	159	67 (42.2)
1976	25	9 (36.0)
Total	870	283 (32.5)

TABLE 2   Examined Cases of Gastric Cancer

Age	Early Cancer M	F	Total	Advanced Cancer M	F	Total	Total
-29	2	3	5(1.8%)	17	12	29(4.9%)	34(3.9%)
-39	20	8	28(9.9)	25	12	37(6.3)	65(7.5)
-49	50	24	74(26.2)	62	35	97(16.5)	171(19.7)
-59	56	16	72(25.4)	98	53	151(25.7)	223(25.6)
-69	63	14	77(27.3)	140	61	201(34.2)	278(31.9)
70-	25	2	27(9.5)	49	23	72(12.4)	99(11.4)
Total			283(100%)			587(100%)	870(100%)

but it is noticeable that five cases (1.8%) of early gastric cancer and 29 (4.9%) of advanced one were found in the younger than thirty year old. Moreover, early gastric cancer was ten years younger in patient's age than advanced gastric cancer. The Japanese Society of Gastroenterological Endoscopy divided early gastric cancer into three types, that is, protruded type (Type I), superficial type (Type II) and excavated type (Type III). The superficial type was further subdivided into superficial elevated, type II_a, superficial flat, type II_b and superficial depressed, type II_c.

Table 3 shows the incidence of different types of early gastric cancer. The depressed type (types II_c, II_c+III, $III+II_c$, etc) is most common (232 cases (82.3%) of all cases) and the majority of them are located at the angulus, the antrum or the lower corpus of the stomach, especially at the lesser curvature or the posterior wall. The incidence of elevated type (types I, II_a, II_a+II_c) is highest in "A" region defined in Table 3.

TABLE 3   Macroscopic Types and Location of
          Early Gastric Cancer

Location Types	C	M	A	Total
I, II$_a$	1 (3.3)	12 (40.0)	17 (56.7)	30
II$_a$+II$_c$	1 (6.2)	3 (18.8)	12 (75.0)	16
II$_b$	–	3 (60.0)	2 (40.0)	5
II$_c$	3 (3.2)	56 (60.2)	34 (36.6)	93
II$_c$+III	4 (2.9)	99 (71.2)	36 (25.9)	139
Total	9 (3.2)	173 (60.8)	101 (36.0)	283 (100%)

Significance of Roentgenography and Endoscopy

In general, routine diagnosis of gastric diseases is first made by general upper G-I series, and endoscopic examination is recommended as a second step in detailed examination. Though endoscopic examination may provide some informations which escape from the roentgenographic examination, it requires many years' experience to detect such intragastric lesions.
Figure 1 compares diagnostic accuracy between roentgenography and endoscopy in 212 cases of early gastric cancer, to which both techniques have been done in our hospital. All cases underwent roentgenographic examination first. Of 120 cases diagnosed as cancer by roentgenography, successive endoscopic examination estimated 9 cases as suspicious and 4 cases as not cancer. Moreover, it should be pointed out that 43 of 58 cases suspicious of cancer and 16 of 34 cases diagnosed not cancer by roentgenography were later diagnosed as cancer by endoscopy. However, 14 cases could not be diagnosed as cancer by both methods, mainly located on the posterior wall or the lesser curvature of the antrum and the gastric angle. Eleven out of them were experienced for six years from 1958 when early gastric cancer was first experienced. There is no characteristic trend in the type or location of gastric cancer in these 11 cases. However, the remainder had different meanings from them, that, is, these 3 misdiagnosed cases consisted of two cases of II$_c$ type

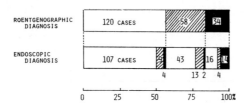

☐   Cancer

▨   Suspicious of cancer

■   Not cancer

Fig. 1   Relationship between roentgenographic and
         endoscopical disgnosis

TABLE 4   Comparison of Endoscopy and X-ray in the Diagnosis of
          Upper G-I Tract Lesions (219 lesions in 134 cases)

Location & Diseases	No. of Lesions	X-ray	Endoscopy
Esophagus			
Esophagitis	4	0	4
Diverticulum	4	4	4
Polyp	3	2	3
Ulcer	1	1	1
Varices	1	1	1
Total	13	8(61.5%)	13(100%)
Stomach			
Ulcer or scar	79	73	78
Cancer	22	19	22
Polyp	13	11	13
Others	34	25	34
Total	148	128(86.5%)	147(99.3%)
Duodenum			
Ulcer or scar	49	42	48
Polyp	4	2	4
Diverticulum	3	3	2
Duodenitis	2	1	2
Total	58	48(82.8%)	56(96.6%)
Total	219	184(84.0%)	216(98.6%)

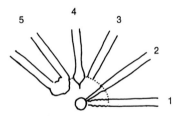

Fig. 2   Specific findings of mucosal folds

and one case of type II$_b$, all of which were accompanied with one or two typical
cancerous lesions at another part of the stomach. From another point of view,
diagnostic accuracy of upper G-I tract between roentgenography and endoscopy are
compared in Table 4, concerning 219 lesions in 134 cases, to which these two
techniques are adopted independently by specialists. In general, diagnostic accuracy of endoscopy was superior to roentgenography, especially for detecting small
and slight depressed or elevated lesions. However, in some cases on the posterior
wall of the corpus and the duodenal bulb, endoscopic diagnosis was inferior to
roentgenographic one. From these data, it is noticeable that accurate diagnosis
results from a combination of these two techniques, since the endoscopic and
roentgenographic diagnostic abilities have a limit by themselves.
Moreover, it is important for us to differentiate an ulceration whether it is malignant or benign. Firstly peptic ulcer in the carcinomatous mucosa shows several
specific findings concerning converged mucosal folds; 1, stiffness of mucosal
folds, 2. narrowing of proximal mucosal folds, 3. abruption of mucosal folds, 4.
thickening of proximal end of abrupted mucosal folds and 5. confluence of mucosal
folds (Fig. 2).
Table 5 shows a comparison of these findings between malignant and benign ulcers
of the stomach. These findings are more frequently observed in malignant ulcer,

but in some kinds of benign ulcer, especially of type Ul-IV, they can be seen even though not so frequently.
Secondly, malignant ulcer has a specific configuration, that is, the shape of ulcer is irregular with zigzag edges and its base is uneven in almost all cases of malignant ulcers, while almost benign ulcer is round with smooth edge (Table 6). Furthermore, on differentiating benign ulcer from malignant one, we must pay our attention to the fact that peptic ulcerations are easy to occur on the cacinomatous mucosa of the stomach and to heal up. This phenomenon is called "Malignant cycle" of gastric cancer (Fig. 3).

TABLE 5   Differentiation of Gastric Ulceration (1)

	mucosal folds				
	rigidity (1)	narrowing (2)	abruption (3)	thickness (4)	confluence (5)
benign ulcer (Ul-IV) 60 cases	9 15%	7 12	4 7	12 20	3 5
malignant ulcer 40 cases	10 25%	10 25	20 50	31 78	32 80
peptic ulcer of carcinomatous mucosa, 20 cases	16 80%	20 100	13 65	7 35	2 10

TABLE 6   Differentiation of Gastric Ulceration (2)

	ulcer					
	configuration		base		edge	
	round	irregular	flat	uneven	regular	zigzag
benign ulcer (Ul-IV) 60 cases	34 57%	26 43	29 48	31 52	52 87	8 13
malignant ulcer 40 cases	1 3%	39 97	3 7	37 93	1 3	39 97
peptic ulcer of carcinomatous mucosa, 20	2 10%	18 90	9 45	11 55	5 25	15 75

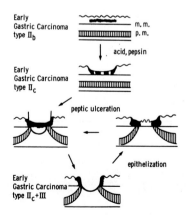

Fig. 3 Malignant cycle of gastric cancer

Significance of Dye Spraying Method in Endoscopy

As was stated in Table 3, the most common type of early gastric cancer is a super-ficial depressed type (type II_c, II_c+III, or $III+II_c$). These lesions are sharply demarcated and central uneven depression surrounded by abnormal mucosal conver-gency. These findings are easily demonstrated by double air contrast technique in roentgenography, and easily confirmed by endoscopy. But the shallower and smaller a lesion becomes, the more difficult to be identified the lesion is. Besides in such a case, the mucosal folds don't show frequently characteristics of peripheral thickening, narrowing and abruption. Gastroscopy frequently reveals only uneven or coarse mucosal patterns and spotty abnormality in colour of the mucosal surface. Up to date, these alterations have been confirmed to be cancer not only by roent-genography but also by endoscopy with the aid of biopsy.

Recently, dye spraying method was deviced as a subsidiary method in endoscopy for recognizing minute granular changes of the gastric mucosa. There are two ways of dye spraying method. The first is a contrast method. When we use an unabsorbed reagent such as indigocarmine, granular areal pattern is contrasted on the mucosal surface of the stomach by this blue dye. The diagnostic accuracy is compared be-tween conventional endoscopy and dye spraying method using indigocarmine, as shown in Table 7. With conventional endoscopy, 54 out of 69 cancerous lesions are cor-rectly diagnosed, 13 lesions are reported as doubtful and two small type II_c le-sions are missed. However, using the dye spraying method, 68 lesions are cor-rectly diagnosed and only one type II_b lesion remained doubtful. Thus, this meth-od is superior to routine endoscopy in diagnosing and detecting minute shallow or slightly elevated cancerous lesions. And also it is useful for delineating can-cerous circumference of minute depressions. Furthermore, with this method the de-veloping site of gastric cancer is recognized from the difference of areal pat-terns in the pyloric gland mucosa and the fundic one. Table 8 shows a comparison of the developing site and histological patterns of gastric cancer. It is notice-

TABLE 7   Comparison of Diagnosis by Routine and Dye Spraying Method

Diagnosis	Routine Method	Spraying Method
Cancer	54	68
Suspicious of cancer	13	1
Overlooked	2	

TABLE 8   Developing Site and Histological Patterns of Early Gastric Cancer

Hist. Pattern / Location	Well Diff. Adeno. Ca.	Poorly Diff. Adeno. Ca.	Undiff. Ca.	Total
pyloric zone	31 (52%)	14 (24%)	14 (24%)	59 (100%)
F-P border	1 (14%)	5 (72%)	1 (14%)	7 (100%)
fundic zone	−	−	3 (100%)	3 (100%)

able that all three cases found in the fundic zone, are of undifferentiated carcinoma, while in the pyloric zone, 45 out of 59 cases are of well or poorly differentiated adenocarcinomas. Undifferentiated carcinoma is observed only on 14 cases
in the pyloric zone.
The second type of dye spraying method is an absorptive dyeing, that is, a functional endoscopy. Using methylene blue as a sprayed dye, we can succeed in observing a staining of the gastric mucosa in vivo. Unlike the normal gastric mucosa, the intestinalized gastric mucosa can absorb methylene blue and is easily
stained blue. Its mucosal surface is very similar to that of the duodenal mucosa,
having intestinal villi. These strikingly interesting facts are useful for know-
ing the relation between histology and the developing site of cancer (Fig. 4).
As above mentioned, with these dye spraying methods, we can not only make an
easier and earlier diagnosis of gastric cancer, but also know the developing site
of cancer. However, in the beginning stage, type II_b, gastric cancer may be covered with the normal gastric epithelium. How can we diagnose such type II_b as
malignancy ? That is a problem awaiting solution.

Significance of Gastric Acid Secretion

From another point of view, when we estimate the gastric acid secretion stimulated
by tetragastrin, the secretory capacity is different acoording to the depth of
gastric cancer infiltration (Fig. 5). Namely, it is worthwhile that almost narmal

FIG. 4   Relationship between Intestinal Metaplasia and
          Histological Pattern of Gastric Cancer

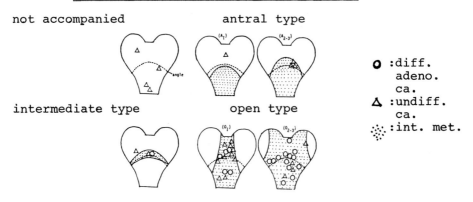

not accompanied   antral type

intermediate type   open type

O :diff.
  adeno.
  ca.
Δ :undiff.
  ca.
:int. met.

FIG. 5   Gastric Acid Secretion in Gastric Cancer
          (stimulated by AOC-tetrapeptide 4γ/kg)

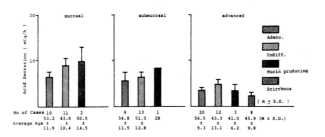

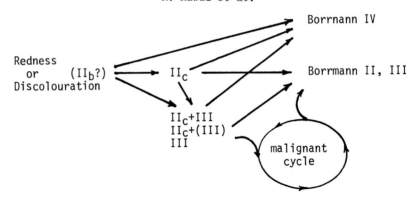

Fig. 6   Natural history of gastric cancer

gastric secretory capacity is preserved in many cases of early gastric cnacer. Further, it is an interesting fact that a protruded type of early gastric cancer has a low secretory capacity, while an ulcerating type including type II_b, the earliest stage of gastric cancer, has almost normal gastric secretory capacity.

Natural Course of Gastric Cancer

We cannot notice clinically the presence of gastric cancer in its initial stage until the mucosa overlying cancer cells is eroded or ulcerated to show some change in colour tint of the mucosa. We know almost nothing about the natural history of real type II_b, because the number of cancer of type II_b have been too small to analyse its clinical course. However, until now we happened to experience some cases of gastric cancer, mainly of depressed type, in which the change in the type of cancer could be observed endoscopically or radiologically from several months to a few years. They are summarized in Fig. 6. A cancer of type II_b takes over two years to grow into a cancer of type II_c or II_c+III which can be easily detected with conventional examinations. It may remain early cancer for several years independent of coincident peptic ulcer with it, and al last it invades into the proper muscle layer to grow into so-called advanced cancer. In some cases of type II_c+III or III, the coincident peptic ulcer with them repeats healing and relapsing (malignant cycle) to advance to Borrmann II or III. As a particular pattern, you can see in Fig. 6 that the change from type II_b to Borrmann type IV (scirrhus) takes comparing short time (average time of six cases is 19 months).

REFERENCES

1. Ida, K., Y. Kohli, K. Shimamoto, Y. Hashimoto and K. Kawai (1973). Endoscopical findings of fundic and pyloric gland area using dye scattering method. Endoscopy, 5, 21-26.
2. Ida, K., Y. Hashimoto, S. Takeda, K. Murakami and K. Kawai (1975). Endoscopic diagnosis of gastric cancer with dye scattering. Am. J. of Gastroent. 63, 316 -320.
3. Kawai, K., Y. Akasaka, F. Misaki, K. Murakami and M. Masuda (1970). Gastrofiber scopic biopsy on early gastric cancer. Endoscopy, 2, 82-87.
4. Kawai, K. (1971). Diagnosis of early gastric cancer. Endoscopy, 3, 23-27.
5. Kawai, K. (1971). Validity rate of concerned diagnosis using various methods. In T. Murakami (Ed.), Monograph on Cancer Research 11, University of Tokyo Press, Tokyo. pp. 273-282.
6. Kawai, K., Y. Akasaka and Y. Kohli (1973). Endoscopical approach to the "ma-

lignant change of benign gastric ulcer" from our follow-up studies.   <u>Endoscopy</u>, <u>5</u>, 53-60.

Gastric Cancer Mass Screening by Ear-puncture Tetracycline Test

Coordinating Group for Detection of Gastric Cancer by Tetracycline Tests, The People's Republic of China

ABSTRACT

The authors planned and carried out an ear-puncture tetracycline test (EPTT) based on tetracycline fluorescence for mass screening of gastric cancer. Of 446 cases of gastric carcinoma, 74.4% were positive. However, the positive rate became 79.5%, if cardiac carcinoma was excluded. In a mass survey of 57,164 persons, 22 cases of gastric carcinoma were found, among which 17 gave positive results in the test. Among them, 3 of 5 cases of early gastric carcinoma were positive. The positive rate for the general population was 1.1-3.4%. This test is simple, inexpensive and painless. It is practical for mass screening of gastric cancer. It may be of significance in the screening of "high risk population" in an endemic area.

METHOD

EPTT depends upon the affinity of tetracycline for cancer tissue. In a healthy subject, the concentration of tetracycline in the blood reaches its maximum 3 hours after oral administration of the drug, while in cancer patients, the blood tetracycline concentration is diminished, because tetracycline is taken up by cancer tissue.

Tetracycline is a fluorescent substance. It gives yellow-green fluorescence with the wave length 515-520 mμ under the excitation of ultraviolet light with the wave length 375-380 mμ. Thus its blood concentration can be measured by observing the intensity of fluorescence.

The examinee takes one tablet (250 mg) of tetracycline with 200 ml of water in the morning when fasting. Three hours later 50 μl of ear blood is taken with a glass capillary. One end is sealed up, centrifuged, and 20 μl of supernatant serum dropped on fluorescent detection paper and, after drying, compared with the known standards (1 μg/ml and o.5 μg/ml) in a dark room under 6W fluorescent light. The test is considered positive if the tetracycline level in the serum is equal to or less than 1 μg/ml in concentration, and negative if the level is above this concentration.

RESULTS

472 patients with malignant gastric tumors were studied. Most of
them had been diagnosed pathologically, and only a few by operation,
fiberscope or cytologic examination. The positive rate of EPTT was
79.5% for gastric carcinoma, 50% for cardiac carcinoma, and 74.4% for
both (Table 1). The positive rates for other malignant tumors was
as high as 88.5%.

EPTT gave some positive results on malignant tumors other than gastric carcinomas. As shown in Table 2, the positive rate for 11 kinds
of malignant tumors (108 cases) averaged only 38.8%.

TABLE 1   Positive Rates of Gastric Cancer

Classification of gastric cancers	Cases	Positive cases	Positive rate (%)
Gastric carcinoma in total	446***	332	74.4
Gastric carcinoma (excluding cardiac carc.)	370*	294	79.5**
Cardiac carcinoma	76	38	50.0**
Other gastric malignant tumor in total	26***	23	23/26(88.5)
Lymphosarcoma	10	10	10/10
Reticulocytic sarcoma	13	11	11/13
Leimyosarcoma	3	2	2/3

*Among 10 cases of early stage, 6 were positive.
**The difference between gastric carcinoma and cardiac carcinoma
  was statistically significant (P < 0.005 by χ^2 test).
***Of the 472 cases, 362 were tested by fluorescence method and 110
  cases by biological assay.

TABLE 2   Positive Rates of Malignant Tumors other than Gastric Carcinoma

Malignant tumors other than gastric carcinoma	Cases	Positive cases	Positive rate
In total	108	42	38.8%
Esophagus carcinoma	21	6	6/21
Colon and rectal carcinoma	7	2	2/7
Liver carcinoma	6	4	4/6
Nasopharynx carcinoma	2	2	2/2
Lung carcinoma	6	3	3/6
Malignant lymphoma	12	9	9/12
Thyroid carcinoma	5	0	0/5
Breast carcinoma	16	8	8/16
Cervix carcinoma	17	3	3/17
Vagina carcinoma	2	1	1/2
Other malignant tumors	14	4	4/14

*All the cases were diagnosed pathologically after operation.

This test also gave some positive results with benign gastric diseases (Table 3). They were as a rule quite low except in atrophic
gastritis with a striking false positive rate of 43%.

TABLE 3 Positive Rates among Benign Gastric Diseases

Benign gastric diseases	Cases	Positive cases	Positive rate
Gastric ulcer	6	2	2/6
Duodenal ulcer	3	0	0/3
Atrophic gastritis	21	9	9/21
Superficial gastritis	8	2	2/8
Chronic gastritis	2	0	0/2
Nearly normal*	3	1	1/3

*All cases except these three were diagnosed by biopsy with fiber-
scope.

To prevent missing the diagnosis, we use a 3-step or 4-step method
for screening (Figs. 1 and 2).

History and physical examination.

Laboratory exam. including EPTT.

Exfoliative cytologic exam. of stomach.

Gastrofiberscope and pathological exam.

Fig. 1. Sketch of 3-step method.

History and physical examination.

Laboratory exam. including EPTT.

Exfoliative cytologic exam. of stomach.

Gastrofiberscope and pathological exam.

Fig. 2. Sketch of 4-step method.

In a mass survey of 57,164 persons in some communes and factories
(rural and urban districts), 22,999 received EPTT, and in positive
cases the test was repeated seven days later. The results are as
Table 4.

In the mass survey, 22 cases of gastric carcinoma were detected, of
which 17 were positive in the test, thus giving a positive rate of
77.3%. Five of the 22 cases were in the early stage. Among them 3
cases were positive. Besides, there were five other cases of severe
atypical hyperplasia of stomach, and 3 of them were positive too.

During the mass survey in Tao-tsun Commune, one hundred more cases
were screened and given fiberscope. There was higher positive rate
in cases of severe intestinal metaplasia, atrophic gastritis, and
severe atypical hyperplasia (Table 5). It seems that tetracycline
test may be significant not only for discovering the precancerous

lesions of the stomach but also for screening "high risk population" in an endemic area.

TABLE 4   Positive Rates of Mass Screening

Type	Name of units	No. of examinees	Positive rate (%)	
			1st test	Repeated test
3-step	Peking Fur Factory	2,527	4.6	1.1
	Peking Medical Supplies Co.	987	3.8	1.4
	The Capital Steel Works	2,069	–	3.4
	Four Factories in Tientsin	1,867	15.1	3.2
	Nan-huang Commune	966	6.8	–
	Tao-tsun Commune	2,567	16.0	2.1
4-step	Tao-tsun Commune	3,331	16.0	6.7
	Kao-ling Commune	811	14.7	6.3
	Out-patients of Peking Oncology Institute	624	21.1	5.3

TABLE 5   Positive Rates of Tetracycline Test in Some Stomach Lesions

Lesions of stomach	No. of persons	No. of positive cases	Positive rate (%)
Atrophic gastritis	34	23	67.6
Severe atypical hyperplasia	5	3	60.0
Moderate " "	17	11	64.7
Severe intestinal metaplasia	21	16	76.2
Moderate " "	12	9	75.0
Mild " "	39	21	53.8
Gastric ulcer	6	1	16.7

Besides, in order to clarify the mechanism of EPTT detecting gastric cancer, we studied the postoperative specimen of the gastric cancer patient, who was given one tablet of tetracycline (250 mg) 3 hrs before operation. The post-operative specimen was observed in a dark room with common and fluorescent light. The results demonstrated that the distribution of the tetracycline fluorescence and the location of the cancer were nearly the same (Fig. 3).

We observed the mice implanted with fore-stomach squamous cell carcinoma in axillary region. with $7-^3H$-tetracycline and autoradiography. $7-^3H$-tetracycline was injected i.p. 30 µCi/mouse, and the tumor mass was removed after 48 hours. The tetracycline was distributed chiefly over the parakeratostic, low-viable cells in the epithelial pearls (Fig. 4).

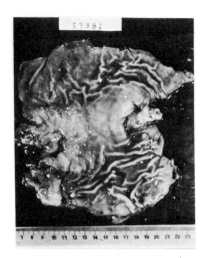 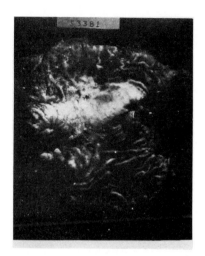

Fig. 3. Patient Luo, female, aged 55. Pathological
diagnosis: adenocarcinoma of gastric antrum.

Left: showing position of gastric cancer.

Right: (fluorescent photograph) showing position of distribution of tetracycline.

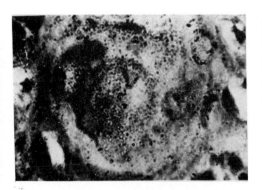 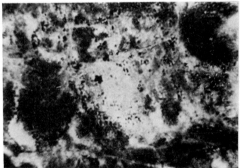

Fig. 4. Autoradiogram of distribution of ^{3}H-7-tetra-
cycline in fore-stomach squamous cell carcinoma of mice.

Developed silver grains distributed over parakeratostic cells.

The Role of Immunological Methods in the Diagnosis of Cancer of the Stomach*

E. D. Holyoke, T. M. Chu, H. O. Douglass, Jr. and M. H. Goldrosen

Roswell Park Memorial Institute, 666 Elm Street, Buffalo, New York 14263

ABSTRACT

Early diagnosis is possible using techniques brought to an advanced state of
efficiency by studies in Japan. However, with the prevalence of the disease in the
United States such a massive endoscopic program does not seem feasible. We need a
better method, a less troublesome method of early diagnosis. CEA and AFP, carcinoembryonic antigen and alphafetoprotein have not seemed useful. Other markers which
are discussed include Serum Basic Fetoprotein (BFP), Tissue Polypeptide Antigen (TPA)
Serum C_3DP) and Poly-L-lysine. It is suggested that some modification of the Leukocyte Adherence Inhibition (LAI) technique of assay may be useful.

INTRODUCTION

In most countries of the world at present the diagnosis of gastric cancer is
ordinarily made at such a late stage of disease than an overall five year survival
of 10 percent is the outlook. Part of the basic problem lies in the fact that early
symptoms may be quite vague. These may include "fullness", belching, heartburn, bad
taste, capricious appetite. These are, of course, similar to symptoms which occur
with benign or functional disease.

Recent progress in our diagnostic capability once we are suspicious of malignancy
has been considerable. Double-contrast radiography, and the use of careful coating
and air contrast techniques have improved x-ray diagnosis, although there is
difficulty with small but "eye-visible" tumors which will escape detection. (Sherman
1967) These minimal lesions include superficial erosions, carcinomas insitu, superficial spreading lesions and polypoid lesions of rugal size. Endoscopic capability
has been revolutionized by the development of the new all-flexible fiberoptic endoscopes. (Colcher 1974) By gross appearance alone, there is an 85 percent chance of
accuracy of decision between benign or malignant ulceration. Endoscopy and contrast
radiography, combined with multiple biopsy push the ability to make a diagnosis cor-
rectly above 98 percent. Cytology has also improved and is a useful technique although
because of its difficulty, complexity, and the cost in time of obtaining necessary
samples, it is not useful for general screening. (Kasugi 1968) Gastric secretion
analysis for acid output, basal and maximal, using pentagastrin or histamane has
limited discrimination. Severe hyposecretion does occur with benign ulcer. This
is also true for measurement of organic acids, B-glucuronidase and protein measurements in gastric juice.

+ Supported in part by U.S.P.H. Contract #N01-CM-43782

Other efforts and suggestions which have not found their way into wide use
include combined aspiration biopsy and angiography and ^{99m}Te scanning although we
expect both to be unsatisfactory particularly in small lesions.

IMMUNODIAGNOSIS

Carcinoembryonic Antigen

Carcinoembryonic Antigen was originally believed to be specific for colon cancer
tissue, but we now know that it is produced in a number of tumors. (Reynoso 1972)
At one point, it appeared that CEA might eventuate as useful in the diagnosis of
cancer of the stomach with a report that 73 percent of patients with distant
metastases were positive in one series. The work by Ravry et al. (1974) sums up
figures later borne out by more extensive comparative evaluation.

Table I

COMPARATIVE EVALUATION
CEA AND AFP IN GASTRIC CANCER*

Extent Gastric Cancer	Serum CEA and AFP		
	CEA > 2.5 ng/ml	AFP > 40 ng/ml	Both Elevated
Regional	1/8**	0/8	0/8
Distant Metastasis	37		
Liver	7/20	8/20	1/20
Other	2/17	4/17	0/17

* Ravry, J.N.C.I. 52, 1019, 1974
** Number Positive/Number Tested

CEA is greater than an accepted cut off level of 2.5 ng/ml in one of eight
individuals tested with regional disease when measured in plasma. This means
that CEA cannot ordinarily be expected to be of use in the diagnosis let alone
screening of gastric cancer. (Holyoke 1976)

For more widespread disease, CEA is still not useful. It is true that 9 of 37
patients with known metastatic disease show an elevated CEA, but this is a low
sensitivity. For non-hepatic metastases the detection rate using CEA is 2 of 17
patients which is certainly not above that found in a similar group of patients
with benign disease. Seven of 20 patients with hepatic metastases were positive
but this is a low number for any practical clinical use.

Alpha Feto Protein

This oncofetal antigen has also been studied by Ravry as can be seen in the
table. Actually, using radioimmunoassay to measure AFP, Ravry reported a greater
sensitivity to hepatic metastases than that for CEA. There were largely additive
and overall 54 percent of patients with metastatic gastric cancer demonstrated
either AFP, CEA or both to be elevated. This suggested to the authors that during
neoplastic formation in gastric cancer as in others, a number of tumor associated
antigens may be produced. This concept is supported by the earlier demonstration that CEA can be identified in primary gastric cancer and that CEA and AFP
can be identified in metastases from gastric cancer.

Interesting as these findings are, it is apparent that these two major oncofetal antigens even when assayed for in combination simply do not allow a sensitivity, let alone a specificity which will suggest they might be even useful for application as a diagnostic adjuvant in gastric cancer.

Table II

CEA IN BENIGN DISEASE

DISEASE	PERCENT POSITIVE CEA
Emphysema	57
Alcoholics	65
Ulcerative Colitis	31
Ileitis	40
Transplants	56
Pneumonia	46
Pancreatitis	53

After Galen, Hosp. Phys. 1976

Table II reports on a basic difficulty with this type of marker. (Galen 1976) The oncofetal antigens and to a greater extent the non-specific biochemical markers are severely limited because they represent only a quantiative change from normal and often are altered in the presence of any proliferative change.

BFP Assay

As reported by Ishii (1978), Serum Basic Fetoprotein is associated with stomach cancers as well as others. It is assayed by using radioimmunoassay, as with other "tumor associated" antigens false positives, i.e. >120 ng/ml occur in over 40 percent of patients with cirrhosis. Overall, 30 percent of individuals tested with gastric cancer are positive. Obviously, this is not a high enough number for screening. And when we consider marker level versus stage, we find that it is unfortunately only elevated in more advanced disease, disease so advanced that there is little opportunity for gain in therapeutic effect through diagnosis by marker.

Tissue Polypeptide Antigen (TPA)

We have anlayzed our patients with gastric cancer for serum TPA as described by Bjorklund (1976). In our hands, TPA is about as effective as CEA when considered as a possible diagnostic agent. There may actually be a slight superiority to TPA over CEA, but it is not marked.

Menendez-Botet (1975) reported on urinary TPA, since as was pointed out by Chu the relatively small molecular weight of this marker indicates that it might be possible to detect its elevation in urine, since it will filter. Twenty-three of thirty-one patients with gastric cancer had an elevated level of TPA in serum, and overall, 64 percent or 49/67 patients with a vareity of tumor demonstrated elevated TPA in urine, while for patients with benign disease, the rate was 24 percent or 7 of 29 patients. We would like to see this facet examined further.

Serum C3 DNA-Binding Protein (C3DP)

This is a portion derived from human complement component C3. Elevated levels of
C3DP have been found to be associated with a wide range of tumor types. (1977)
This fragment has been shown to be elevated in several patients in initial in-
vestigation in gastric cancer.

Summarizing the oncofetal and other marker proteins as they might be used for
evaluating patients with gastric cancer, three major aspects stand out. First,
we have identified several markers, many of which can be antigenic. Second,
all suffer as clinical tools in that they have too low a specificity or sensitivity to be of use, especially in screening, or even in diagnosis of gastric cancer.
Third, none has been identified in this group which has a marked shift towards
sensitivity or specificity for gastric cancer although somewhat different
spectra of frequency in serum for different neoplasma have been identified.

CANCER ASSOCIATED PROTEINS IN EFFUSION FLUIDS

One possible use of CEA as a diagnostic aid is in the presence of ascites fluid.
Booth (1977) has demonstrated that in patients with GI cancer including gastric
cancer, CEA in ascites fluids tends to be quite high compared to serum CEA
levels. The reverse is true for cirrhosis. We can see this in Figure 1.
This helps diagnose the problem of ascites, but it is of little benefit to the
overall problem of the diagnosis of gastric cancer.

Figure 1

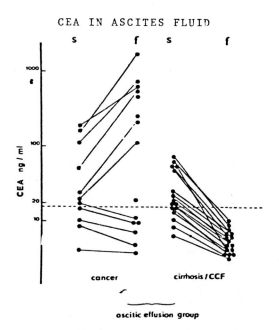

Fig. 1 *Serum (S) and effusion fluid (f) CEA*
After Booth, S.N. et al.: J. Clin.
Path. 30, 537, (1977)

Fetal Sulfoglycoprotein (FSA)

Hakkinen (1976) has described an antigen which is a fetal sulfoglycoprotein (FSA) and is found in gastric juice, using micro-ouchterlony assay. The marker is found regularly in gastric cancer cells, but not exclusively since mucosa cells with FSA can be found in non-cancerous areas. Apparently, FSA is a product of active secretion. The amount of FSA in a sample of gastric juice always exceeds the mucosal content. FSA is a regular component of fetal gut.

FSA In Gastric Cancer

In extensive screening of a population aged 40 to 70 years, Micro-Ouchterlony revealed 6-9 percent FSA positives up to 1974. The latest presentation of this data indicates that most of these are false positive values on further study. The problem as pointed out by Hakkinen is to determine when and how frequently FSA production starts in the gastric mucosa and what is the correlation to FSA positivity with the development of gastric malignancy. To date, as we stated, a positive group of 6-9 percent is found on screening. We would have to say that this assay which depends on passage of an N.G. tube, is although the most interesting immunodiagnostic modality we have discovered to date, still is of obvious limited usefulness primarily because of a "high" false positive rate.

LYMPHOCYTE RESPONSES TO HUMAN TUMOR ANTIGENS

Structuredness of the Cytoplasmic Matrix Test

Moore and Lajtha (1977) discussed the structuredness of the cytoplasmic matrix (SCM) Test. Takaku et al. (1977) reported on the possible use of this test in gastric cancer. They performed two preliminary studies, one involving gastric cancer and benign disease, as well as normal control individuals and one involving ten patients with early cancer that is with mucosal or submucosal penetration by tumor only. Essentially, the assay measured changes in cytoplasmic structure using spectrophotometric analysis. Lymphocytes from healthy donors and patients with non-malignant diseases responded to PHA stimulation with a decrease in SCM of 25 percent on the average. In contrast, patients with malignant disease demonstrated no change in SCM value or at least >5 percent change. On the other hand, lymphocytes from healthy donors and from benign disease patients did not respond to Cancer Basic Protein whereas there was a 20 percent decrease in SCM seen in patients with malignancy. Changes in the SCM response and of lymphocytes to CA BP and PHA are presented as the SCM response ratio RR SCM = P_{CaBP}/P_{PHA}. The RR_{SCM} values usually range from 1.06-1.55 for patients with benign disease and from 0.66 to 0.99 for patients with cancer. It is of interest that the highest value seen for gastric cancer "early" of the 10 tested was 0.91. Subsequent work by Cerek, however, in this area suggests some difficulty in repetition.

Poly-L-lysine Induced Agglutination Test

As described by Schottler et al. (1978) and others (Bauer et al.1977), the PAL, Poly-L-Lysine agglutination test may be of interest. Results are too early to say. They reported the detection through positive test of 10 of 12 gastric cancers. Ordinarily in a healthy population, a false positive is rare. However, as high as 25 percent positivity may occur in benign disease.

Other Lymphocyte Assays

These include lymphoproliferative tests in microculture to PHA, CON A, etc. Our
experience (Evans 1977) with patients with benign disease, let alone with normal
individual patterns particularly in studying this type of analysis as a possible
predictor for outcome in colon cancer indicates to us that usefulness is unlikely.
This type of assay might be of more significance using specific tumor antigens as
suggested by Dean (1976) for lung cancer. Leukocyte migration inhibition as
discussed by McCoy (1978) at the recent Washington Marker Conference may be tried.
As a matter of fact, several migration inhibition assays are available. All
suffer as biological tests and in our hands in a detailed study of colon cancer
were not useful for early Stage A or B diagnosis.

Dermal Antigen Testing

We will first consider non-specific antigen testing. We find no possibility for
detection of cancer of the stomach using non-specific recall antigens. These
skin tests are not depressed or altered until disease is advanced. Concannon
et al. (19) reported generally favorably on the Makri Dermal Antigen Assay.
But for gastrointestinal cancer other than colon cancer only 2 of 6 were
positive and for peptic ulcer 1 of 3. This would suggest that with the antigens
used in their studies at least, there is not much likelihood of a fruitful sceen-
ing or diagnosis program being developed using this assay.

The Search for Specificity

It is apparent that what is needed for gastric cancer is a technique, an assay
preferably of blood or urine which will allow early diagnosis. We need this
capability in the asymptomatic individuals or individual with very minimal
symptoms. Once symptomatology develops to the point where medical assistance is
sought, our success rate in diagnosis is quite high.

It may be that a specific TAA for gastric cancer can be identified and following
the lead of Hollinshead applied to gastric malignancy as it has been for lung,
this might be useful, but is speculation at the moment.

Leukocyte Adherence Inhibition Assay is our approach to the problem. We believe
the requirements for a useful assay for gastric cancer are quite stringent and
for a new attempt, an assay with far more specificity than those employed to
date is needed. In this assay, leukocyte adherence to a plastic surface is
measured in the presence or absence of tumor antigens prepared from tumor
membrane. We have studied patients with pancreatic tumor extensively with this
assay. Those with gastric cancer are now being studied.

The LAI Index as we record it as measures.

$$\frac{\text{Experimental Counts} - \text{Mean Control Counts}}{\text{Mean Control Count}}$$

Figure II presents our data to date. We wish to present this evidence that
relatively specific antigenic groups may exist for gastric cancer. It is in
the direction of trying to identify these antigens that we should go.

Figure 2

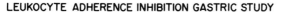

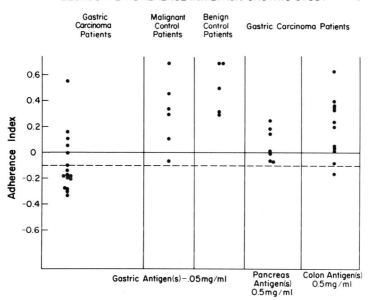

LEUKOCYTE ADHERENCE INHIBITION GASTRIC STUDY

After Goldrosen et al. In Press

CONCLUSION

We have come at this p oint in time to the following conclusions:

a. The problem in gastric cancer is really that, because we can diagnose more advanced established disease, we need a good screening method.

b. None of the non-specific glycoprotein and protein fragments are specific or sensitive enough, or at least have been demonstrated specific enough or sensitive enough to be of use in gastric cancer diagnosis.

c. Most lymphocyte assays of structure and function are probably non-specific and not sensitive enough to be of use either in screening diagnosis.

d. More effort must be made to identify specific antigens and then MIF assay or Hollingshead antigen testing may increase our sensitivity and specificity.

e. We present the LAI assav as evidence that there may indeed be such antigens and as our unit approach.

REFERENCES

Ax, W., Schottler, S. and Bauer, H.W. (1978). The PAL Test for Malignant Disease in Man. Brit. J. Can. 37. 319-321.

Bauer, H.W. and Ax, W. (1977) Detection of Sensitized Human Blood Lymphocytes by Agglutination with Basic Peptides. A Possible Test for Malignant Disease. Brit. J. Can. 36. 708-712.

Bjorklund, B. (1976). Tissue Polypeptide Antigen (TPA) in Cancer and Other Conditions. Onco-Developmental Gene Expression. Fishman W.H. Sell S. EDS. N.Y. Acad. Press. 501-508.

Booth, S.N., Lakin, G., Dykes, P.W., Burnett, D. and Bradwell, A.R.(1977). Cancer-Associated Proteins in Effusion Fluids. J. Clin. Path. 30. 537-540.

Colcher, H. (1974) Cancer of the Gastrointestinal Tract. c. Gastric Cancer Diagnosis, Diagnostic Fiberoptic Gastroscopy. J.A.M.A. 228. 891-892

Concannon, J.P., Blace, K.E., Brodmerkel, G.J., Zemel, R., Liebler, G.A., Nambrisan, P.T.N. Evaluation of the Makari Intra-dermal test in the Diagnosis of Cancer . Ann. NY Acad. Sci. 276, 97-105.

Dean, J.H., Jerrells, T.R., Cannon, G.B., Baumgardner, B., McCoy, J.L., Suslov, I., Herberman, R.B. (1978) Microculture Lymphocyte Proliferation (LP) Assay Using Autologous Lung Tumor Cell Preparations. N.C.I. Conference on Tumor Markers. In Press.

Evans, J.T., Goldrosen, M.H., Han, T., Minowada, J., Howell, J., Mittelman, A., Chu, T.M., Holyoke, E.D. (1977). Cell Mediated Immune Status of Colon Cancer Patients. Evaluation By Dermal Antigen Testing, Measurement of Lymphocyte Stimulation and Counts of Peripheral Blood Rosette-Forming Cells. Cancer 40. 2716-2725.

Galen, R.S. (Oct.1976). "What is Normal". Hosp. Physician 12 p. 22 only.

Hakkinen, I.P. (1976) The FSA Reaction in Early Detection of Gastric Cancer. Bostrom, H. et al. Almquist and Wiksell. Stockholm. 105-117.

Hollingshead, A.C. (1978). Specific Active Immunotherapy of Lung Cancer. Proc. XII Internation Congress (U.I.C.C.) In Press.

Holyoke, E.D. (1976) Cancer of the Stomach. The Aged and High Risk Surgical Patient. Seigel, J.H., and Chodoff, P.D. Grune and Stratton, Inc. 767-775.

Ishii, M. (1978). Serum Basic Protein. (BFP) National Cancer Institute Conference on Tumor Markers. (Sept. 1978) In Press.

Kasugi, T. (1968). Gastric Lavage Cytology and Biopsy for Early Gastric Cancer Under Direct Vision by the Fiber gastroscopy. GastroIntestinal Endoscopy 14. 205-208.

McCoy, J.L. (1978) Direct Capillary Tube Leukocyte Migration Inhibition. N.C.I. Conference on Tumor Markers. In Press.

Mendez-Botet, C.J., Schwartz, M.K. (1975) A Preliminary Evaluation of Tissue
(TPA) in Serum and/or Urine of Patients with Cancer. A Preliminary Evaluation.
Clin. Chem. 21. 985.

Moore, M. and Lajtha, L.G. (1974). Lymphocyte Responses to Human Tumor Antigens
Their Role in Cancer Diagnosis. Int. Rev. Exp. Pathol. 17. 97-142.

Parsons, R.G., Longmire, R.L., Hoch, S.O. and Hoch, J.A. (1977). A Clinical
Evaluation of Serum C3DP Levels in Individuals with Malignant Diseases. Can.
Res. 37. 692-695.

Ravry, M., McIntire, K.R., Moertel, C.G., Waldmann, T.A., Schutt, A.J., and Go,
V.L.W. (1974) Carcinoembryonic Antigen and Alpha-Fetoprotein in the Diagnosis
of Gastric and Colonic Cancer: A Comparative Clinical Evaluation. J.N.C.I.-
52. 1019-1021.

Reynoso, G., Chu, T.M., Holyoke, E.D., Cohen, E., Nemoto, T., Wang, J.J., Chuang,
J., Guinan, P. and Murphy, G.P. (1972). Carcinoembryonic Antigen in Patients
with Different Cancers. J.A.M.A. 220. 361-365.

Sherman, R.S. (1967). Roentgenologic Diagnosis of Genetic Tumors. Neoplasms
of the Stomach; J.B. Lippincott Co. EDS. NcNeer and Pack. 129-179.

Takaku, F. and Yamanaka, T., Hashimoto, Y. (1977) Usefulness of the SCM Test
in the Diagnosis of Gastric Cancer. Brit. J. Can. 36. 810-813.

Long Term Results of Surgical Treatment for Gastric Cancer

K. Kato

The 3rd Dept. of Surgery, Aichi Cancer Center Hospital,
Nagoya, Japan

ABSTRACT

Two thousand and two patients who underwent laparotomy for carcinoma of the stomach at the Aichi Cancer Center Hospital were studied. Of these 2002 patients, 1253 underwent curative gastrectomy. Twenty (1.5%) of the 1253 patients died within 30 days after operation. Excluding these 20 patients, the five-year survival rate for the patients undergoing curative gastrectomy was 64.1%, computed by the actuarial method without correction for age. In 368 patients (29.8 %), carcinoma involved the mucosa or submucosa but did not reach the muscularis propria. This type of lesion is termed an "Early Gastric Cancer". The five-year survival rate of 368 patients with early gastric cancer was 93.5%, reflecting the very favorable survival rate in this group. Thus, the surprisingly improved survival rate for patients with gastric cancer in recent times seems partly due to the high incidence of these early cancer cases among our patients. Three hundred and forty-eight patients underwent noncurative gastrectomy. One half of these 348 patients died within 1 year and five-year survival rate of them was 11.4%. One hundred and forty-one had a gastrojejunostomy, 30 a gastrostomy or jejunostomy and 230 an exploratory laparotomy. All but 1 of these patients who could not have a gastrectomy died within 2.5 years. A retrospective analysis of recurrence rates for the patients undergoing curative gastrectomy revealed some evidence of drug benefit in patients receiving Mitomycin C postoperatively as an adjuvant chemotherapy.

Keywords: Gastric Cancer, Surgery, Survival Rate, Curative Gastrectomy, Early Gastric Cancer, and Adjuvant Chemotherapy.

PREFACE

Gastric cancer in Japan accounts for about 40% of all malignancies, and about 20% of the male population over thirty years of age dies of gastric cancer in Japan. The most effective method of present treatment for gastric cancer is surgery. Therefore, it is important to improve surgical results for gastric cancer in order to further

lower the mortality rate of this disease. This paper presents surgical results of patients with gastric cancer with special reference
to prognoses of patients with early gastric cancer following gastrectomy.

MATERIALS AND METHODS

From January 1965 through December 1975, 2040 patients underwent
laparotomy for gastric cancer at the Aichi Cancer Center Hospital.
Of these 2040 patients, 38 were excluded for this study because of
unknown histopathological categories, unknown lymph node metastases
or having undergone polypectomy. Of the remaining 2002 patients in
this study, 1253 underwent a curative gastrectomy (total gastrectomy
202; partial gastrectomy, 1051). These 1253 patients had no distant
metastases and underwent gastrectomy along with removal of the regional lymph nodes. The lymph nodes which are removed in curative gastrectomy in our clinic are the perigastric nodes and the lymph nodes
located along the left gastric artery, celiac artery, common hepatic
artery, splenic artery and the hepatoduodenal ligament(Fig. 1).
Splenectomy and partial pancreatectomy are routinely performed with
total gastrectomy or proximal gastrectomy.

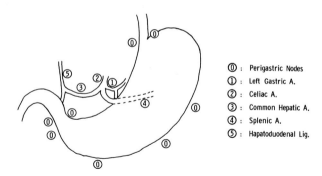

Fig. 1.   The lympn nodes removed with curative gastrectomy.

TABLE 1   Operatios for Gastric Cancer

Curative Gastrectomy	1253
Total Gastrectomy	202
Pattial Gastrectomy	1051
Noncurative Gastrectomy	348
Gastrojejunostomy	141
Gastrostomy or Jejunostomy	30
Exploratory Laparotomy	230
Total	2002
Excluded Cases	38

Three hundred and forty-eight underwent noncurative gastrectomy. Some of these 348 had a palliative gastrectomy and histopathological findings revealed the rest had tumor cells remaining after operation. One hundred and forty-one had a gastrojejunostomy, 30 a gastrostomy or jejunostomy, and 230 an exploratory laparotomy. All of the patients underwent follow-up observation.

RESULTS

Early Postoperative Deaths

Twenty(1.5%) of the 1253 patients who underwent curative gastrectomy died within 30 days after operation. Of these 20 patients, 9 succumbed to peritonitis, 3 to acute heart failure, 2 to acute renal shut-down, 2 to myocardial infarction, 2 to pneumonia, 1 to intestinal obstruction, and 1 died of an unknown cause.

TABLE 2   Early Postoperative Deaths in 1253 Patients
Undergoing Curative Gastrectomy

Peritonitis	9
Acute Heart Failure	3
Acute Renal Shut-down	2
Myocardial Infarction	2
Pneumonia	2
Intestinal Obstruction	1
Unknown Cause	1
Total	20

Survival Rate for Patients Undergoing Curative Gastrectomy

Excluding the 20 patients died within 30 days after operation, the five-year survival rate for the patients undergoing curative gastrectomy was 64.1% and ten-year survival rate was 54.2%, computed by

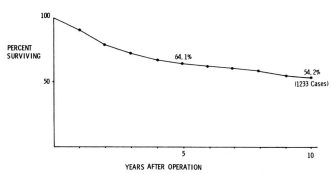

Fig. 2.   The survival curve for patients undergoing curative gastrectomy (excluded 20 deaths within 30 days of operation).

the actuarial method without correction for age. The survival curve
for the patients is shown in Fig. 2.

Five-year survival rates according to histopathological categories
for the patients are shown in Table 3. The distribution of the patients according to histopathological categories is also shown in
the same table. Cases (m) in which carcinoma was limited to the
mucosa were found in 132 patients, the survival rate was 94.3%.
Carcinoma involved the submucosa in 236 patients (sm) and the survival rate was 93.1%; the carcinoma reached the muscularis propria
in 212 cases (pm), and 76.2% survived; it attained the subserosa
in 24 cases (ss), and 72.7% survived; the carcinoma involved the
serosa, the tissues adjoining the stomach or a neighboring organ in
629 cases (s), and the survival rate was 42.9%.

TABLE 3   Five-year Survival Rates for Patients Undergoing
          Curative Gastrectomy
          (Excludes 20 deaths within 30 days of operation)

Histopathological Category	No. of Patients	5-year Survival
m	132	94.3%
sm	236	93.1%
pm	212	76.2%
ss	24	72.7%
s	629	42.9%
Total	1233	64.1%
m and sm ("Early Gastric Cancer")	368(29.8%)	93.5%

In 368 patients (29.8%), carcinoma involved the mucosa or submucosa
but did not reach the muscularis propria. This type of lesion is
termed an "Early Gastric Cancer". The five-year survival rate of
368 patients with early gastric cancer was 93.5%, reflecting the
very favorable survival rate in this group.

Deaths in Patients with Early Gastric Cancer

Unfortunately, a few patients with early gastric cancer died after
operation. In order to improve results in the surgical treatment
of gastric cancer, it is important to analyse the causes of death
with these patients. Until April 1977, 33 of 368 patients with
early gastric cancer had died later than 30 days postoperatively
(Table 4).Three of these 33 patients died of unknown causes and one
had another primary cancer, making it impossible to determine which
of the cancers caused her death. Twenty-three patients died of other
diseases, 6 of another cancer (sites of these 6 malignancies: 2 in
the liver, 1 in the lung, 1 in the maxillary, 1 in the stomach and
1 in the hypalarynx), 4 of liver cirrhosis, 3 of acute heart failure
3 of a cerebro-vascular accident, 2 of myocarcial infarction, 2 of
intestinal obstruction, 1 in a traffic accident, and 1 of pneumonia.
This distribution of the causes of death was not significantly different from that of the nation as a whole, as calculated from the
statistical table of causes of death in Japan In 1970.

TABLE 4   Causes of Death in Patients with Early Gastric Cancer

```
 5 : early postoperative deaths (within 30 days)
        3 : peritonitis
        1 : acute renal shut-down
        1 : myocardial infarction
33 : deaths later than 30 days
        3 : unknown cause
        1 : co-existing primary cancer
       23 : other diseases
                6 : other primary cancer
                4 : liver cirrhosis
                3 : acute heart failure
                3 : cerebro-vascular accident
                2 : myocardial infarction
                2 : intestinal obstruction
                1 : peritonitis
                1 : pneumonia
                1 : traffic accident
        6 : recurrent gastric cancer
```

Six of the 33 patients succumbed to recurrent gastric cancer. In 4 of the 6, there were hematogenous metastases of the liver, lung or bone; in 1 there were metastases attaining the lymph nodes and a local recurrence in the remaining patients. It seems to be natural for the hematogenous metastases to be more frequently the causes of recurrence in early gastric cancer than in more advanced gastric cancer in the pm, ss and s category (Table 5).

TABLE 5   Patients with Recurrent Tumor (Early Gastric Cancer)

Case	Histopath. Category	Lymph node Metastases	Survival Period	Form of Recurr.
55 yrs. M	sm	n+	1 yr. 11 mos.	hepatic meta.
56 yrs. M	sm	n-	1 yr. 9 mos.	hepatic meta.
55 yrs. M	sm	n-	6 yrs. 7 mos.	pulmonary meta.
56 yrs. M	m	n-	3 yrs. 1 mo.	bone meta.
50 yrs. M	sm	n+	2 yrs. 7 mos.	lympn node meta.
55 yrs.	sm	n-	5 yrs. 6 mos.	local recurr.

Survival Rates for Patients Undergoing Noncurative Gastrectomy

Three hundred and forty-eight patients underwent noncurative gastrectomy. Two hundred and eighty of them had hematogenous metastases peritoneal disseminations or distant lymph node metastases and had a palliative gastrectomy; 68 of the 348 were found by histopatholog to have tumor cells remaining postoperatively. The five-year survival rate of these patients, excluding the 6 who died within 30 days after operation, was 11.4%(Fig. 3).

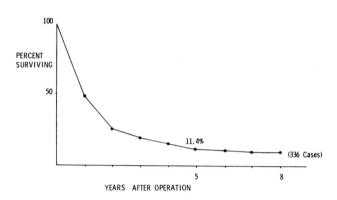

Fig. 3. The survival curve for patients undergoing noncurative gastrectomy (excluded 6 deaths within 30 days of operation).

Ten of the 348 patients were those with early gastric cancer. One of these 10 had distant lymph node metastases and died 17 months after operation. Another of the 10 had bone metastases and died 4 months after operation. Two of the 10 showed inadequate removal of the lymph nodes but are both still alive, a years and 11 months after operation and 2 years and 6 months after operation. The remaining 6 patients had tumor cells at the lines of resection, cause by inadequate resection of the distal or proximal margin. Of these 6 patients, one died of bile duct cancer, but no tumor was found in

TABLE 6   Patients with Early Gastric Cancer Undergoing Noncurative Gastrectomy

Reason Gastrectomy Noncurative	No. of Patients	Post-op. Course
distant lymph node metastases	1	died of recurr.
bone metastases	1	died of recurr.
inadequate removal of lymph nodes	2	both alive without recurr.
tumor cells at the lines of resection	6	1 : died of bile duct c 1 : died of pneumonia 4 : alive without recur

the stomach at autopsy; 1 died of pneumonia, 7 years and 7 months
after operation without evidence of recurrence; 4 were alive without evidence of recurrence as of April 1977.

Survival Rate for Patients without Gastrectomy

Four hundred and one patients were unable to undergo gastrectomy
because of much advanced tumors. In some of them, the tumor was attached to the neighbouring organ or to the retroperitoneal wall and
was unable to be resected. In the rest, abdominal carcinomatosis
was in high grade. Of these 401 patients, 141 had a gastrojejunostomy, 30 underwent gastrostomy or jejunostomy and 230 had an exploratory laparotomy. All of them died within 2 and one-half years.
The survival curve for the 401 is shown in Fig. 4.

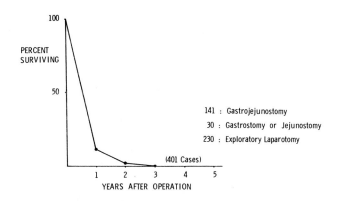

Fig. 4. Survival curve for patients without gastrectomy
(excluded 27 deaths within 30 days of operation).

Adjuvant Chemotherapy with MMC for Patients in "pm" Category

From January 1965 through December 1972, 148 patients with gastric
cancer in the pm category underwent curative gastrectomy. Excluding
the 2 patients who died within 30 days of operation, all of the remaining 146 patients were studied. Sixty-one of them were administered Mitomycin C (MMC) as an adjuvant chemotherapy. Most of the 61
were given MMC 0.08 mg/kg twice a week intravenously postoperatively
and ten times in total, so the total dose was 0.8 mg/kg. The remainder of the 61 were given MMC 0.4 mg/kg in the celiac artery and 0.1
mg/kg in the peritoneal cavity at the time of operation. The other
85 patients were administered no antitumor drugs. Of the 61 patients
undergoing adjuvant chemotherapy, 8(13.1%) died of recurrent tumor;
of the 85 not undergoing adjuvant chemotherapy, 17(20.0%) died of
recurrent tumor. This difference in recurrence rate between the
adjuvant and non-adjuvant groups is not statistically significant,
but it suggests a beneficial drug effect from the use of MMC as an
adjuvant chemotherapy.

TALBE 7   Patients with Gastric Cancer in the "pm" Category
          Undergoing Curative Gastrectomy (1965--1972)

	No. of Patients	No. of Patients Died of Recurrent Tumor
Adjuvant MMC*	61	8 (13.1%)
No Drugs	85	17 (20.0%)

* MMC 0.08 mg/kg i.v. 2/w x 10
  or MMC 0.4 mg/kg i.a. + MMC 0.1 mg/kg i.p.

COMMENT

The surprisingly improved survival rate for patients with gastric
cancer in recent times seems partly due to the high incidence (29.4
%) of these early cancer cases among our patients, thanks to the
recent progress in the diagnosis of gastric diseases. On the other
hand, the lower mortality observed in patients with early gastric
cancer suggests that gastrectomy with removal of the aforementioned
lymph nodes is indicated for treatment of gastric cancer. The distribution of the causes of death in patients with early gastric cancer
having curative gastrectomy was not significantly different from
that of the nation as a whole, as calculated from the statistical
table of death in Japan In 1970. This evidence seems that curative
gastrectomy with removal of the lymph nodes itself does not influence the mortality rate of other diseases following recovery from
operation.

None of the 6 patients with early gastric cancer having tumor cells
at the lines of resection died of recurrent tumor. These cases sug-

TABLE 7   Patients with Gastric Cancer Having Tumor
          Cells at the Lines of Resection

	No. of Patients	Post-operative Course
Early Gastric Cancer	6	4 : alive
		1 : died of pneumonia after 7 yrs. 7 mos. of op.
		1 : died of bile duct ca. after 1 yr. 8 mos. of op.
Advanced Gastric Cancer	62	10 : alive
		52 : died of recurr.
		(Median Survival Period: 17 Mos.

gest that early gastric cancer grows slowly and that it may result
in late apperance of signs of recurrence. In some cases no remaining

tumor cells may be found in the stump, in spite of the resected surgical specimen. An early gastric cancer patients with tumor cells at the lines of resection seldom dies shortly after operation and should not taken for a hopless prognosis. Patients with advanced gastric cancer are in quite a different category. During the past 11 years, 62 patients with advanced gastric cancer who underwent gastrectomy in our clinic were found to have tumor cells at the lines of resection. All but 6 died within 5 years and the median survival period are 17 months (Table 7).

In order to improve surgical results for gastric cancer, it is most effective to operate in the early stages. On the other hand, for the improvement of surgical results for gastric cancer in its advanced stages, I am quite interested in the application of adjuvant chemotherapy, using Mitomycin C (MMC). In patients with gastric cancer in the pm category, the incidence of hematogenous metastases is more than 50% among those showing evidence of a recurrence, and it is expected that the effectiveness of the adjuvant chemotherapy would be proved clearly. This is a retrospective study of adjuvant chemotherapy for gastric cancer in pm category. The difference in recurrence rate between the adjuvant and non-adjuvant groups is not statistically significant, but it suggests a beneficial drug effect from the use of MMC as an adjuvant chemotherapy.

CONCLUSIONS

1) The overall five-year survival rate for patients who underwent curative gastrectomy was 64.1%. This favorable result seems partly due to the fact that the incidence of early gastric cancer was 29.8 % of all operated cases, owing to recent progress in endoscopy and radiology in the diagnosis of gastric diseases as well as our mass survey campaign. 2) For patients with early gastric cancer, the mortality rate of other diseases after recovery from surgery was no different from people without gastric cancer. 3) In early gastric cancer, no evidence of recurrence has been observed so far in 6 patients who had cancer cells at the lines of resection. The reason for this finding is not clear. Early gastric cancer may behave in a benign fashion than advanced gastric cancer. 4) A retrospective analysis of recurrence rates for the patients with gastric cancer in the pm category undergoing curative gastrectomy revealed some drug benefit in the patients receiving Mitomycin C as an adjuvant chemotherapy.

REFERENCES

Imanaga, H. and H. Nakazato (1977). Results of surgery for gastric cancer and effect of adjuvant Mitomycin C on cancer recurrence. World J. Surg., 1, 213-221.
Japanese Reserch Society for Gastric Cancer (1973). The general rule for the gastric cancer study in surgery. Jap. J. Surg., 3, 61.
Kato, K., T. Kito, H. Nakazato, S. Miyaishi, and E. Yamada (1975). Gastric cancer: survival rates with special reference to "early gastric cancer". Nagoya J. med. Sci., 38, 35-42.
U. S. Public Health Service (1964). Computation of survival rates. National Cancer Institute Monogragh, 15, 381-385.

Yamada, E., H. Nakazato, A. Koike, K. Suzuki, K. Kato, and T. Kito
     (1974). Surgical results for early gastric cancer. J. Int.
     Surg., 59, 7-14.

Surgery and Intraoperative Irradiation for Gastric Cancer

T. Tobe*, Y. Hikasa*, K. Mori** and M. Abe***

*Department of Surgery, **Anesthesiology and ***Radiology
Kyoto University Medical School, Kyoto, Japan

ABSTRACT

In order to increase the cure rate of stomach cancer, we have developed "intraoperative radiotherapy" in which resectable lesions are
removed surgically and the remaining cancer nests sterilized by
irradiation with a single massive dose during laparotomy. In
cooperation with surgeons, radiogists and anesthesiologists, effective
doses of irradiation of 3,000-4,000 rads were administered in 88 cases
of advanced cancer. After resection of the stomach and removal of
regional lymph nodes and before gastrojejunostomy, the celiac axis is
irradiated in order to destroy regional microscopic metastasis which
cannot be removed surgically. The cure rate of 88 cases with intraoperative radiotherapy was analyzed. The irradiation field includes
celiac axis, its branches and about a half of pancreas. No serious
complications occurred except for an increase of serum amylase. These
results as well as experimental radiotherapy on canine pancreas were
discussed.

KEYWORDS

Stomach cancer, Surgery, Intraoperative radiotherapy, Technique,
Results, Complication

INTRODUCTION

During the period from January 1931 to December 1975, 3802 cases of
carcinoma of the stomach were operated on in the second surgical
department of Kyoto University.
During the same period there were 1195 cases of breast cancer and 678
of carcinoma of the rectum. Carcinoma of the stomach accounted for
50% of all malignant tumors.
The overall 5-year survival rate of breast cancer was 74.8% and that
of carcinoma of the rectum was 58.2% in our department. These results
are comparable to those of other institutions at home and abroad.
The 5-year survival rate of carcinoma of the stomach, however, is as
low as 26.6% because of the large number of advanced cases, such as
S_2 (invasion through the serosa) and/or N_2 (lymph metastasis along the

247

vessels of the celiac axis).
The problem for Japanese surgeons in cancer therapy is to increase
the cure rate in these patients with advanced gastric cancer.

INTRAOPERATIVE RADIOTHERAPY

Recent advances in diagnostic radiology and endoscopic technique have
led to more gastrectomies at an early stage and higher survival rates.
However, the percentage of cases of early gastric cancer in which
cancerous invasion is limited to the mucosa or submucosa is still
very small. In the large majority of patients the tumor has already
reached the muscularis propria and extends to or into the serosa with
perigastric lymph node metastasis.
For the treatment of these advanced gastric cancers, surgeons have
exerted much effort in performing larger, more extensive resections.
However, the 5-year survival rate of patients subjected to curative
operation is only about 40%. The main reason that the success of
gastric cancer surgery remains poor is that the incidence of metastasis to the lymph nodes along the left gastric and common hepatic
arteries and around the celiac axis is high, and complete elimination
of cancer cells around these blood vessels is hard to attain by surgical procedures.
Radiotherapy has not played a major role in the treatment of gastric
cancer, since adenocarcinoma is radioresistant and external irradiation to the gastric region causes intestinal damage. This damage is
often a serious limiting factor in the delivery of a complete course
of radiotherapy.
In order to overcome these limitations of surgery and radiotherapy,
we have developed "intraoperative radiotherapy" in which resectable
lesions are removed surgically and the remaining cancer nests are
sterilized by irradiation with a single massive dose during laparotomy.
These were reported in various reports (Abe 1975, 1976; Tobe 1976).

ITS PROCEDURE AND TECHNIQUE

Laparotomy is performed under general anesthesia. The duodenum is
mobilized by Kocher's manuever. Lymph nodes No. 13 (posterior
pancreatic), No. 12 (hepatoduodenal ligament), No. 14 (mesenteric
radix), No. 15 (middle colic artery) and No. 16 (periaortic) are
explored in succession.
If a metastasis is found in any of these lymph nodes or P(+) (peritoneal dissemination) and or H(+) (liver metastasis), intraoperative
radiotherapy is not indicated.
If no metastasis is found in these lymph node groups, subtotal
gastrectomy is performed with cleaning of the lymph nodes along the
vessels of the celiac axis.
Black silk sutures are placed in the duodenal stump and the celiac
axis as markers for radiotherapy. The abdomen is closed temporarily.
The patient is transfered to the radiation room on a stretcher
expecially designed by our department. (Fig. 1)
In the radiation room, the abdomen is opened and the treatment cone
tube is inserted into the abdomen.
The surgeon and the radiologist make sure of the radiation field.
This Fig. (Fig. 2) shows the pentagonal irradiation field after
subtotal gastrectomy with cleaning of the regional lymph nodes but
before gastrojejunostomy. It encompasses the lymph node groups
around the major blood vessels, such as the celiac axis and common
hepatic artery, and the pancreas which is often invaded when gastric

cancer penetrates through the serosa.
The Fig. 3 (Fig. 3) shows that the treatment cone is inserted into
the abdomen, at an angle of about 15°, so that the celiac axis is
sufficiently covered.
In this radiation therapy, radiation damage to normal structures is
minimized, since normal organs adjacent to the stomach can be shifted
from the field so that the lesion may be exposed directly to irradiation. Thus, a sufficient dose can be delivered to the lesions without
affecting the small intestine or liver.
The Fig. 4 (Fig. 4) shows the patient during intraoperative irradiation on the irradiating table after removal of the stomach.
The patient is anesthetized by inhalation of nitrous-oxide-oxygen-
halothane. Respiration is controlled with Bird's ventilators.
Optimal electron energy is selected according to the depth of the
lesion. Usually a level of 8 MeV electron energy is selected.
In intra-operative irradiation a concerocidal dose must be delivered
at one session. Out clinical results indicate that a dose ranging
from 3,000 - 3,500 rads is adequate.
The patient is observed by anesthesiologists in the control room on
closed curcuit television. The electrocardiogram is monitored
continuously on a heartscope and the adequency of ventilation is
monitored by the respiratory movement of the thorax.
The arterial blood pressure is monitored intermittently by the Riva-
Rocci method.
In order to deliver 3,500 rads, about 10 minutes are required. After
irradiation, retrocolic gastrojejunostomy is performed.

RESULTS

We call this procedure intraoperative irradiation or intraoperative
radiotherapy, and 88 patients with gastric carcinoma have been treated
with this procedure. These 88 patient can be divided into three
groups.
I.   patients with peritoneal or liver metastasis -- 14 cases
II.   patients who received non-curative surgery -- 15 cases
III.   patients who received curative surgery -- 59 cases
The mean survival time in group I was 6.2 months. Postmortem examinations revealed that a single dose of at least 4,000 rads is
necessary to eradicate the primary tumor, but 3,000 rads is sufficient
for lymph node metastasis. No serious complications were noted except
for a temporary increase in serum amylase, suggesting acute subclinical pancreatitis.
Of the 15 patients in group II, non-curative surgery.
Two patients have survived for more than 9 years and have returned to
work with no signs of recurrence.
In the case of Fig. 5 metastatic nodes were cleaned. The area of
invasion into the pancreas was not resected but was irradiated. This
patient is alive and well more than 9 years later. (Fig. 5)
In the case of Fig. 6 gastrectomy with cleaning of the lymph nodes
for advanced stage carcinoma was performed, but there was no resection
for invasion of the pancreas. This patient also is alive and well
more than 9 years after intraoperative radiotherapy. (Fig. 6)
Group III consists of 59 patients who received curative resection.
The patients who received intraoperative radiotherapy and survived
for more than 5 years were compared with those who received gastrectomy and surgical cleaning only. In all stages the irradiated group
showed better results than that which received surgery alone.

COMPLICATIONS

Electron beam irradiation has resulted in no serious complications.
The pancreas, however, is always situated in the field, and the
possibility of acute pancreatitis is always present. Trasirol 200,000
to 600,000 units/day is administered prophylactically for several
postoperative days.

As can be seen in Fig. 7 in some cases there was sudden rise of serum
amylase but no clinical manifestations of pancreatitis, and the serum
amylase returned to normal within a few days. This may be called
iatrogenic subclinical acute pancreatitis.

Leucocytosis is not marked.

We investigated the effect on the pancreas of a single massive dose of
irradiation.

Under general anesthesia, the abdomen of an adult mongrel dog was
opened and the pancreas irradiated with 2,000 to 8,000 rads in a
single massive electron beam. The pancreas was examined for more than
one year with electron microscopy, and no serious change was seen
after doses of 3,000 to 4,000 rads.

SUMMARY

In order to increase the cure rate of stomach cancer, we have developed "intraoperative radiotherapy" in which resectable lesions are
removed surgically and remaining cancer nests sterilized by irradiation with a single massive dose during laparotomy. With surgeons,
radiologists and anesthesiologists working in cooperation, effective
doses of irradiation of 3,000 - 4,000 rads were administered in 88
cases of gastric cancer.

The cure rate of 88 cases with intraoperative radiotherapy was
analyzed. The irradiated group showed a better cure rate in all
stages.

No serious complications occurred.

REFERENCES

Abe, M., Yabumoto, E., Takahashi, M., Tobe, T., and Mori, K. (1975).
  Intraoperative radiotherapy of gastric cancer. Cancer, 34,
  2034-2041.
Abe, M., Takahashi, M., Yabumoto, E., Onoyama, Y., Toritsuka, K.,
  Tobe, T., and Mori, K. (1976). Techniques, indications and results
  of intraoperative radiotherapy of advanced cancer. Radiology,
  116, 693-702.
Tobe, T., Kaneko, I., Hikasa, Y., Abe, M., and Mori, K. (1976).
  Surgery and intraoperative radiotherapy for gastric cancer.
  Cancer clinics, 22, 1074-1090.

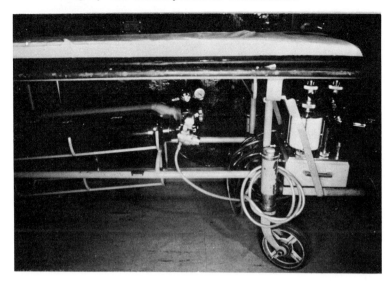

Fig. 1

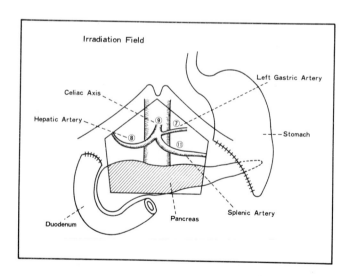

Fig. 2

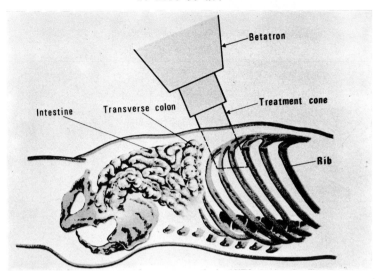

Fig. 3

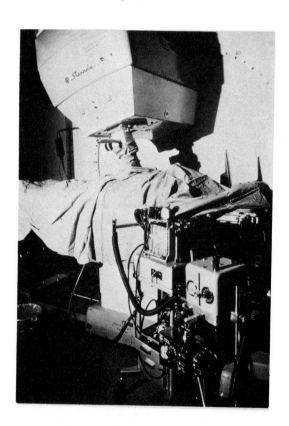

Fig. 4

Case 21   Y.N.   64Y. M

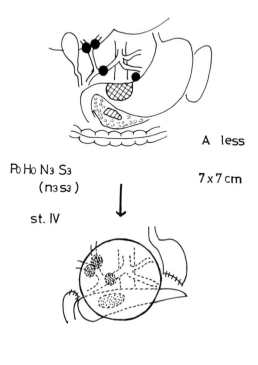

A less

P0 H0 N3 S3
   (n3 s3)

7 x 7 cm

st. IV

Fig. 5

Case 22   T. I.   64 Y.   M.

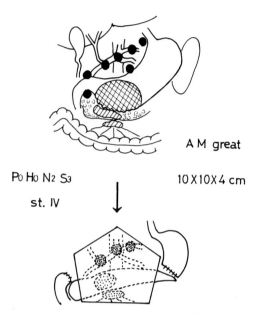

A M great

P0 H0 N2 S3

st. IV

10 X 10 X 4 cm

Fig. 6

Preventive Chemotherapy after Radical Operations in Stomach Cancer

Tadashi Kimura and Yoshiyuki Koyama

*National Medical Center Hospital (Ex-First National Hospital of Tokyo),
Tokyo, Japan*

ABSTRACT

Chemotherapy as an adjuvant to surgery was studied in 2516 cases of gastric carcinoma that had never undergone chemotherapy prior to these studies.   These cases
were collected from the Cooperative Research Unit of National Hospitals in
Japan.   The study was started on July 1, 1959, and consisted of six consecutive
studies.   Mitomycin C, thio-TEPA, cyclophosphamide, chromomycin A3 and 5-FU were
used.   For these controlled clinical trials, patients were randomised into chemotherapy groups and control groups using the Fisher-Yates' table of random numbers
and the envelope method, and calculation of the complete survival curves was
applied to these studies.   Significantly higher survival rates were observed in
the mitomycin C group of the third study, 5-FU group of the fifth study and in the
preoperative mitomycin C + postoperative 5-FU group of the sixth study.
Relatively higher survival was also obtained in the high dose of mitomycin C
group of the fourth study.

KEYWORDS

Adjuvant chemotherapy, gastric carcinoma, cooperative study, controlled clinical
trial, mitomycin C, 5-FU

INTRODUCTION

The Stomach Cancer Study Group of the Cancer Chemotherapy Cooperating Research Unit
of National Hospitals in Japan investigated therapeutic and side effects of chemotherapy as an adjuvant to surgery in stomach cancer.   The first study was started
on July 1, 1959, and continued to October 31, 1961; the second was carried out from
November 1, 1961, to December 31, 1963; the third was from January 1, 1964, to June
30, 1966; the fourth was from December 1, 1966, to March 31, 1969 (UICC 68-31(c));
the fifth was from June 1, 1969, to November 30, 1971, (UICC 69-23); the sixth was
from August 1, 1972, to March 31, 1975, (UICC 72-35); the seventh was from May 1,
1975, to June 30, 1978, and eighth is currently studying from July 1, 1978.
Nine National Hospitals participated in the first and in the second, further three
National Hospitals were added.   Another two National Hospitals were added in the
third study (total 14), eighteen National Hospitals participated in the fourth,
seventeen in the fifth, nineteen in the sixth, twenty in the seventh and eighth.
Therefore, these studies were carried out on a nationwide scale of cooperative
research (Fig. 1).

Fig. 1   Location of 22 National Hospitals on the Map of Japan

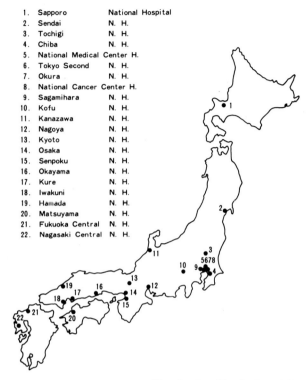

1. Sapporo   National Hospital
2. Sendai   N. H.
3. Tochigi   N. H.
4. Chiba   N. H.
5. National Medical Center H.
6. Tokyo Second   N. H.
7. Okura   N. H.
8. National Cancer Center H.
9. Sagamihara   N. H.
10. Kofu   N. H.
11. Kanazawa   N. H.
12. Nagoya   N. H.
13. Kyoto   N. H.
14. Osaka   N. H.
15. Senpoku   N. H.
16. Okayama   N. H.
17. Kure   N. H.
18. Iwakuni   N. H.
19. Hamada   N. H.
20. Matsuyama   N. H.
21. Fukuoka Central   N. H.
22. Nagasaki Central N. H.

Fig. 2. Age Distribution of Gastric Cancer Patients.

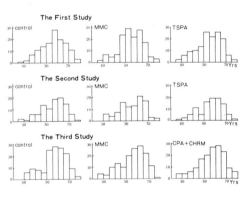

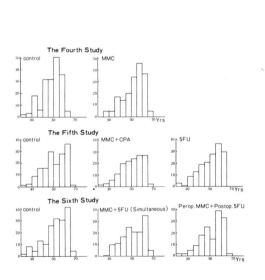

MATERIALS AND METHODS

At each hospital, patients participating in these program were histologically diagnosed as carcinoma. Only new cases that had never undergone chemotherapy were
selected, and randomized into chemotherapy groups and control group by using the
Fisher-Yates' table of random numbers and the envelope method.
The following chemotherapeutic   regimens were tried in six studies: (Table 1)
In the first study, 4 mg of mitomycin C (MMC) or 5 mg of thio-TEPA (TSPA) were
intraperitoneally administered during the operation. Then, daily doses of 0.08
mg/kg of body weight of MMC or 0.2 mg/kg of TSPA were intravenously administered
from the day of the operation, – the total dosage of MMC was more than 0.8 mg/kg
and TSPA was more than 1.0 mg/kg. (The average dosage of MMC was 1.0 mg/kg and
TSPA was 1.6 mg/kg.) This was the moderate dosage study.
In the second, the chemotherapeutic procedure was the same, except that the daily
dose of MMC and TSPA was reduced to one-half that used in the first study, and
the total dosage of MMC was 0.8 mg/kg and that of TSPA was 2.0 mg/kg. This was
a small dosage study.
In the third study, we devided two different chemotherapy groups. One was MMC-
group, another was cyclophosphamide (CPA) + chromomycin A3 (CHRM) group. In MMC-
group, 4 mg of MMC was given intraperitoneally during the operation, then 0.2 mg/
kg of MMC was intravenously given twice a week by the one shot method (totaling
0.8 mg/kg). In CPA + CHRM group, 200 mg of CPA was given intraperitoneally
during the operation, then mixture of 2.0 mg/kg of CPA and 0.01 mg/kg of CHRM were
intravenously administered every day for following 30 days (total dose was 60 mg/
kg of CPA and 0.3 mg/kg of CHRM). This was a large dosage study regarding MMC
treatment.
In the fourth study, 4 mg of MMC was intraperitoneally given during the operation.
Then 0.4 mg/kg of MMC was intravenously administered by the one shot method on
the day of surgery and 0.2 mg/kg of MMC was given on the following day, totaling
0.6 mg/kg. This was a push therapy study of MMC.
In the fifth study, we also used two different chemotherapy groups. One was MMC +
CPA group, another was 5-FU group. In MMC + CPA group 8 mg of MMC was intraperitoneally and 0.2 mg/kg of MMC was intravenously administered during the operation
and then 4 mg/kg of CPA was intravenously given daily for the following fifteen
days, totaling 60 mg/kg of CPA (combination therapy of MMC). In 5-FU group,
5 mg/kg of 5-FU was intravenously injected on the day of surgery and the following five days, and then 10 mg/kg of 5-FU was given every other day for four weeks,
totaling 150 mg/kg of 5-FU.
In the sixth study, there were two different chemotherapy groups. One was consist
of MMC and 5-FU which were simultaneously administered. Another was peroperative
MMC and postoperative 5-FU treatment group. In the former group, 4 mg of MMC was
intraperitoneally administered during the operation, then 0.12 mg/kg of MMC and
10 mg/kg of 5-FU were intravenously given twice a week for three weeks-totaling
0.72 mg/kg of MMC and 60 mg/kg of 5-FU. In peroperative MMC and postoperative
5-FU group, 0.2 mg/kg of MMC was intravenously injected on the day of surgery and
then 10 mg/kg of 5-FU was given every other day for following three weeks-totaling 0.2 mg/kg of MMC and 90 mg/kg of 5-FU.
In each study intravenous chemotherapies were started on the day of the operation.
A follow-up observation was conducted, as a rule, 3, 6, 9 and 12 months after
initiation of chemotherapy or surgery and cnce every six months for five years
thereafter, and then once a year for ten years. Each member of the study group,
using the designated forms, sent the following reports to the chairman concerned:
registration, treatment, follow-up, discontinuance and death reports, and reports
of cytological and histological diagnosis and autopsy. Evaluation on X-ray and
histological diagnosis and the overall evaluation were rendered by the respective
committees concerned, in all cases.

T. Kimura and Y. Koyama

Table 1 Method of Chemotherapy in Gastric Carcinoma

Study	Drug	During the operation (i.p.)	During and after surgery (i.v.)	
			Daily dosage	Total dosage
First (July 1959~ Oct. 1961)	MMC	4 mg	0.08 mg/kg daily	over 40 mg
	TSPA	5 mg	mg/kg daily	over 50 mg
	Control	–	–	–
Second (Nov. 1961~ Dec. 1963)	MMC	4 mg	0.04 mg/kg daily	0.8 mg/kg
	TSPA	5 mg	0.1 mg/kg daily	2.0 mg/kg
	Control	–	–	–
Third (Jan. 1964~ Jun. 1966)	MMC	4 mg	0.2 mg/kg twice a week	0.8 mg/kg
	CPA–CHRM	CPA 200 mg	CPA 2.0 mg/kg daily	60 mg/kg
			CHRM 0.01 mg/kg daily	0.3 mg/kg
	Control	–	–	–
Fourth (Dec. 1966~ Mar. 1969)	MMC	4 mg	0.4 mg/kg on the day of surgery	0.6 mg/kg
			0.2 mg/kg on the following day	
	Control	–	–	–
Fifth (Jan. 1969~ Nov. 1971)	MMC–CPA	MMC 8 mg	MMC 0.2 mg/kg on the day of surgery	0.2 mg/kg
			CPA 4 mg/kg daily	60 mg/kg
	5–FU		5 mg/kg daily, and 10 mg/kg every other day	150 mg/kg
	Control	–	–	–
Sixth (Aug. 1972~ Mar. 1975)	MMC–5–FU (Simul- taneous)	MMC 4 mg	MMC 0.12 mg/kg 5–FU 10 mg/kg twice a week simultaneously	0.72 mg/kg 60 mg/kg
	perop.MMC– postop.5–FU	–	MMC 0.2 mg/kg on the day of surgery 5–FU 10 mg/kg every other day	0.2 mg/kg 90 mg/kg
	Control	–	–	–

RESULTS OF THE STUDIES

In the first study, evaluable cases were 129 cases using MMC, 123 cases using
TSPA, 107 cases of the control making a total 359 cases. In the second 95 cases
of MMC, 95 cases of TSPA, 95 cases of the control, making a total of 285 cases.
In the third 141 cases using MMC, 155 cases using CPA with CHRM, 139 cases of the
control, a total of 435 cases. In the fourth study, there were 186 cases of MMC,
195 cases of the control, making a total of 381 cases. In the fifth study, there
were 191 cases of MMC-CPA, 195 cases of 5-FU and 210 cases of the control, 596
cases in total. In the sixth study, there were 144 cases of MMC-5-FU simultaneous
administration group, 145 cases of peroperative MMC and postoperative 5-FU therapy
group, 171 cases of the control, 460 cases in total. The age distribution of
patients in each treatment group was approximately the same in these six studies.
(Fig. 2).
Some results of from the first to fifth studies have been reported at the 8th, 9th,
10th and 11th International Cancer Congress. All cases were divided into four
groups, classified according to the stage of the disease by the Japanese Research
Society for Gastric Cancer (the 8th edition of the "General Rules for Gastric
Cancer Study" renewed in 1971), (Table 2), and curatively operated cases were also
classified by the degree of the differentiation of cancer: well differentiated
type, moderately differentiated type and poorly differentiated type, and degree
of the infiltrative tendency: sharply demarcated type, intermediate type and ill-
definited type.   Nearly all cases of stage Ⅳ, included in early five studies,
were relatively non-curative resection cases according to the Japanese General
Rules for Gastric Cancer. These are the cases with possible complete removal of
the cancer in the cases beyond the definition of the curative resection. For
example, cases has a few resectable disseminating metastasis to the adjacent peritoneum and resected completely are relatively non-curative operated cases. (Table
3). The relative survival rates were calculated and the statistically significant differences were presented only where there was 95% confidence. In this
report, five years follow-up study was completed in early five studies, but it was
not yet completed in the sixth study.
a. Results of curatively operated cases in the first, second, third, fourth,
fifth and sixth studies.
The survival rate of the MMC-group in the fourth study was higher than that of the
controlled group after five to ten years. The survivals among 5-FU-group of the
fifth study was higher after four to seven years, and also higher in peroperative
MMC + postoperative 5-FU group of the sixth study after two years. On the other
hand, survival rate of the chemotherapy groups of the first study and MMC-group
of the second study was low. But these were not statistically significant. (Fig.
3,4)
The longitudinal line in two, five and ten years of the figures shows the 95%
confidence limit.
b. Results in stage I, Ⅱ and Ⅲ
In stage I, survival rates of the controlled group were slightly higher in the
third, fourth and fifth studies, but these were not statistically significant.
In the stage Ⅱ, the survivals of the chemotherapy groups of the sixth study were
relatively high, but there were no differences in the first to fifth studies.
In the stage Ⅲ, a significantly high 5 year survival with 5-FU was obtained
among the 113 cases of the fifth study. (5 year survival rate of the 5-FU group
was 66% and that of the control was 35%) (Fig. 6) A relatively high one and two
year survival with MMC were observed in 51 cases of the first study, but there
were no differences between MMC-group and control thereafter. Five year survival
with MMC among the 91 cases of the fourth study was relatively higher than control,
and peroperative MMC + postoperative 5-FU group also had slightly high two year-
survival among the 128 cases of the sixth study. (Fig. 5,7)
c. Results of the cases classified by the degree of the differentiation of
cancer.

Table 2   Staging of Gastric Cancer

Items / Stage	Peritoneal metastasis	Liver metastasis	Lymph node metastasis	Degree of serosal metastasis
I	P_0	H_0	n_0	s_0
II	P_0	H_0	n_1, n_2	s_1
III	P_0	H_0	n_3	s_2
IV	more than P_1	more than H_1	n_4	s_3

P_0 No dissemination to peritoneum

P_1 Dissemination to adjacent peritoneum without distant metastasis

H_0 No liver metastasis

H_1 Metastasis limited to one of the liver lobes

n_0 No lymph node metastasis

n_1 Metastasis to lymph nodes of group 1

n_2 Metastasis to lymph nodes of group 2

n_3 Metastasis to lymph nodes of group 3

n_4 Metastasis to lymph nodes of group 4

s_0 No invasion to the serosa

s_1 Slight invasion to the serosa

s_2 Definite invasion to the serosa

s_3 Infiltrate to the other organ

From the General Rules for the Gastric Cancer Study in Surgery and Pathology (the 8th edition, 1971).

Table 3   Difinition of curative and relatively non-curative resection

Curative Resection

No metastasis to liver and peritoneum.

No cancer infiltration to the cut margin.

Complete removal of the gastric cancer and lymph nodes metastasis.

Relatively non-curative resection

The case with possible complete removal of the cancer, in the case beyond the definition of the curative resection.

(According to the General Rules of the Japanese Research Society for Gastric Cancer)

Fig. 3 **Relative Survival Rate of Gastric Carcinoma Chemotherapy as an Adjuvant to Surgery**

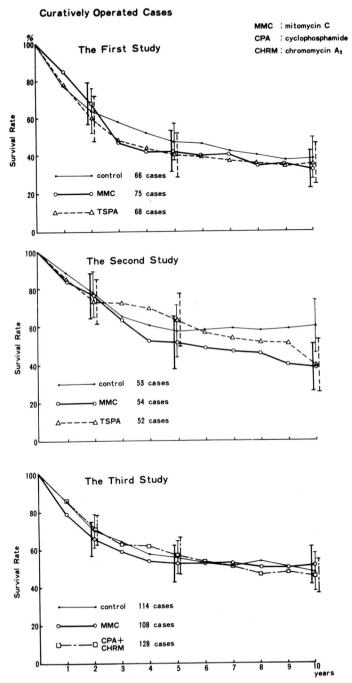

Curatively Operated Cases

MMC : mitomycin C
CPA : cyclophosphamide
CHRM : chromomycin A₃

The First Study

control 66 cases
MMC 75 cases
TSPA 68 cases

The Second Study

control 53 cases
MMC 54 cases
TSPA 52 cases

The Third Study

control 114 cases
MMC 108 cases
CPA+CHRM 128 cases

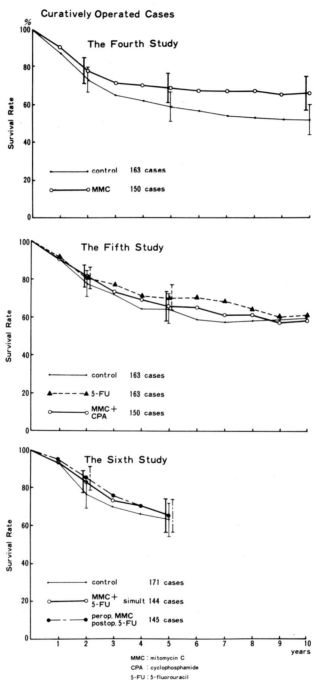

Fig. 4   Relative Survival Rate of Gastric Carcinoma
         Chemotherapy as an Adjuvant to Surgery

Curatively Operated Cases

The Fourth Study

control   163 cases
MMC   150 cases

The Fifth Study

control   163 cases
5-FU   163 cases
MMC+   150 cases
CPA

The Sixth Study

control   171 cases
MMC+   simult 144 cases
5-FU
perop. MMC   145 cases
postop. 5-FU

years

MMC : mitomycin C
CPA : cyclophosphamide
5-FU : 5-fluorouracil

Fig. 5 **Relative Survival Rate of Gastric Carcinoma Chemotherapy as an Adjuvant to Surgery**
Curatively Operated Cases

Classified by the Stage of the Disease

The Fourth Study

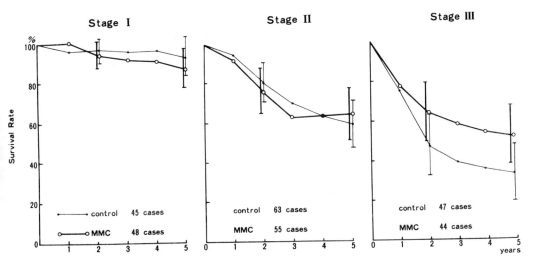

Fig. 6 **Relative Survival Rate of Gastric Carcinoma Chemotherapy as an Adjuvant to Surgery**
Curatively Operated Cases

Classified by the Stage of the Disease

The Fifth Study

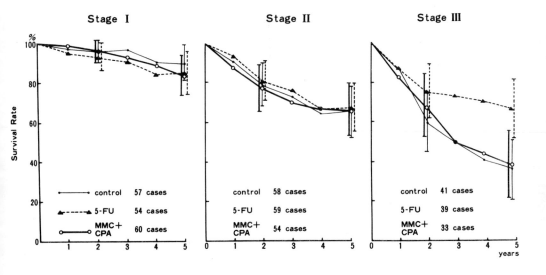

Fig. 7 **Relative Survival Rate of Gastric Carcinoma** Chemotherapy as an Adjuvant to Surgery
Curatively Operated Cases

Classified by the Stage of the Disease

The Sixth Study

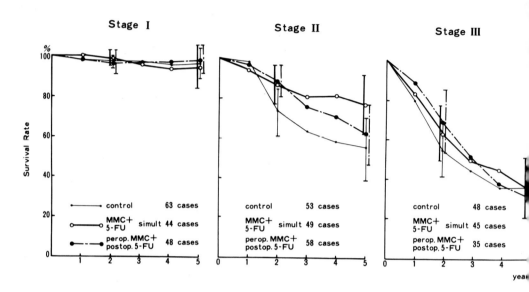

Fig. 8

Relative Survival Rate of Gastric Carcinoma
Chemotherapy as an Adjuvant to Surgery
Relatively non-curative Resection Cases
(According to the General Rules of the Japanese
Research Society for Gastric Cancer)

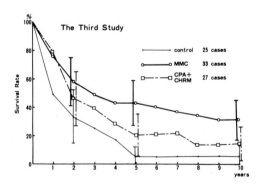
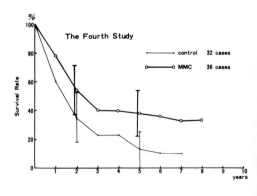

Cases of the well differentiated type were few.

In the moderately differentiated type, peroperative MMC + postoperative 5-FU group consist of 196 cases of the sixth study showed a significantly high survival rate after two years (two year survival rate of peroperative MMC + postoperative 5-FU group was 97%, and that of the control was 76%). Relatively high survival rate were observed in the TSPA-group in the second study, MMC-group in the third and fourth studies, as well as both chemotherapy groups of the fifth study and in the MMC + 5-FU simultaneously administered group of the sixth study.

In the poorly differentiated type, relatively high survival rate were observed in the MMC-group of the second and fourth study and also in the 5-FU group in the fifth study. On the other hand, survivals of the MMC-group of the third study was relatively low.

d. Results of the cases classified by the degree of infiltrative tendency.

In the sharply demarcated type, survival rate of the chemotherapy groups in the fifth study was lower than that of the controlled group.

In the intermediate type, the survival rates were relatively high in the MMC-group of the third and fourth studies, 5-FU-group and MMC + CPA group of the fifth study, and in the peroperative MMC + postoperative 5-FU group of the sixth study.

In the ill-definited type, the relatively high survival rates were obtained in the MMC-group of the first and fourth studies, and also in the 5-FU-group of the fifth study.

e. Results of the relatively non-curative resected cases in the first, second, third, fourth and fifth studies.

The MMC-group showed a significantly high survival rate in 85 cases of the third study. (5 year survival rate of the MMC-group was 33%, the CPA + CHRM-group was 20% and the control group was 4%) Relatively high survival rates were observed in the CPA + CHRM-group of the third study and the MMC-group of the fourth study. (Fig. 8)

In seventh and eighth studies, another combination chemotherapy regimen were under investigation (Table 4) and results are still pending.

SIDE EFFECTS

Leukopenia, thrombocytopenia, anemia, hemorrhagic diathesis, disturbance of liver function, albuminuria, loss of appetite, nausea, vomiting, diarrhea and epilation were studied for side effects. Table 5 shows the incidence of leukopenia, thrombocytopenia, disturbance of liver function and albuminuria. Leukopenia of less than 3,000 was found in 24.6% with MMC, and 18.3% with TSPA in the first study, in 24.7% with MMC, and in 25.8% with TSPA in the second, in 21.7% with MMC, and in 19.2% with CPA-CHRM in the third, in 32.0% with MMC in the fourth, in 36.3% with MMC-CPA in the fifth and 28.8% with MMC-5-FU simultaneously administered group in sixth study. These side effects were statistically significant ($P<0.05$). Thrombocytopenia of less than 50,000 was observed in 12.5% with MMC in the second study, this was also statistically significant. No significant differences were found in disturbance of liver functions and albuminuria among treated groups of these six studies. (Table 5)

Diarrhea was occurred in 16.3% with 5-FU and epilation was in 26.5% with MMC-CPA in the fifth study.

Cases in which chemotherapy was stopped because of leukopenia or thrombocytopenia were 6 out of 129 cases using MMC in the first study, 5 out of 95 using MMC and 7 out of 95 using TSPA in the second, and 2 out of 141 cases using MMC in the third, these were not significant. Chemotherapy was stopped because of leukopenia in 14 out of 191 cases with MMC-CPA in the fifth study. Cases in which chemotherapy was stopped because of nausea, vomiting or diarrhea were 23 out of 155 using CPA-CHRM in the third study and in 17 out of 192 cases with 5-FU in the fifth. They were statistically significant ($P<0.05$). (Table 5)

Table 4   **Method of Chemotherapy as an adjuvant to Surgery in Gastric Carcinoma**
            (Co-operative Study of National Hospitals)

Study	Drug	Dosage			Total dosage
		During the operation (i.p.)	During and after surgery		
			Daily dosage		
Seventh (May 1975~ Jun. 1978)	MMC+5-FU	MMC 4 mg	MMC 0.2 mg/kg on the day of surgery and 3 days after		0.4 mg/kg
			5-FU 10 mg/kg three times a week		90 mg/kg
	5-FU+CQ	—	5-FU 5 mg/kg		50 mg/kg
			CQ 0.04 mg/kg simultaneously twice a week		0.4 mg/kg
	control	—	—		—
Eighth (July 1978~)	ADM+ 5-FUds or FT	—	ADM 0.2 mg/kg daily three times 5-FUds 4 mg/kg or FT 12 mg/kg p.o. 8 weeks		0.6 mg/kg
	NCS+ 5-FUds or FT	NCS 4 mg	NCS 0.04 mg/kg daily 10 days 5-FUds 4 mg/kg or FT 12 mg/kg p.o. 8 weeks		0.4 mg/kg
	MMC+5-FU	MMC 4 mg	MMC 0.2 mg/kg on the day of surgery and 3 days after		0.4 mg/kg
			5-FU 10 mg/kg three times a week		90 mg/kg

MMC : mitomycin C   5-FU : 5-fluorouracil   CQ : carbazilquinone   ADM : adriamycin   NCS : neocarzinostatin
5-FUds : 5-FU dry syrup   FT : Ftrafur

Table 5   Side Effects of the Adjuvant Chemotherapy to
            Surgery in Gastric Carcinoma
            (The first, second, third, fourth, fifth and sixth studies)

Side effects	First study			Second study			Third study			Fourth study		Fifth study			Sixth study		
	Cont. %	MMC %	TSPA %	Cont. %	MMC %	TSPA %	Cont. %	MMC %	CPA-CHRM %	Cont. %	MMC %	Cont. %	MMC-CPA %	5-FU %	Cont. %	MMC-5-FU (simult.) %	Perop.MMC-Postop. 5-FU %
Leukopenia (less than 3,000)	2.6	24.6*	18.3*	4.4	24.7*	25.8*	1.6	21.7*	19.2*	2.9	32.0*	3.2	36.3*	8.2	3.5	28.8*	8.0
(less than 1,000)	0	1.5	0.8	0	1.1	1.1	0	0	0.7	0	0.6	0	1.4	0	0	0	0
Thrombocytopenia (less than 5x10⁴)	0	4.7	2.9	0	12.5*	8.8	0	7.9	1.5	0	3.9	0	0.8	1.4	0.7	5.7	1.5
(less than 3x10⁴)	0	1.9	0	0	5.0	2.5	0	4.0	0	0	0	0	0.8	0	0	1.4	0
Disturbance of liver function	15.8	17.3	11.7	18.6	10.8	9.4	4.0	4.9	4.9	5.0	6.7	3.3	4.9	7.1	3.0	10.6	5.4
Albuminuria	1.7	8.9	7.3	2.0	6.7	3.3	3.3	3.8	0.9	4.1	3.9	0.7	0	1.3	2.7	3.9	1.6
Cases in which chemotherapy was stopped because of side effects	0/107	6/129	0/123	0/95	5/95	7/95	0/139	2/141	23/155*	-/195	0/186	0/210	14/191*	17/195*	0/171	5/144	6/145

*P<0.05

SUMMARY AND CONCLUSION

Chemotherapy as an adjuvant to surgery was studied in 2516 cases of gastric carcinoma that had never undergone chemotherapy prior to these studies. These cases
were collected from the Cooperating Research Unit of National Hospitals in Japan.
The study was started on July 1, 1959, and consisted of six consecutive studies
which lasted from 26 months to 32 months. Mitomycin C, thio-TEPA, cyclophosphamide, chromomycin A3 and 5-FU were used as chemotherapeutics. For this controlled
clinical trials, patients were randomized and divided into different treatment
groups, and calculation of the complete survival curves was applied to these studies. From results of six studies, the following conclusion were obtained:
1. There were significant differences in the survival rates between the control
and the chemotherapy groups in the stage III of the 5-FU-group of the fifth study,
in the moderately differentiated type of the perop. MMC + postop. 5-FU group of
the sixth study, and in the relatively non-curative resected cases of the MMC-
group of the third study. Relatively high survival was also obtained in the high
dose of MMC-group of the fourth study.
2. In the stage I group, chemotherapy as an adjuvant to surgery may not be necessary, because it decreased in the survival rates in the third, fourth and fifth
studies.
3. Total doses of more than 0.6 mg/kg of MMC is necessary to obtain significant
differences in the survival rate between the control and the treated groups.
4. As for side effects,the incidence of thrombocytopenia was higher in the daily
administration of small dosage of MMC in the second study. The incidence of
leukopenia, less than 3,000 was higher in almost all chemotherapy groups, but no
significant difference was observed in the incidence of leukopenia, less than
1,000.
Further controlled clinical studies are necessary to determine the effects of a
long-term and multiple combined chemotherapy as an adjuvant to surgery of gastric
cancer, and we are studying these subject in the on-going projects.

REFERENCES

1) Ohara, T.: Chemotherapy of gastric cancer (1964), Acta Unio Internationalis
    Contra Cancrum, 20, 1.

2) Koyama, Y.: Experiences with chemotherapy as an adjuvant to surgery and radio-
    therapy (1967), UICC Monograph Series, Vol.10: Nineth International Cancer
    Congress, 209-220, Springer-Verlag, Berlin, Heidelberg, New York.

3) Koyama, Y., T. Ohara, T. Kimura and T. Ogura : Chemotherapy of Surgically
    treated cancer (1967), Vth International Congress of Chemotherapy, Vol. III,
    501-513, (B 11/8), Verlag der Wiener Medizinischen Akademie, Wien, Austria.

4) Japanese Research Society for Gastric Cancer: The general rules for the gastric
    cancer study in surgery and pathology , the 8th edition(1971), 4-25, 28-35,
    the 9th edition(1974), 4-25, 28-61, Kanehara Printing Co., Tokyo-Kyoto.

5) Koyama, Y., T. Kimura and Y. Takemasa : Chemotherapy as an adjuvant to surgery
    in stomach cancer (1970). Progress in Antimicrobial and Anticancer Chemothe-
    rapy, Vol.II , 242-249, University of Tokyo Press, Tokyo. Proceedings of the
    VI th International Congress of Chemotherapy.

6) Flamant R.: Controlled therapeutic Trials in Cancer (1972), UICC Technical
    Report Series, Vol.8, UICC, Geneva.

7) Koyama, Y.: Chemotherapy in operable and disseminated gastric cancer (1978).

Advances in Cancer Chemotherapy, H. Umezawa et al. (EDS.), 151–165, Japan Scientific Society Press, Tokyo/University Park Press, Baltimore.

8)   Koyama, Y.: The current status of chemotherapy for gastric cancer in Japan with special emphasis on mitomycin C (1978).   Recent Results in Cancer Research, S.K. Carter et al. (EDS.), Vol.63, 135–147, Springer-Verlag, Berlin, Heidelberg, New York.

Chemotherapy in the Management of Gastric Carcinoma

P. V. Woolley, J. S. Macdonald and P. S. Schein

Division of Medical Oncology, Vincent T. Lombardi Cancer Research Center
Georgetown University Medical Center, Washington, D.C. U.S.A.

ABSTRACT

Several cytotoxic drugs show definable activity in gastric carcinoma and the use of drug combinations produces improvement in the results achieved with single agents. The combination of 5-fluorouracil, adriamycin and mitomycin-C (FAM) has produced a 50% partial response rate in 36 patients treated at this institution. Median survival for responders was 13 months, compared to 2.5 months for non-responders. Toxicity consisted mainly of myelosuppression and was moderate. A second trial that substituted the 5-FU analogue Ftorafur for 5-FU produced substantial non-myelosuppressive toxicity without increasing the therapeutic benefit. Further trials are presently underway to investigate the use of nitrosoureas such as chlorozotocin in this combination.

Carcinoma of the stomach is an important cause of cancer mortality in the United States and in other areas of the world. While its incidence in the United States has declined in recent years, countries such as Japan and Chile show very high occurrence rates.

Recent evidence shows that gastric cancer is responsive to treatment with cytotoxic drugs. While experience is still limited, several trials have generated encouraging results. The individual agents of most importance are 5-fluorouracil, the lipid-soluble chloroethyl nitrosoureas such as BCNU and methyl CCNU, adriamycin and mitomycin C.

The fluorinated pyrimidines, particularly 5-FU, have been the mainstay of therapy for gastrointestinal carcinoma for 20 years. 5-Fluorouracil has been given in a variety of schedules, both orally and parenterally, but there is not a marked schedule dependence of this drug. The superiority of intravenous to oral 5-FU is clear, but weekly bolus injection, loading course therapy and continuous infusions do not produce substantial variations in response rates. In combination with other drugs, either weekly bolus or loading course 5-FU may be used with benefit. This subject has been well reviewed by Comis and Carter (1974).

The lipid-soluble nitrosoureas have definite single agent activity in gastric cancer. Moertel (1973) observed a response rate of 15% for BCNU and 29.5% for

5-FU in a randomized comparison of the two drugs. The average duration of response to BCNU was 4.7 months and that to 5-FU was 5.3 months. Combinations of 5-FU and BCNU or methyl CCNU have also been used successfully, with increased patient survival compared to treatment with single agents. Kovach (1974) reported a 41% response rate with the combination of 5-FU and BCNU as opposed to 29% for 5-FU alone and 17% for BCNU alone. BCNU as a single agent did not prolong survival in that study but both 5-FU and 5-FU plus BCNU did, yielding median survivals of 7.4 and 7.7 months, compared to 4.0 months for retrospective controls.

The Eastern Cooperative Oncology Group, has confirmed and extended the validity of these observations. Moertel (1976) reported a 4 arm study of methyl CCNU alone or with 5-FU, and either preceded or not preceded by an induction course of cyclophosphamide. The response rate to 5-FU plus methyl CCNU was 40% and superior to the other combinations. Methyl CCNU as a single agent was ineffective therapy. Cytoxan induction added only toxicity and actually detracted from the therapeutic efficacy of the other drugs.

Since 1975 the Division of Medical Oncology at Georgetown University has used either a combination of 5-fluorouracil, adriamycin and mitomycin C (FAM) or a modification of this regimen for the treatment of gastric cancer. The initial FAM combination is shown below (Macdonald, 1978):

	Week 1	2	3	4	5	6	7	8	9
5-Fluorouracil 600mg/m^2 IV x1	x	x			x	x			R
Adriamycin 30mg/m^2 IV x1	x				x				E P E
Mitomycin C 10mg/m^2 IV x1	x								A T

Over a period of 2 years, this regimen was used to treat 36 patients with advanced measurable gastric cancer. These included patients with large abdominal masses and with extensive metastatic liver disease. There was a partial response in 18/36 patients (50%), based on the reduction in size of measurable disease. Regression was observed in disease metastatic to the liver in 8 patients, as well as in local masses and nodal metastases. The median duration of remission was 9.5 months and median survival of responding patients was 13 months, while median survival of non-responding patients was 2.5 months.

Several variables may influence the response of the advanced cancer patient to chemotherapy. These include performance status, resectability of the primary tumor, and histologic grade of the malignancy. An analysis of these factors for this patient population revealed that there was no significant difference between responding and non-responding patients with respect to initial performance status. The median pretreatment performance status for responders was 1 but there were several who were either 3 or 4 and showed good response. There was not a preponderance of poor performance status patients among the non-responders.

Similarly the degree of histologic differentiation of the tumor did not correlate with either response to therapy or overall survival. Patients with poorly differentiated tumors showed as good response and survival as those with well differentiated tumors, and the responding and non-responding groups did not differ in their composition with respect to histologic grade of tumor.

The resectability of the primary tumor was also a factor of possible significance to prognosis. About half of these patients had had the primary respected and their distribution was balanced between responders and non-responders. The responding group did not contain an excess of patients with resected primaries.

The regimen was well tolerated and only moderate myelosuppression was observed. Median white count nadirs in partial responders was 2300 cells/mm3 and median platelet nadir was 75,000 cells/mm3.

This trial indicated a major responsiveness of gastric carcinoma to this combination of drugs. A second trial was then designed that incorporated the 5-FU analogue Ftorafur into the FAM combination in place of 5-FU (FAM II). Ftorafur consists of 5-FU conjugated to a furanyl ring and was originally synthesized in the Soviet Union. It is metabolized in the body to the parent compound 5-FU and thus acts as a slow release form of 5-FU. It has been shown in Phase I trials to be relatively non-myelosuppressive and can be given intravenously in doses up to 2.0g per day for 5 days (Valdivieso, 1976). The FAM II combination was given as follows (Woolley, 1978):

	Week	1	2	3	4	5	6	7	8	9	
Ftorafur 1.5g/m^2 IV daily x5		x				x					R E
Adriamycin 40mg/m^2 IV x1		x				x					P E
Mitomycin C 10mg/m^2 IV x1		x									A T

This combination was tested in 15 patients with advanced measurable gastric cancer. Responses were observed in 3 patients, all of whom lived in excess of 12 months. Progression was observed in 7 patients who had a median survival of 2.5 months. Hematologic toxicity was moderate in severity. The median white blood cell count nadir was 3500 cells/mm3 and the median platelet nadir was 187,000 cells/mm3. The treatment limiting toxicity was non-hematologic in the form of nausea, vomiting, dizziness and vertigo. These symptoms were most marked in an initial group of patients who received Ftorafur at a dose of 2.0 g/m^2/day. In subsequent patients the dose was lowered to 1.5 g/m^2. This produced fewer symptoms but was still associated with significant nausea and vomiting in about 50% of cases. Because of the toxicity, because of the inconvenience of administering the drug in 5 day courses, and most importantly because the FAM II combination failed to produce responses that were equivalent in either quantity or quality to those of FAM, the trial was terminated after 15 patients.

At the present time, the FAM combination appears to represent the most effective known therapy for advanced gastric cancer. Comparison of this regimen with methyl CCNU/5-FU and 5-FU/adriamycin/methyl CCNU is underway in cooperative group studies. Analysis of data from the Gastrointestinal Tumor Study Group indicates that FAM is superior to 5-FU/methyl CCNU. Further Phase II trials are underway at Georgetown. At the present this involves addition of a new chloroethyl nitrosourea, chlorozotocin, to the FAM combination. In conclusion, gastric cancer is responsive to therapy with combinations of cytotoxic agents and is a major target for clinical research today. Further improvements in response rate and survival should be sought using new combinations of agents.

REFERENCES

1) Comis, R.L. and S.K. Carter (1974). A Review of Chemotherapy in Gastric Cancer. Cancer 34:1576-1586.
2) Kovach, J.S., C.G. Moertel, A.J. Schutt, R.G. Hahn, and R.J. Reitemeier (1974). A Controlled Study of 1,3-bis-(2-chloroethyl)-1-nitrosourea and 5-Fluorouracil Therapy for Advanced Gastric and Pancreatic Cancer. Cancer 33:563-567
3) Macdonald, J.S., P.V. Woolley, T. Smythe, W. Ueno, D. Hoth and P.S. Schein (1978). 5-Fluorouracil, Adriamycin and Mitomycin-C (FAM) Combination

Chemotherapy in the Treatment of Advanced Gastric Cancer. _Cancer_ (In Press).

4) Moertel, C.G. (1973). Therapy of Advanced Gastrointestinal Cancer with the Nitrosoureas. _Cancer Chemother. Rep_. 4:27-34.

5) Moertel, C.G., J.A. Mittelman, R.F. Bakemeier, P. Engstrom and J. Hanley (1976). Sequential and Combination Chemotherapy of Advanced Gastric Cancer. _Cancer_ 38:678-682.

6) Valdivieso, M., G.P. Bodey, J.A. Gottlieb and E.J. Freireich (1976). Clinical Evaluation of Ftorafur (Pyrimidine-deoxyribose N1-2'-Furanidyl-5-Fluorouracil) _Canc. Res_. 36:1821-1824.

7) Woolley, P.V., J.S. Macdonald, T. Smythe, D.G. Haller, D.F. Hoth, S. Rosenoff and P.S. Schein (1978). A Phase II Trial of Ftorafur, Adriamycin and Mitomycin-C (FAM II) in Advanced Gastric Adenocarcinoma. _Cancer_ (Accepted)

Cancer of the Stomach—An Introduction to the Panel Discussion on Management

Toriola F. Solanke

Department of Surgery, University of Ibadan, Ibadan, Nigeria

ABSTRACT

Stomach cancer presents a singularly resistant challenge to medicine as 5 year survival rates have barely increased in 25 years and yet all measures of incidence show a decline in many but not all countries. The major problem confronting workers in the management of this disease is the control be it primary or secondary. The present status of the various treatment modalities is discussed and some areas of future research identified.

COMMENTS

Cancer of the stomach remains a common disease and the overall prognosis is bad. The absolute 5 year survival rate has been reported by various workers to range between 5 and 19 per cent (White et al, 1975). Brookes et al, (1965) for example, in a survey of 5441 cases in the Birmingham Regional Cancer Registry, found a total five-year survival of just under 5%. A quarter of the patients had had radical "curative" surgery, and their five-year survival was 15.6%. For the 16% of patients submitted to palliative operations the five-year survival fell to 1.4%; and survival dwindled to near zero for the remaining patients - over half the total - who were subjected to laparotomy only or to no surgical procedure whatsoever. Hawley et al (1970) in a study of 205 resections for cancer of the stomach, found a crude five-year survival of 19.4%; this fell to 11% in those patients with lymph node invasion, and no patient with resection for linitis plastica survived for more than two years after gastrectomy.

A contributory factor to the relatively lower 5-year survival rate in some institutions may be that the majority (over 80%) of the patients present with stages III or IV of the disease (TNM staging). The disease is often far advanced before histological diagnosis is made and subsequent therapy instituted because gastric cancer is associated with vague complaints and can be easily misdiagnosed. It has been reported in a large series of patients that 46 per cent (Svennevig and Nysted, 1976) had advanced disease at the time of their initial clinical examination.

Happily the incidence is falling particularly in highly endemic areas like Japan and the United States of America where it is still a leading cause of cancer death. A clear cut decrease is observed both in age specific morbidity and death rates. Detection rate of stomach cancer by mass screening is observed to have come down during the past 15 years. Relative frequency in autopsy statistics also came down. The available figures derived from cancer registry show that a major part of the decrease is due to the reduced morbidity rather than mortality.

Various methods of treating patients with carcinoma of the stomach have been utilized. These include gastrectomies ('curative' and non-curative) palliative surgical procedures, chemotherapy, radiotherapy and immunotherapy. A number of authors have reported that total gastrectomy carries a mortality rate of 8-37 per cent as compared with 7 to 17. 9 per cent for subtotal gastrectomy. Patients with incurable disease who underwent palliative subtotal gastrectomy had an average survival rate of 9. 5 months and compared with 4. 6 months for patients subjected to laparotomy alone. Other palliative surgical procedures for nutritional purposes such as gastroenterostomy, gastrostomy and jejunostomy have a relatively high mortality rate, do not significantly relieve symptoms, and therefore are doubtful therapeutic value for late stage gastric cancer. When the patient returns with further symptoms after radical resection of a gastric tumour the prognosis may seem very gloomy indeed, but this is not invariably so (Ellis and Jayasekara, 1975).

Once operability has been determined, the possibility of resectability must be ascertained. When all macroscopic disease cannot be excised by means of a curative operation resections should be conservative. Mere size of the tumour alone should not be contraindication to curative resection because some polypoid growths of gastric cancer can achieve massive size yet still be confined to the stomach and its immediately adjacent nodes (Cady 1968). The chief reasons for unresectability at operation are diffuse peritoneal seeding, ascites, direct extension into unresectable adjacent strictures and massive involvement of coeliac and other adjacent lymph nodes. Certainly if all macroscopic disease can be removed, radical surgery is selected with every attempt to preserve at least a small cuff of disease free-proximal stomach because of the marked decrease in operative mortality that results by using stomach rather than oesophagus for anastomosis.

Because 'cure' in gastric cancer is directly related to the size of the primary lesion and the number of lymph nodes involved, attempts to excise large masses of lymphatic tissue radically are of no benefit. Resection of stomach, duodenum, and oesophagus to insure liberal but not excessive disease free margins is far more important. The use of oesophagastrectomy for cancers of proximal stomach or cardia is becoming necessary as incidence of these lesions is increasing, both absolutely and relatively for reasons that are unclear. Here judgement as to course of treatment demands an extra measure of concern because of the infrequent cure rate and the high mortality rate. However, relief of dysphagia and obstruction is a worthwhile therapeutic goal and, if technically possible, should be attempted. There are several reports on the end results of early gastric carcinoma (Ikeguchi et al 1972, Fujii et al 1973) detected by mass survey in Japan expressed in the conventional 5 year survival rateswhich are usually over 95 per cent.

The chemotherapy of cancer was born when Faber (1948) first succeeded in producing remission in acute lymphoid leukaemia with aminopterin, the first on-costatic agent to be synthesized. For two decades chemotherapy gave disappointing results. Progress has however come from three directions (a) an increase in the number of drugs with an oncostatic action, at present there are more than 40 available, (b) improved operational use in the light of better understanding of the kinetics of cells and of pharmacology and (c) their administration to forms of cancer susceptible to their action and at periods when they are cyto-toxically effective (Mathé 1975).

Chemotherapy is a major weapon in the treatment of cancer. It is effective not only against leukaemias and haematologic malignancies but also against the majority of solid tumours. It is now apparent that gastric cancer is more responsive to cytotoxic drug therapy. Current trials fall into the categories of treatment of advanced disease, treatment of locally unresectable disease and the treatment of surgical adjuvant case. The role of chemotherapy in the management of early gastric cancer has still to be determined and compared with other modalities now in use. The practitioner can no longer neglect to consider the place due to chemotherapy and the results he may expect from it before he commences treatment.

There are three series of these compounds which are the focus of great interest at the present time. These are (a) the series of podophyllotoxin derivatives, which comprises of two agents 4 demethyl-epipodophyllotoxin-β-D thenylidene glucoside (VM26) and 4-demethyl epipodophyllotoxin β-D ethylidene glucoside (VP 16213) (b) the series of ellipticine derivatives 9 methoxy-ellipticine having proved its efficacy against certain myeloblastic proliferations and shown itself to be probably capable of crossing the blood-brain barrier, and (c) the nitro-sourea derivative drugs which are of great value because of their ability to cross the blood-brain barrier and their potent oncostatic effect, but handicapped by immunosoppresive and thrombo-cytotoxic properties.

Many studies have revealed (a) that the cytostatic agents do not all act at the same phases of the cycle (b) the phase or phases at which each of them acts and (c) that none of them acts on cells in G_0 phase gap which follows phase of DNA synthesis). Drugs with single activity in gastric cancer include 5 fluorouracil, BCNU, methyl CCNU, adriamycin, and mitomycin C. Beneficial effects of combination of these drugs have been reported by some workers.

The reasons why an attempt has been made to replace the continuous administration of small doses of anticancer agents by large intermittent doses are as follows:

(a) such a regimen allows the blood to regenerate during the intervals (the absence of the agent in the organism allows a compensatory proliferation without risk to the haemopoietic cells) and

(b) one and the same total dose of a compound has been observed in experiments to be more active when administered in one single injection than when spread over ten more.

It has been noticed that intermittent doses are much less frequently immuno-suppresive than continuous administration: which is explained by the fact that the lymphocytes, which are immunologically competent cells and in G_0 phase, enter the cycle to form immunoblasts only under the influence of an antigenic stimulus.

The experience of antibacterial antibiotics naturally led to the use of combinations of oncostatics. One such combination depends on the differing action of the various drugs at the different phases of the cell cycle and this led to the concept of recruitment by cellular synchronization. The second type of interaction is based on multiple and complex mechanisms which can be summarised under the concept of potentiation. The combination of two drugs may (a) result in the addition of their effects (b) result in their mutual inhibition (e.g. asparaginase and methotrexate) and (c) produce a result which is greatly superior to the addition of their effects. The effectiveness of chemotherapy is equivoval. Response rates of 15-29 per cent have been reported with a response duration of 4-5 months with a single agent chemotherapy. Combination chemotherapy has yielded only slightly better results.

Radiotherapy to the abdomen may offer some palliation to patients with carcinoma of the stomach. However, it is often unsuccessful because of the biological characteristics of carcinoma of stomach. The work of Moertel et al (1969) has been instrumental in developing new combined treatment programmes; although Moertel was able to demonstrate figures of improved duration and quality of life with combinations of 5 fluorouracil and supervoltage radiation therapy that were of statistical significance, yet dramatic clinical results were small and very few patients survived for long periods. At Hammersmith Hospital London workers have been interested in the palliative treatment of the advanced disease with fast neurons. In a series the mean survival was 5 months and the longest survival was 2 years. Many patients died from metastases. Neutron therapy may have a place in the palliative treatment of advanced gastric cancer. It may have a curative role combined with operation and/or chemotherapy in early cases especially when beams of higher energy and penetration become available.

Skipper's demonstration of the reasons for the failure of chemotherapy to eradicate tumours has fostered interest since 1962 in the direction to invoke the immune machinery. Immunotherapy and immuno-intervention are to intensify the immune reactions rejecting cancer cells and thus to increase the number of cells that these reactions can eradicate. The most potent form of immuno-intervention is obtained by the simultaneous administration of a specific stimulus (tumour cells which carry the same tumour antigens as the cancer to be treated and are treated by irradiation) and a non specific stimulus induced by a series of agents referred to as immunity adjuvants, the most efficacious being BCG. Of particular interest is the fact that BCG administered alone is effective after another therapy be it chemotherapeutic, radiotherapeutic, cell reductive, or surgical.

The major problem confronting workers in the management of gastric cancer is the control of the disease. Effective control is only possible if the biology of the disease is fully understood, and this is far from being so. Control can either be primary at the period prior to the onset of pathology and secondary during the presymptomatic period of the disease. At the moment, there appears to be no clear steps towards primary prevention apart from the elimination of known carcinogens from the diet and health education. The relative inaccessibility of the stomach to investigate procedures (like direct visual examination and biopsy, exfoliative cytology and chemical analysis) supports the notion that primary prevention will in the long run be more productive than secondary prevention which is based on a number of assumptions about the natural history or biology of the disease. The assumption that there is a progression of the disease with time presupposes that there are points in time when intervention would stop or delay the disease. Some of the assumptions are in themselves unscientific. It is generally assumed by most workers in the clinical areas of this disease that early intervention is more likely to prolong life. "Does earlier mean better?" The answer for stomach cancer could be "possibly".

It does appear that in the management of carcinoma of the stomach no single treatment modality is wholly effective against the disease and that consideration must be given to treating all categories of patients for the modest gains now achievable with the hope that newer drugs, and drug combinations will offer better results. Aggressive multimodality therapy is well worth considering even for the early cases. This audience will have to discuss and evaluate the development in experimental research, surgery, adjuvant therapy, radiotherapy and immunotherapy in the management of cancer of the stomach.

Brookes, V.S., Waterhouse,J.A.H.,and Powell,D.J.(1965).
Carcinoma of Stomach: a 10-year survey of results and of factors
affecting prognosis. Brit. med.J 1, 1577-1583.

Cady, B. (1968).
Complicated problems in cancer management. Surg. Clin.North
America 48 679-699.

Ellis, H. and Jayasekara, G. (1975).
Is 'second look surgery' justified in suspected recurrences of
Cancer of the Stomach   Bri.J. Surg.62 226-230.

Faber, S., Diamond, L.K., Mercer, R.D., Sylvester, R.F. and
Wolff, J.A. (1948). Temporary remission in acute leukaemia in
children produced by folic acid antagonist, 4 aminopteroyl-
glutamic acid (aminopterin). New Engl.J.Med.238, 787-793.

Fujii, A., Saito,T., Fuchigani,A., and Nishi,M. (1973)
End results of gastic carcinoma detected by gastric mass survey.
Japanese Journal of Cancer Clinics 19 852-858.

Hawley,P.R., Westerholm,P.,and Morson,B.C. (1970).
Pathology and prognosis of carcinoma of the stomach.
Br.J.Surg.57 877-883.

Ikeguchi,S., Matsuzawa,Y.,Arakawa,S., Mono,L.,Takamura,T.,Tsuda,H.,
Yasui,A., Sawada,Y., and Shida, S. (1977).
End results of gastric carcinoma detected by gastric mass survey.
Gastric Cancer 23, 57.

Mathe,G.,Kenis,Y. (1975).
La chimiotherapie des cancers: leucemies, hematosaromes et tumeurs
solides 3rd ed Expansion Scientifique Francaise Paris.

Skipper,H.E., and Schabel,F.M. (1962).
Experimental evaluation of potential anticancer agents, VII. Cross
resistance of alkylating agent-resistant neoplasms.
Cancer Chemother Rep. 22 1-22.

Stern,J.L.,Denman,S.,Elias,E.G.,Didolkar,M.,Holyoke,E.D., (1974).
Evaluation of palliative resection in advanced carcinoma of the
stomach. Surgery 77, 291-298.

Svennevig, Jan-L., and Nysted,A. (1976)
Carcinoma of the Stomach.
Acta Chir Scand 142, 78-81.

White,R.G.,Mackie,J.A.,Fitto,W.T. (1975).
An analysis of twenty years experience with operations for carcinoma
of the stomach. Ann. Surg. 181, 611-615.

Possibilities of Immunotherapy in Prevention of Recurrences and Metastases after Radical Surgery in Stomach Cancer *

E. Douglas Holyoke

Roswell Park Memorial Institute, 666 Elm Street, Buffalo, New York 14263

ABSTRACT

Animal and human studies which provide a basis for believing immune therapy possible are reviewed. Pertinent assays of immune function are briefly discussed. Pertinent observations concerning tumor antigens are reviewed. Active Non-Specific, Contact, Passive, Active Specific, and Active Transfer Immunotherapy are discussed. Possible avenues of study are suggested, and a look ahead to the type of second generation information needed for furtehr progress is undertaken.

INTRODUCTION

Survival for gastric caneer, as it is still encountered in most countries, is quite low. As Stated by Rubin (1974), perhaps 10 percent five year survival free of disease is an overall reasonable figure. An international study under the auspices of the International Federation of Surgical Colleges reported that at 12 months, only 4 percent of patients with non-resectable cancer were alive, similarly, 28 percent of patients with palliative resection and 49 percent of patients following radical resection still lived.

The first point to be made is that staging is of key importance. At present, we use the TNM Classification familiar as the American Joint Commission staging system. For the primary tumor, we consider depth of penetration and degree of spread. The basic evaluation of lymph node spread is essentially a consideration of the location, number, or multiple locations of lymph nodes. It is important to present precise staging data in all therapeutic trials. But it is particularly so in reporting immunotherapy studies because it appears that immunotherapy may have its best prospects for success in adjuvant treatment and in proper combination with other therapy. (McKhann and Gunnarson 1974) Since variation in survival may be greater in a chemotherapy treated group of patients, and since immunotherapy effect may be small or added to drug effect, we must be accurate in defining our treated populations.

* Supported in part by U.S.P.H., N.C.I. Contract N01-CM-43782

279

Other parameters which in our experience and that of many others bear on survival are the location of the primary and the histologic type of tumor, (Lewin 1960) and (Lauren 1965) In addition, Hawley (1970) has reported that plasma cell infiltration may be prognostic. This may indicate a need to look at the potential for immunotherapy in gastric cancer, but it also is another possible staging parameter. There is also the need to evaluate lymph nodes histologically for the presence of tumor as shown by Cantrell (1971). Similar findings have been reported for other diseases as breast or melanoma, and the point is that a surgical report of involved nodes will not do, sans histological confirmation, in staging. Furthermore, one occasionally hears claims for success in treating gastric cancer with large nodes left behind. Without histologic diagnosis, these reports are not helpful.

THE BASIS FOR POSSIBLE IMMUNOTHERAPY

In animal studies, tumor antigens, that is, antigens available for immunologic recognition in tumor cells but not found in analogous normal cells, have been demonstrated. As early as 1943, Gross demonstrated that partially syngeneic mice which had been immunized with a chemically induced sarcoma were resistant to the subsequent subcutaneous transplantation of the same tumor. Foley (1953) using syngeneic mice demonstrated that immunization against a fully syngeneic methochloanthrene-induced fibrosarcoma produced resistance against further grafting of the same tumor. Prehn and Main (1957) also contributed evidence for tumor antigenicity. Chemical carcinogen induced tumors have been shown to have individual specific (tumor unique antigens) antigens. (Baldwin 1978) Common antigens have been demonstrated between some of these tumors. (Herberman 1977) Some of these are embryonic antigens reexpressed in "dedifferentiated" tumor cells. In some tumor models individual specific antigens have been related to host control, mainly through cell mediated immunity, and a variety of immunotherapy approaches have been successful in these models. (de Landazuri et al. 1974)

Several neoantigens have also been described for virus induced tumors. In general, these are related to the inducing viruses. (Aoki 1973) These may relate to the virus envelope or to the virus genome. Burkitts lymphoma virus induced tumors may also express embryonic antigens. Individual specific antigens may also occur in these tumors. De Landazuri et al. (1974) also reported evidence that antibody dependent cell mediated cytotoxicity is a major method of host control for these tumors. Virus induced animal tumors can be prevented by vaccination with virus. (Hersh et al. 1973)

STUDIES IN MAN

As reviewed by Everson and Cole (1966) occasional "spontaneous" regression of tumor is seen in man. This is a very rare event, but it is finite. Perhaps the best documented patients occur with melanoma. Southam et al. (1973) demonstrated that the transplantability of tumor cells in man could be altered by patient lymphocytes or serum. Hughes (1966) studied in vivo delayed hypersensitivity to tumor extract in man. About a third of patients demonstrated a positive delayed reaction to such extracts. It was necessary to use control extracts to be sure a tumor response was seen. It is interesting and sobering that Hughes (1970) later demonstrated an instance where delayed tumor recurrence indicated a different immunogenicity to that of melanoma tumors occurring early. Oren and Herberman (1971) studied patients with lymphomas, leukemias, and carcinomas. Positive delayed hypersensitivity reactions to autochthonous cell membrane extracts were found in 50 percent of non-anergic patients. Some normals did produce non-specific response. With purification, Hollinshead et

al. (1972) obtained a fraction from tumor tissue which gave positive skin reactions in 16 of 18 patients with colon cancer. None was positive when antigen was
obtained from adjacent normal tissue.

These in vivo efforts to demonstrate tumor immunogenicity in man have been
supplemented by numerous techniques to demonstrate this immunogenicity in man in
vitro. The methods used which we will not elaborate here include fluorescent
antibody studies used in several modifications to demonstrate serum antibodies
against melanoma, sarcoma, and leukemia cells. (Eilber and Morton 1970) (Morton
et al. 1969) The latter found that families and social contacts of patients
with osteogenic sarcoma demonstrated an increased presence of antibody over unrelated controls. Other in vitro assays which have been studied include Macro-
phage Inhibition, Lymphoblastogenesis Assay, and Cytotoxicity Assay among
others. (Hersh and Oppenheim 1967) (Mavligit et al. 1974) Herberman et al.
1975) All of these methods have been used to detect changes in host immune
response in the presence of tumor in man. Many of the changes described, however, are suppressive and develop late after tumor is well established which
may not help our prospects for immune therapy. But from these studies, comple-
menting ongoing animal studies has come a great deal of information concerning
what we now know to be a very complex response, cellular and humoral, which is
the immune response in man. In particular, the demonstration of "serum blocking"
has been of significance. (Hellstrom et al. 1973)

TUMOR ANTIGENS

In recent years a search for tumor antigens in man has indicated many different
tumor associated antigens. (Gold and Freedman 1965) Thus, many human tumors
may have relatively specific antigens (Banwo 1974) Unfortunately, for our
purposes, many of these are carcinoembryonic antigens which may imply a priori
a limited usefulness in developing immunotherapy. But they are present nevertheless and further search should be encouraged. Table I presents a partial list
of these antigens.

Table I :   CARCINOEMBRYONIC ANTIGEN AND COMPARABLE SUBSTANCES
                              IN THE
                     DIAGNOSIS OF HUMAN CANCER

                         TUMOR MARKERS

        Carcinoembryonic Antigen   CEA
        Alpha Fetoprotein   AFP
        Tissue Peptide Antigen   TPA
        Serum Basic Fetoprotein   BFP
        Serum Alpha Subunit αCG
        Serum Chorionic Gonadotrophin   CG
        Serum C^3 DNA-binding Protein   C3DP
        Thomsen-Friedenreich Specific Substances   T
        Serum B_2-Microglobulin
        Human Sarcoma Antigens $S_1 S_2 S_3$

IMMUNOTHERAPY

For discussion, we will consider five main categories of immunotherapeutic approach.

Active Non-Specific Therapy. This attempts to boost the general immunocompetance of the patients; either the cell mediated, humoral immunity or the reticulo-endothelial system, or all three. The most extensive experience to date is with BCG. (Eilber et al. 1976) (McKneally et al. 1976) As we all know, this is an attenuated form of tuberculosis organism. In animal models where BCG treatment is successful, we have found that many factors play a role; these include viable BCG count, innoculation of BCG directly into tumor, or within the area of regional node drainage, tumor mass, animal immunocompetance, dose, genetic strain of animal, and the method of preparing BCG. (Zbar et al. 1972) (Baldwin and Pimm 1973) (Hanna et al. 1973)

Table II   TIME OF ADMINISTRATION OF BCG AND TUMOR TAKE

AGENT	-7D	PROTOCOL OD	+7D	MST	T241 Sign.	N	MST	B16 Sign.	N
BCG	BCG	Tumor -	--	51.6	p<.01	5	45.2	N.S.	5
	--	Tumor-BCG	--	22.8	N.S.*	4	24.6	N.S.	5
	--	Tumor	BCG	41.2	p<.01	5	30.3	N.S.	4
Control	--	Tumor-HBSS	--	28.0	-	5	28.2	-	5
C.Parvum	CP	Tumor -	--	36.8	N.S.	4	38.2	N.S.	5
	--	Tumor-C.P	--	29.0	N.S.	5	32.6	N.S.	5
	--	Tumor -	C.P	29.4	N.S.	5	34.0	N.S.	4
Control	--	Tumor-HBSS	--	28.0	-	5	28.2	-	5
MER	MER (14 d)	Tumor -	--	26.6	p<.01	7	39.5	N.S.	7
	MER	Tumor -	--	14.6	N.S.	6	37.8	N.S.	6
		Tumor-MER	--	15.5	N.S.	6	34.6	N.S.	6
		Tumor -	MER	20.5	N.S.	6	41.0	N.S.	6
Control	--	Tumor -	--	16.8	-	6	39.0	-	7

*Very close to significance T=15, Need T<11:showing trend toward Enhancement

To illustrate a potential problem inherent in this method which we encountered in the laboratory in a study we carried out after talking with Baldwin, see Table II above. These brief studies were done in mice with the Lewis T-24 sarcoma and the B-16 melanoma. The BCG used was Cannaught, C-Parvum was from Burroughs Wellcome. BCG was administered i.v. 1.0 mg in 0.1 ml of water. C-Parvum was given 0.4 mg CP in 0.1 ml saline i.v., MER was given i.v. in 0.1 ml, 0.5 mg per dose. Mean mouse survival time after tumor injection was recorded in days. Tumor cell suspensions were injected intravenously on day 0. There was no significant effect on B-16 melanoma. However, BCG inhibited the T-241 sarcoma given either a week before or a week following intravenous tumor injection. On the other hand, BCG given within an hour following tumor cell injection demonstrated probable enhancement. It is interesting that C-Parvum was not effective against pulmonary take whereas MER given far in advance of tumor may have been. Timing of dose is critical.

BCG can be injected directly into cutaneous lesions and cause regression. We have occasionally seen distant lesions also regress. Regional therapy may also be effective. (Gutterman et al. 1974) The study of McKneally (1976) with the intrapleural injection of BCG in low dose, Tice Strain, after pneumonectomy for bronchogenic carcinoma appears to delay recurrence and prolong survival.

A few years ago, we examined the possible use of intralesional BCG from a toxicity point of view. Karakousis et al. (1976) in our Department injected dogs and baboons with Glaxo BCG into the wall of the bowel, liver and pancreas at laparotomy, 3.6×10^7 organisma were injected per animal. Two thirds of the animals were preimmunized with BCG. The animals were killed up to 14 weeks after injection for pathologic study and straining for organisms. There was some persistance of acid fast organisms about half of the time in liver and pancreas. No lesions appeared grossly except for slight induration in the pancreas. Histologically inflammation was more pronounced in the pancreas. Small granulomas regularly occurred in the liver. There was no greater or less response in the preimmunized animals. In 24 dogs and 6 baboons studied, there were no instances of clinical hepatitis, pancreatitis, or perforation of the bowel or stomach. This information suggests the feasibility of regional injection of BCG for gastric cancer.

Ambus (1978) has reported one of the more interesting studies to date using immunotherapy for gastric cancer. BCG was given intraperitoneally, 2 mgm of Cannaught, at surgery and followed by 120 mgms orally monthly. 5-FU was loading and weekly thereafter at 15 mgms per kg. The gastric and pancreas patients were treated as above. The colon study was treated with BCG, 120 mgms p.o. q 2 weeks for three months and then monthly. No significant advantage was seen. The 54 patients treated for gastric cancer are reported in Figure I. The study was randomized with 24 receiving 5-FU alone and 30 receiving 5-FU with BCG. Ten in the BCG group underwent resection, but only 5 in the 5-FU group. Although median survival time was 48 weeks for combined therapy compared to 24 for 5-FU alone, there is not a significant difference. Two abdominal granulomas required excision and drainage. Five patients continued febrile until given antituberculous therapy with good results. There were two non-tuberculous abscesses. Oral BCG usually produced no effect except for occasional mild nausea and cramps.

C-Parvum is another bacterial product which may cause non-specific active immunization. There is currently a great deal of interest in intravenous C-Parvum. We cannot speak for C-Parvum and gastric cancer, but we recently completed an adjuvant study using intravenous C-Parvum for treatment of melanoma. The experience taught us several valuable lessons. C-Parvum was given in increasing doses monthly for 12 months with an esculator dose technique. We found that the treatment was quite unpleasant, and we encountered one life threatening toxicity in the form of a hypotensive episode. This was in spite of the fact that if symptoms were severe, the dose was either not given the next day or not escalated. We noted some variation in different lots of material. As seen in Table III on page 6, there were 29 patients randomized to the control group. Thirty-two individuals were treated with C-Parvum. We attempted accurate staging by Clark's method. For Clark's level, the groups were similar. In our studies, we do prophylactic node dissection. We later identified more patients with histologically positive nodes in the treatment group than in the control group, 13/5. Recurrence in the group treated with DTIC and C-Parvum was also 13

Figure 1

5FU and BCG in gastrointestinal cancer

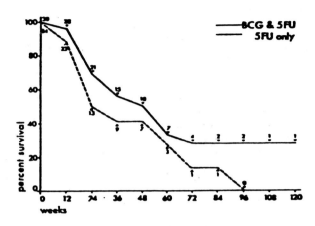

Adenocarcinoma. Stomach.

After Ambrus, U. et al. Int. Symp. Biol.
Prep. in Cancer, S. Karger, Basel, 38,
541,(1978)

Table III

ADJUVANT CHEMOIMMUNOTHERAPY IN MALIGNANT MELANOMA[1]

	No. Patients	Clark's Level Primary Lesion				L.N. Status			Recurrence			Present Status			
		3	4	5	U	+	–	U	0	Reg. Alone	Hem.	AND	DWD	AWD	U
Control	29	11	17	1		5	21	2	22	1	5(4*)	25	4		
DTIC + C. Parvum	32	15	13	2	2	13	15	4	17	2	13(8*)	19	10	2	1

*Patients with both hematogenous and regional recurrence.

[1] AND – Alive, no evidence of recurrent disease.
DWD – Dead with disease.
AWD – Alive with disease
U – Unknown

After Karakousis In Press

against 5 in those patients who only underwent surgery. Certainly we can't say
from our study that the DTIC was helpful. We can't say that it was helpful in
these Level III, IV, or V patients or patients with nodes clinically involved
because it appears that the presence of histologically positive nodes far out
weighed any therapeutic effect of DTIC and C-Parvum as a factor. At any rate,
the importance of careful staging is to be emphasized here.

Levamisole is another non-specific immune stimulant. It may be effective in
lung, breast, and head and neck cancer. (Miwa 1977) (Amery 1977) (Amery et al.
1977) It probably will find its way into relatively early trial because of its
virtues of low toxicity and availability.

Summing up prospects for active non-specific immunotherapy for gastric cancer, we
can say that regional node treatment with BCG might provide an acceptable treatment approach. For C-Parvum or MER in gastric cancer, there is little information
but our experience with the former intravenously and consideration of other results when it was given cutaneously, would make us put it low on any list.
Levamisole remains untried and available.

CONTACT IMMUNOTHERAPY

As we have noted already, there is evidence of increased efficacy of BCG injected
directly into a tumor mass. (Baldwin et al. 1978) (Salomon et al. 1976)
(Zbar et al. 1972)

Dykes (1978) injected C-Parvum up to 7.0 mgms per dose twice over a two week
period directly into gastric cancer. Surgery was carried out two weeks later.
There was pyrexia up to 39°C from 8-18 hours. No other result such as ulceration
or bleeding was seen. There was a varied lymphocyte response, but usually a
greater blastogenic potential was seen after the first injection. The response
may later diminish, but at least some transient response is seen. There is
animal data to suggest that such local therapy may have potential and there is
some rationale. At any rate, it appears feasible as an approach which might be
tried.

PASSIVE IMMUNOTHERAPY

The first successful report of passive immunity goes back to Gorer and Amos.
(1965) Immune serum would prevent growth of cells of leukemia injected 48 hours
prior to therapy. But there are many potential problems. Among these is enhancement reported early for sarcoma by Moller. (1964) Several principles have
evolved. The amount of antibody is critical. Furthermore, serological specificity has been a problem in the past. However, there are some possibilities and
one of these is use of a good highly specific antibody as a carrier of drug. We
also would have to consider the use of "deblocking antibody". This would reduce circulating tumor antigen and/or antigen antibody complex in such a way
that it might no longer be blocking. (Baldwin et al. 1972) (Sjogren et al. 1971)
(Noonan et al. 1977) Also, specific antibody tested active in antibody specific
cytotoxicity reactions might be used.

ACTIVE SPECIFIC IMMUNOTHERAPY

This is largely explored except quite empirically. There is evidence that
ordinarily the patient is receiving all the possible immunization from his own
tumor. Allogeneic tumor cells may be used, usually killed or inactivated. This
approach has produced limited results. (Nadler and Moore 1969) The explanation
for effect here is that the immune activity of tumor cells is increased by the
immune activity generated by HL-A antigens providing increased stimulus. Tumor

Tumor cell antigenicity may be modified by coupling with a strong antigen as BSA or by treatment with neuraminidas which alters the cell surface and may increase immunogenicity. Soluble antigens offer another possibility, but blocking is possible. (Hollingshead and Stewart 1977) (Hollingshead 1978)

ACTIVE TRANSFER OF IMMUNITY

The pioneering work of Moore suggested that lymphocytes might be used or perhaps immune RNA. Moore in his studies clearly demonstrated some therapeutic effect using murine lymphocytes. Transfer factor has been shown to transfer immunity from immune lymphocytes to a recipient. (Hitzig and Grob 1974) It is non-immunogeneic and of great importance, and seems to affect cellular immunity and not antibody production. (McKhann 1974)

Figure 2 shows the method of preparing sheep immune RNA used by Ramming (1977).

Figure 2

PREPARATION OF IMMUNE RNA

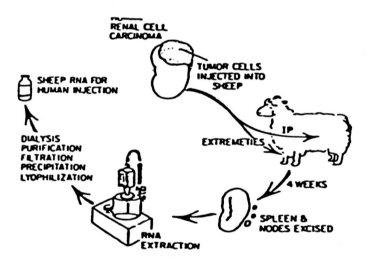

After Ramming, K., Ann. Surg. <u>186</u>, 459, 1977.

In Figure 3, the survival difference between the RNA treated group and the matched control group as a whole are not significant at all points. For just those patients wtih pulmonary metastases the differences are significantly greater.

Figure 3

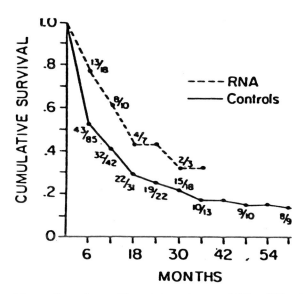

IMMUNE RNA FOR RENAL
CELL CARCINOMA

After Ramming, K., Ann. Surg. **186**, 459, 1977.

DISCUSSION

What are our possibilities for immunotherapy of gastric cancer at present? We
have some partially rational leads to continue. Intra-tumor or intra-nodal
non-specific immunostimulation with BCG offers a possible approach. Levamisole
may be tried. Information on solid tumors in man of a critical nature is lacking
in this area. But one possible approach for active specific immunotherapy may
still be with cells treated with neuraminidase. Vaccines must be used with care
because of the potential danger of disadvantageous stimulation of antibodies
with   soluble antigens. Adoptive Transfer may prove useful with immune RNA
although evidence for success with this therapy or with transfer factor in man is
uncertain or absent.

We have to review and add to the new molecular biological knowledge of antigen
and antibody function and structure as seen in Figure 4. We have to work back to
identifying precise genetic defects and from these enzymatic and structural
alterations which may uncover potential areas of immune therapy not now apparent.
In the interim, more empiric search for antigens, especially those which might be
immunogens, should continue in a variety of tumor systems including gastric cancer.
This approach might provide a partial short cut. It should be recognized that
these are highly sophisticated areas of study. I believe that it is desirable to
try to form small groups who work well together linking molecular biology, biochemistry and immunology to the clinician and to each other.

Figure 4

MODERN ANTIBODY STRUCTURE

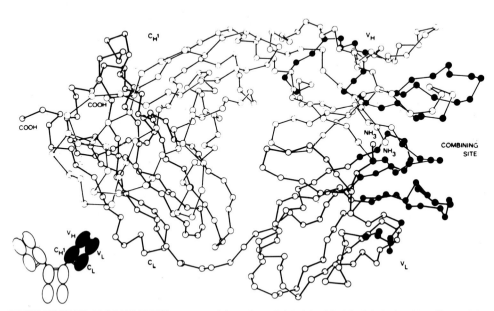

CARBON SKELETON OF Fab FRAGMENT (one prong of the antibody molecule) from a mouse myeloma protein designated McPC 603 shows how the entire fragment is divided into closely packed constant and variable regions composed of paired domains from the heavy chain (*color*) and the light chain (*black*) and joined by extended segments called "switch" regions. The combining site at the tip of the fragment is made up entirely of adjacent loops of hypervariable amino acid units (*filled-in balls*) contributed by both polypeptide chains.

After Capra and Edmundson, Sci. Amer. 236, 50-59, (Jan. 1977)

Clinical testing is a difficult and underrated scientific endeavor. We have already emphasized staging, but careful follow up is necessary. The most meaningful area to study for immunotherapy is, because of the need for small tumor load, in adjuvant treatment programs. The possibility of adverse effects and possible evidence of enhancement of tumor can be observed in patients with residual disease, or even moderate amounts of tumor who appear immunologically intact in first trial. But, unfortunately, failure in this group does not rule out completely the possibility for adjuvant success.

Possibly the best likelihood of success at present would be in the application of non-specific immunotherapy to try to offset concommittant damage to the immune system from chemotherapy or radiation therapy. More reports studying the changes in animals and in man undergoing such combination treatment to determine possible optimal sequences of therapy are desirable. (Tagliabue 1977) Such a treatment program is self defeating unless we are sure timing allows immunostimulation to take place.

At our Institution, we believe that unless very marked effects are seen, adjuvant studies must be prospective and randomized. A large number of patients will be needed because stratification has to be precise and in addition, study over several years is necessary to see results.

We all know the dilemma in evaluating immunotherapy. It is still possible to ask if immune therapy against tumor in man exists at all, at least in the solid tumors. At a national conference in 1976, (Immunotherapy of Cancer) some 40 reports covering immunotherapy trials in man in various stages of execution were discussed. About half of these indicated that immune therapy had effect, and in about half that there were none. The negative half included a majority of the prospective randomized studies. Because of the complexities involved, it is quite easy to criticize many of the negative studies indicating, for example, the dose, timing, or manufacture of BCG is incorrect. I believe the evidence indicates immunologic treatment effect, and in particular the intrapleural treatment in lung with BCG, if it continues, is valid. Hollingshead's data with lung cancer is another instance which appears sound. But many positive results reported are uncertain. Nevertheless, most of us have seen patients cured of present disease with only immunotherapy in a few instances. So we know it is a finite treatment. The approach to the problem posed in our laboratory at the present time is to encourage a search for gastric antigens which may be specific. We have identified gastric LAI specific activity, and we are following that lead.

REFERENCES

Ambus, U., Falk, R.E., Landi, S., Bugala, R., and Langer, B., (1978). Randomized Trial of Chemoimmunotherapy for Resectable and Non-Resectable Gastrointestinal Cancer. Develop. Biol. Stand. 38, 541-545.

Amery, W.K. (1977). Levamisole as an immunotherapeutic agent in the treatment of cancer. World J. Surg. 1(5) 597-604.

Amery, W.K. (1977). Adjuvant treatment with Levamisole in cancer, a review of experimental and clinical data. Can. Treat. Rev. 4(3) 167-194.

Aoki, T. (1973). An Analysis of Antigens on the Surface of Murine Leukemia Viruses and Cells.in Dutcher R.m., Chicco-Biachi. C.   Unifying Concepts of Leukemia (Basel: Bibl Haematology).

Baldwin, R.W., Price, M.R., and Robins, R.A. (1972) Blocking of Lymphocyte Mediated Cytotoxicity for Rat Hepatoma Cells by Tumor Specific Antigen--Antibody Complexes. Nature New Biol. 238, 185-187.

Baldwin, R., Primm, M.V. (1973) BCG Immunotherapy of Local Subcutaneous Growths and Post-surgical Pulmonary Metastases of a Transplanted Rat Epithelioma of Spontaneous Origin. Int. J. Cancer 12, 420-427.

Baldwin, R.W., Hopper, P.G., Pimm, M.V. (1976) Bacillus Calmette-Gyerin. Contact Immunotherapy of local and metastatic deposits of Rat Tumor. Am. N.Y. Acad. Sci. 277, 124.

Baldwin, R.W. (1978) Immunological Adjuvants in Cancer Immunotherapy. Int. Symp. on Biol.Prep. in the Treatment of Cancer. London 1977. Devel Biol. Standards Vol. 38, 3-12. S. Kenger Basal.

Banwo, O. Versey, J. and Hobbs, J.R. (1974) New Oncofetal Antigen for Human Pancreas. Lancet 1643-45.

Cantrell, E.G. (1971) The Importance of Lymph Nodes in the Assessment of Gastric Carcinoma at Operation. Brit. J. Surg. 58, 384-386.

de Landazuri, M.O., Kedar, E., and Fahey, J.L. (1974) Antibody dependent cellular cytotoxicity to a syngeneic gross virus-induced lymphoma. J.N.C.I. 52, 147-152.

Dykes, P.W. and Trejdosiewicz, L.K. (1978) Intra-Tumor C-Parvum Therapy in Gastric Carcinoma. A Pilot Study. Devel. Biol. Stand. 38, 547-552. S. Karger Basal.

Eilber, F.R. and Morton, D.L. (1970) Immunologic Studies of Human Sarcomas: Additional evidence suggesting an associated sarcoma virus. Cancer 26:588-96.

Eilber, F.R., Morton, D.L., Holmes, E.C., Sparks, F.C., Ramming, K.P. (1976) Immunotherapy with BCG for Lymph Node Metastases from Malignant Melanoma. N.E.J.M. 294, 237-240.

Everson, T.C., Cole, W. (1966) Spontaneous Regression of Cancer. W.B. Saunders Company, Philadelphia.

Foley, E.J. (1953) Antigenic Properties of Methyl-Cholanthrone Induced Tumors in Mice of the Strain of Origin. Can. Res. 13, 835-837.

Gold, P., Freedman, S.O. (1965) Specific Carcinoembryonic Antigens of the Human Digestive System. J. Exp. Med. 122, 467-481.

Gorer, P., and Amos, D.B. (1956) Passive Immunity of Mice Against C57Bl leukosis EL4 by Means of 180 serum. Can. Res. 16 338-343.

Gross, L. (1943) Intradermal Immunization of C3H Mice against a Sarcoma that Originated in an Animal of the Same Line. Can. Res. 3, 320-333.

Gutterman, J.U., Hersh, E.M., Rodriguez, V., McCredie, K.B., Mavligit, G.M., Reed, R., Burgess, M.A., Smith, T., Gehan, E., Bodey, G.P., Sr., Freirich, E.J. Chemo-immunotherapy of Adule Acute Leukemia, Prolongation of Remission in Myeloblastic Leukemia with Bacillus Calmette-Guerin. (1974) Lancet 2. 1405-1409.

Hanna, M.G., Jr., Snodgrass, M.J., Zbar, B. and Rappo. H.J. Histologic and Ultra structural studies of tumor regression in inbred guineas pigs after intralesional injection of mycobacterium bovis (BCG). Nat. Can. Inst. Monogr. 39. 71.

Hawley, P.R., Westerholm, P., Morson, B.C. (1970). Pathology and Prognosis of Carcinoma of the Stomach. Br. J. Surg. 57, 877-883.

Hellstrom, I., Warner, G.A., Hellstrom, K.E. and Sjogren, H.O. (1973) Sequential Studies of Cell-mediated Tumor Immunity and Blocking Serum Activity in 10 Patients with Malignant Melanoma. Int. J. Cancer 11, 280-292.

Herberman, R.B., Hollingshead, A., Char, P., Oldham, R., McCoy, J., and Cohen, M. (1975) In vivo and In vitro studies of cell-mediated Immune response to Antigens Associated with Malignant Melanoma. Behring Inst. Mitt. 56. 131.

Herberman, R.B. (1977) Immunogenicity of Tumor Antigens. Biochem. & Biophys. ACTA 473, 93-119.

Hersh, E.M. and Oppenheim, J.J. (1967) Inhibition of an In Vitro Lymphocyte Transformation during Chemotherapy in man. Can Res. 27, 98-105.

Hersh, E.M., Gutterman, J.U. and Mavligit, G.M. (1973) Immunotherapy of Cancer. Major Problems of Childhood Cancer. Springfield, Ill. Charter C. Thomas, Publisher.

Hitzig, W.H., Grob, P.J. (1974). Therapeutic Uses of Transfer Factor. Ed. Schwarts, R.S. Progress in Clinical Immunology, N.Y. Greene & Strats. 69-100.

Hollingshead, A.C., McWright, C.S., Alford, T.C., Glew, D.H., Gold, P., and Herberman, R.B. (1972). Separation of Skin Reactive Intestinal Cancer Antigen from the Carcinoembryonic Antigen of Gold. Science 177. 887-889.

Hollingshead, A.C. and Stewart T.H.M. (1977). Lung Tumor Antigens. Proc. In. Symp. on Detect. and Prevent. Cancer. N.Y. Marcel Decker

Hollingshead, A.C. (1978). Specific Active Immunotherapy of Lung Cancer. XII Int. Cancer Congress, Buenos Aires. In Press.

Hughes, L.E., Kearney, R., Tully, M. (1970). A Study in Clinical Cancer. Cancer 26. 269-78.

Hughes, L.E., Mackay. (1966). Immunological Concepts in Malignant Disease. The Medical Journal of Australia. 1741-1745.

Karakousis, C.P., Jager, B.V., Holyoke, E.D., Douglass, H.O.. (1976) BCG Injection in the Alimentary Tract: An Experimental Study. J. Surg. Res. 21. 239-246.

Lauren, P. (1973). The two histological types of gastric carcinoma, diffuse and so called intestinal type carcinoma. Acta Pathol. Microbiol. Scand. 64, 31-49.

Lewin, E. (1954) Gastric Cancer: A Clinical Study with Reference to Total Gastrectomy and Microscopic Grading. Acta Chir. Scand. (Suppl.). 262. 1-104.

Mavligit, G.M., Hersh, E.M., and McBride, C.M. (1974). Lymphocyte Blastogenesis Induced by Autochthonous Human Solid Tumor Cells, Relationship to Stage of Disease and Serum Factor. Cancer 34. 1712-1721.

McKhann, C.F. and Gunnarson, A. (1974). Approaches to Immunotherapy. Cancer 34. 1521-1531.

McKneally, M.F. Implication of Immuno Stimulation in Lung Cancer. Williams, T.E. et al. Ed. Perspectives in Lung Cancer Basal Karger.

Miwa, H., Oritak. (1971). Reactivating effect of levamisole on cell mediated immunity in gastrointestinal cancer patients. Acta. Med. Okagama 31(5) 325-329.

Moller, G. (1964) The effects of tumor growth in syngeneic recipients of antibodies against tumor specific antigens in the methochloanthrene induced Murine Sarcomas. Nature 204. 846-848.

Morton, D.L., Malmgren, R.H., Hall, W.T. et al. (1969). Immunologic and Virus Studies with Human Sarcomas. Surg. 66. 152-161.

Nadler, S. and Moore, G.E. (1969) Immunotherapy of Malignant Disease. Arch. Surg. 99. 376-389.

Noonan, F.P., Halliday, W.J., Wall, D.R., Clonie, G.J.A. (1977) Cell-mediated Immunity and Serum Blocking Factors in Cancer Patients during Chemotherapy and Immunotherapy. Can. Res. 37, 2473-2480.

Oren, M.E. and Herberman, R.B. (1971) Delayed Cutaneous Hypersensitivity Reactions to Membrane Extracts of Human Tumor Cells. Clin. Exp. Immunol. 9. 45-56.

Prehn, R.T. and Main, J.M. (1957) Immunity of the methochloanthrene Induced Sarcomas. J.N.C.I. 18. 769-775.

Ramming, K.P., and deKernion, J.B. (1977). Immune RNA Therapy for Renal Cell Carcinoma: Survival and Immunologic Monitoring. Ann. Surg. 186. 459-467.

Rubin, P. (1974). Cancer of the Gastrointestinal Tract. D. Gastric Cancer; Treatment Principles. J.A.M.A. 228, 1283-1286.

Solomon, J.C., Galinah, A., Lascaux, V., Prim, J., Purin, F., Lynch. N. (1976) Intra-lesional Injection of Stimulants in Bilateral Rat Tumor. Int. J. Cancer 18, 279-91.

Sjogren, H.O., Hellstrom, I., Bansal, S.C., and Hellstrom, K.E. (1971) Suggestive Evidence that the "Blocking Antibodies" of Tumor Bearing Individuals may be Antigen-Antibody Complexes. Proc. Nat. Agad. Sci. (Wash.) 68, 1372-1375.

Southam, C.M.. Marcove, R.C., Levin, A.G., Buchsbaum, H.J., and Mike, V. (1973) Clinical Trial of Autogenous Tumor Vaccine for Treatment of Osteogeneic Sarcoma. Proc. Natl. Cancer Conf. 7. 91-100.

Tagliabue, A., Polentarutti, N., Vecchi, A., Manovani, A., and Spreafico, F. Combination Chemo-Immunotherapy with Adriamycin in Experimental Tumor Systems. Eur. J. Cancer 13. 657-665.

Zbar, B., Berstein, I.P., Bartlett, G.L., Hanna, M.G., Rapp. H.J. (1972) Immuno-therapy of Cancer: Regression of Intradermal Tumors and Prevention of Growth of Lymph Node Metastases After Intradermal Injection of Living Mycobacterium boris.

Current Management of the Gastrointestinal Malignancies

P. V. Woolley, J. S. Macdonald, Daniel F. Hoth, Fred P. Smith and P. S. Schein

Department of Medicine, Division of Medical Oncology and Vincent T. Lombardi Cancer Research Center, Washington. D.C. USA

ABSTRACT

A number of studies have recently been conducted at the Vincent T. Lombardi Cancer Research Center, Georgetown University, in the area of chemotherapy of gastrointestinal cancer. Of particular interest is the combination of 5-fluorouracil, adriamycin and mitomycin C (FAM), which has been effective in gastric cancer and pancreatic cancer as well. The combination of streptozotocin, mitomycin C and 5-fluorouracil (SMF) has also produced beneficial effects in pancreatic cancer. Other trials in pancreatic cancer have included examination of the effects of neutron radiation on locally unresectable disease. Colon carcinoma remains a difficult problem. Neither the combination of 5-fluorouracil, methyl CCNU, vincristine (FMV) or FAM produced a significant improvement in survival of responders over non-responders. These trials illustrate the problems and complexities of dealing with this group of diseases.

INTRODUCTION

The gastrointestinal malignancies are as a group the most common cause of cancer mortality in the United States, and the clinical approach to these diseases remains a major challenge in the field of oncology. While treatment is difficult, current results indicate that combinations of agents and combined modality approaches may produce responses that are associated with prolonged patient survival.

GASTRIC CANCER

Chemotherapy of gastric cancer shows particular promise. Data in the literature, such as those of Kovach (1974) and Moertel (1976) show that 5-fluorouracil (5-FU) plus 1,3-bis(2-chloroethyl)-1-nitrosourea (BCNU) or 1-(2-chloroethyl)-3-(4-methylcyclohexyl)-1-nitrosourea (methyl CCNU) produce objective responses in advanced gastric cancer. In the study by Kovach and colleagues, the response rate of 41% to 5-FU plus BCNU was superior to either drug used alone and the survival of patients treated with the combination was statistically greater at 18 months than those treated with 5-FU alone. The data of the Eastern Cooperative Oncology Group (Moertel, 1976 a) indicate that the combination of 5-FU and methyl CCNU was superior both in response rate (52%) and survival benefit to methyl CCNU alone. Of interest in that study was the observation that an induction course of Cytoxan did not improve the clinical results obtained with the 5-FU/nitrosourea combination.

Both adriamycin and mitomycin C are drugs with single agent activity in gastric cancer. Each shows a response rate of 25-35% (Woolley, 1977). Recent studies at the Vincent T. Lombardi Cancer Research Center at Georgetown University have emphasized the combination of 5-FU with adriamycin and mitomycin C, as well as modifications of this combination with 5-FU analogues or with newer nitrosoureas.

The combination of 5-FU, adriamycin and mitomycin C (FAM) was employed as therapy for 36 patients with advanced measureable gastric carcinoma, in the schedule below (Macdonald, 1978);

	Week	1	2	3	4	5	6	7	8	9
5-Fluorouracil 600 mg/m^2 IV x 1		x	x			x	x			Repeat
Adriamycin 30 mg/m^2 IV x 1		x				x				Cycle
Mitomycin C 10 mg/m^2 IV x 1		x								

There were 18 partial responders (50%) among these patients. The median duration of remission was 9.5 months and the median survival for responding patients was 13 months, while the median survival for nonresponding patients was 2.5 months and all were dead within 6 months of the initiation of therapy. Analysis of such variables as initial performance status, resectability of the primary tumor and histologic differentiation of the neoplasm failed to account for differences in patient response and survival. In addition the regimen was well tolerated and produced only moderate bone marrow suppression.

A subsequent protocol (FAM II) was designed to incorporate the 5-FU analogue Ftorafur into this regimen (Woolley, 1978). Ftorafur is chemically composed of 5-FU conjugated to a furanyl ring and was originally synthesized in the Soviet Union. It is metabolized, at least in part, to 5-FU within the body and thus acts as a slow release form of the parent compound. Its major clinical advantage is that it is less myelotoxic than 5-FU and thus has the potential of providing an improved therapeutic index over 5-FU.

The FAM II combination was administered as follows:

	Week	1	2	3	4	5	6	7	8	9
Ftorafur 1.5 g/m^2/day IV x 5 days		x				x				Repeat
Adriamycin 40 mg/m^2 IV x 1		x				x				Cycle
Mitomycin 10 mg/m^2 IV x 1		x								

In fifteen patients who were treated with the combination, three (20%) showed an objective response, five showed temporary stabilization of disease and seven showed progression while on treatment. All responding patients showed survivals in excess of 12 months. The hematologic toxicity of the regimen was only moderate in severity. However the major and limiting toxicity was non-hematologic in the form of nausea, vomiting, dizziness and vertigo. The combination failed to demonstrate a clinical improvement on the FAM combination and was terminated after 15 patients.

Further clinical trials in the area of gastric cancer are ongoing at Georgetown and at the present time are directed toward incorporating newly developed and relatively non-myelosuppressive nitrosoureas such as chlorozotocin into the FAM combination. Although no definitive conclusions can as yet be drawn from these studies, continued patient accrual should bring results within the next few months.

PANCREATIC CANCER

The treatment of advanced pancreatic cancer with combinations of drugs has been an area of small gains in the past. Kovach (1974) reported improved response rate for the combination of 5-FU and BCNU over the drugs used as single agents. A recent trial at Georgetown (Wiggans, 1978) employed the 3 drugs streptozotocin, mitomycin C and 5-fluorouracil (SMF).

Drug	Dose		Week								
		1	2	3	4	5	6	7	8	9	
Streptozotocin	1.0 g/m^2 IV	x	x			x	x				R
Mitomycin C	10mg/m^2 IV	x									E
5-Fluorouracil	600 mg/m^2 IV	x	x			x	x				P
											E
											A
											T

This combination produced 10 responses in 23 patients treated (43%) and the responders lived to a median of 8 months while the non-responders had a median survival of 3 months. Toxicity was mild, and consisted of reversible myelosuppression and nephrotoxicity.

In a second trial the FAM combination, as described above, was employed as therapy in 25 patients with advanced pancreatic cancer. There were objective responses in 10 patients. These responses lasted a median of 9 months and there is a median 10 month survival in the responding group as opposed to 3 months in the non-responding group.

These trials show that pancreatic cancer is at least marginally responsive to chemotherapeutic agents and that response to therapy may be associated with prolongation of survival. Another approach to this disease has been to employ neutron radiation in the therapy of locally unresectable carcinoma. The background for this study has been the experience that high dose radiation therapy in doses of 4000 or 6000 rads, plus 5-fluorouracil, was more effective than 6000 rads alone in prolonging survival in such patients (Moertel, 1976 b). Seventeen patients with unresectable pancreatic carcinoma were treated with neutron radiation and variable concomitant doses of 5-fluorouracil. Responses were seen in 5 and toxicity was dependent upon the dose of 5-fluorouracil. In 75% of patients there were gastrointestinal symptoms and in half of these cases these symptoms necessitated interruption of therapy. There were 3 cases of hemorrhagic gastritis. The major toxicity was myelosuppression and was most severe at a concomitant 5-FU dose of 500 mg/m^2. It was less severe at 375 mg/m^2 5-FU and least when no 5-FU was given. The value of this approach relative to other regimens needs to be assessed in prospective trial.

COLON CANCER

The chemotherapeutic approach to colon cancer, either in the advanced disease or surgical adjuvant setting, has traditionally employed the fluorinated pyrimidines such as 5-FU as the first line agents. 5-Fluorouracil as a single agent produces an overall response rate of about 20% and this figure is not substantially altered by variations in scheduling such as weekly bolus versus loading course or continuous infusion. A major problem in the chemotherapy of this disease is that the combination of additional active agents with 5-fluorouracil doses not produce large dividends in terms of increasing the response rate. Falkson (1974) described a 43% response rate in advanced disease using the combination of 5-FU, ditriazenoimidazole carboximide (DTIC), vincristine and BCNU. Moertel (1975)

subsequently reported a similar response rate using 5-FU in a loading schedule
with methyl CCNU and vincristine. A trial at Georgetown (Macdonald, 1976) using
5-FU in a weekly bolus schedule, plus methyl CCNU and vincristine also produced a
43% response rate. There was, however, no statistically significant difference
between the survivals of responding and non-responding patients. In a second
trial, the FAM combination produced only a 17% response rate in patients with advanced colon carcinoma (Haller, 1978), which is no better than 5-FU alone. Such
data appear to present a basic biological dilemma, inasmuch as individually active
drugs produce little or no additive effect in colon cancer over 5-FU alone and the
responses that are achieved may have only a marginal effect on survival. As a
result there is ample scientific and ethical justification for proceeding with
trials of new Phase II agents in this disease before 5-FU is used. An ongoing
trial at Georgetown, which is being done conjointly with the Mayo Clinic, is examining the activity of the nitrosourea chlorozotocin in the two dose levels as a
single agent in previously untreated patients with advanced colon cancer. A
second trial is evaluating the two drug combination of 5-FU and chlorozotocin.
Clealy much additional intensive work in this area will be required for significant progress to be made. Phase II trials of new agents are needed with application not only to the advanced disease situation but also to the surgical adjuvant setting.

SUMMARY

The most recent progress in the treatment of gastrointestinal cancer has been in
the area of gastric cancer. Both 5-FU/methyl CCNU and FAM produce responses
which are associated with increases in survival for the responders. Although it
remains to be proven by prospective trial, the FAM combination appears superior
to the 5-FU/nitrosourea combination. Two three drug combinations tested at
Georgetown have produced objective responses in pancreatic cancer. Colon cancer
remains a major therapeutic challenge and the various 5-FU/nitrosourea combinations
in current use have only slight effects on overall survival. Because of their
numerical importance, the gastrointestinal malignancies should be major targets
for clinical research in the next several years.

REFERENCES

1) Falkson, G., E.G. Van Eden, and H.C. Falkson (1974). Fluorouracil, Imidazole
    Carboximide Ditriazeno, Vincristine and Bis-chloroethyl Nitrosourea in
    Colon Cancer. Cancer, 33:1207-1209

2) Haller, D.G., P.V. Woolley, J.S. Macdonald, and P.S. Schein (1978). Phase
    II Trial of FAM in Advanced Colorectal Cancer. Canc. Treat. Rep. 62:563-65.

3) Kovach, J.S., C.G. Moertel, A.J. Schutt, R.G. Hahn and R.J. Reitemeier (1974).
    A Controlled Study of Combined 1,3-bis(2-chloroethyl)-1-nitrosourea and
    5-Fluorouracil Therapy for Advanced Gastric and Pancreatic Cancer. Cancer
    33:563-567.

4) Macdonald, J.S., D.F. Kisner, T. Smythe, P.V. Woolley, L. Smith and P.S.
    Schein (1976). 5-Fluorouracil, Methyl CCNU and Vincristine in Treatment
    of Advanced Colorectal Cancer; A Phase II Study Utilizing Weekly 5-Fluoro-
    uracil. Canc. Treat. Rep. 60:1597-1600.

5) Macdonald, J.S., P.V. Woolley, D.G. Haller, D.F. Hoth, T. Smythe, S. Rosenoff,
    and P.S. Schein (1978). Treatment of Advanced Gastric Cancer with 5-
    Fluorouracil, Adriamcyin and Mitomycin C (FAM) Cancer (In Press).

6) Moertel, C.G., A.J. Schutt and R.G. Hahn (1975). Therapy of Advanced Colo-
    rectal Cancer with a Combination of 5-Fluorouracil, Methyl CCNU and Vin-
    cristine. J. Nat. Canc. Inst. 54:69-71.

7) Moertel, C.G., J.A. Mittelman, R.F. Bakemeier, P. Engstrom and J. Hanley (1976). Sequential and Combination Chemotherapy of Advanced Gastric Cancer. Cancer 38:678-682.

8) Moertel, C.G., J.J. Lokich, D.S. Childs and P.S. Schein (1976). An Evaluation of High Dose Radiation and 5-Fluorouracil Therapy for Locally Unresectable Pancreatic Carcinoma. Proc. Am. Soc. Clin. Oncol. 17:244

9) Wiggans, R.G., P.V. Woolley, J.S. Macdonald, T. Smythe, W. Ueno and P.S. Schein (1978). Phase II Trial of Streptozotocin, Mitomycin C and 5-Fluoro uracil (SMF) in the Treatment of Advanced Pancreatic Cancer. Cancer 41: 387-391.

0) Woolley, P.V., J.S. Macdonald, and P.S. Schein (1977). Chemotherapy of Gastrointestinal Cancer. In G.B. Jerzy Glass (Ed.) Progress in Gastro-enterology, Vol. 3, Grune and Stratton, New York pp. 671-692.

1) Woolley, P.V., J.S. Macdonald, D.G. Haller, D.F. Hoth, T. Smythe, S. Rosenoff and P.S. Schein (1978). Phase II Trial of Ftorafur, Adriamycin and Mito-mycin in Gastric Cancer (Submitted).

Oesophageal Cancer

Epidemiology of Esophageal Cancer in Iran

E. Mahboubi

*Eppley Institute for Research in Cancer, University of Nebraska Medical Center,
Omaha, Nebraska 68105, U.S.A.*

ABSTRACT

Epidemiology of esophageal cancer is reviewed for Iran, which is among the cancer
belt countries in Asia. Data for one-tenth of the population is well-documented, while for the rest of the country, cancer information is mostly based on
the relative frequencies of pathological materials diagnosed in different medical
institutions. Despite lack of data for comparison, it is apparent that esophageal
cancer is a common disease in Iran, where one area records the highest incidence
in the world and constitutes 40% of all registered cancer cases in the country.
Findings from an intense search for its etiology are discussed.

Keywords: Esophageal cancer--etiology--Iran

INTRODUCTION

Epidemiological and geographical pathology studies have tremendously increased our
understanding of certain factors associated in the promotion or cause of some forms
of cancer. Esophageal cancer is one of a few cancer types with an incidence that
varies greatly in different world regions (see Table 1) and is probably dependent
in at least 80% of the cases on environmental factors.

TABLE 1 Annual Age-Adjusted[*] Incidence Rates per 100,000 Population of Esophageal
Cancer in Iran and Selected Countries Around the World, by Sex and Male
Female Ratios

Country	High risk areas		Low risk areas		M/F Ratio	Source Ref. No.
	Male	Female	Male	Female		
Asia						
Iran						
Northern Gonbad	165.5	195.3			.85	Mahboubi et al., 1973
Fouman			10.4	2.7	3.85	
India						
Bombay	15.2	10.8			1.41	Waterhouse et al., 1976

TABLE 1　Annual Age-Adjusted[*] Incidence Rates per 100,000 Population of Esophageal Cancer in Iran and Selected Countries Around the World, by Sex and Male Female Ratios (cont'd)

Country	High risk areas Male	Female	Low risk areas Male	Female	M/F Ratio	Source Ref. No.
Asia						
Israel						
All Jews			2.5	2.1	1.19	Waterhouse et al., 1976
Japan						
Miyagi	12.9	4.1			3.15	Waterhouse et al., 1976
Osaka	9.7	2.9			3.34	Waterhouse et al., 1976
Singapore						
Chinese	20.1	6.4			3.14	Waterhouse et al., 1976
Africa						
Nigeria						
Ibadan			1.5	1.1	1.36	Waterhouse et al., 1976
Bulawayo	63.8	2.2			29.00	Waterhouse et al., 1976
Cape Province	37.5	14.3			2.62	Doll et al., 1970
Natal African	40.9	12.3			3.33	Doll et al., 1970
Natal Indian			5.5	12.9	.43	Doll et al., 1970
Europe						
United Kingdom						
Liverpool			6.8	4.2	1.62	Waterhouse et al., 1976
Ayrshire			5.9	1.9	3.11	Waterhouse et al., 1976
Norway			2.8	0.7	4.00	Waterhouse et al., 1976
Switzerland						
Geneva			8.5	1.3	6.54	Waterhouse et al., 1976
France[**]	14	1.13			12.39	Segi and Kurihara 1972
Americas						
United States						
Detroit (non white)	14.1	3.7			3.81	Waterhouse et al., 1976
Detroit (white)			4	1.1	3.6	Waterhouse et al., 1976
Canada						
Newfoundland			4.7	2.2	2.14	Waterhouse et al., 1976
Maritime Provinces			2.3	0.9	2.56	Waterhouse et al., 1976
Brazil						
Sao Paulo	13.1	2.2			5.95	Waterhouse et al., 1976

*Adjusted to the world population　　　　**Death rates

IRAN IN ESOPHAGEAL CANCER BELT

In Iran, clinical and surgical observations were made of vast numbers of esophageal cancer patients from the Northeastern area of Gonbad. These were mostly
Turkomans who sought treatment at the main cancer center in the capitol Teheran.
The ensuing findings focused increased attention by the medical profession on
the Gonbad and resulted in several reports (Sarkissian, 1960; Armin, 1967; Habibi,
1965) from which little reliable data can be extracted for determining incidence
of the disease. Therefore, the Institute of Public Health Research of the University of Teheran and the International Agency for Research on Cancer (IARC) of
the World Health organization (WHO) jointly established a systematic cancer registry in 1968 for Mazandaran Province to cover approximately two million persons,
including the suspected highly susceptible Turkomans of northern Gonbad. In 1969,
cancer registration was extended to the neighboring provinces of Guilan and
Ardabil in eastern Azarbaijan, with a total of four million inhabitants. This
populace resided in the narrow strip of diverse land around the southern shore
of the Caspian Sea (Kmet and Mahboubi, 1972). This land borders the U.S.S.R. on
the north and the northern slopes of the Alborz Mountains in the south (Fig. 1).

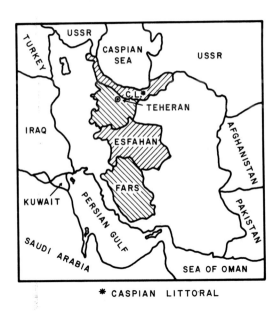

* CASPIAN LITTORAL

Fig. 1. Four study areas in Iran

The results of the first three years of registration are published (Mahboubi et
al., 1973) and it is not the purpose of this paper to further discuss these data,
except to confirm that the northeastern corner of Iran is not only one of the
highest esophageal cancer incidence areas in the world (Fig. 2), but the highest
ever recorded anywhere in the world. Moreover it is part of the vast high incidence area for esophageal cancer that extends from northeastern China to the
Middle East and includes Mongolia, parts of Siberia, Soviet Central Asia and
Afghanistan (Kmet and Mahboubi, 1972; Mahboubi et al., 1974). From western Iran,
the incidence area may extend toward Turkey and Iraq.

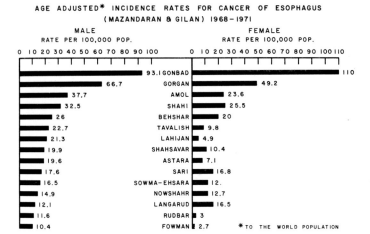

Fig. 2.   Incidence rates in high and low areas by sex

This esophageal cancer belt information is based on different types of evidence. In the Caspian Littoral of Iran the information is very well-documented (Kmet and Mahboubi, 1972; Mahboubi et al., 1973). There are adequate data also from northeastern China and Soviet Central Asia, but the information for other parts of this cancer belt including southern, eastern, western and central Iran, is less reliable and subject to controversy.

As indicated, except for Mazandaran and Guilan provinces, there is no population-based information for the rest of the country (of about 35 million people), with regard to all cancer types. However, there are numerous reports from different geographical areas in Iran (e.g., Esfahan, Mashhad, Tabriz and Shiraz). These data are based on the relative frequencies found in surgical specimens or autopsies performed and examinations in various medical institutions or private pathology laboratories (Habibi, 1965; Haghighi et al., 1971; Sadeghi et al., 1977).

SEX RATIOS

Esophageal cancer is one of the few cancer sites that fascinates epidemiologists, because firstly, its incidence and death rates are very close and vary strikingly from place to place, and the differences between high and low incidence areas may be as great as 100 times. In truncated incidence rates in men (aged 35-64), esophageal cancer is 200 times more common in the Gurjev district of Kazakhstan of the U.S.S.R. than in parts of Canada (Alberta, Manitoba) and the Netherlands (Doll, 1967) or even 250 times more common in parts of Gonbad for females than in Canada (Mahboubi et al., 1973). Secondly, the disease is generally more common in males than in females and the ratio sometimes is as great as 12, e.g. in France (Segi, 1972) and in parts of France is even more than 22 (Kmet, 1974). But in parts of Africa (South Africa, Natal) this ratio is reversed to 0.4 (Doll, 1970) (from 22 in France to 0.4 in Africa). It is of interest to note that in high incidence areas in Iran, Turkoman women get the disease at the same rate as Turkoman men, if not at a slightly higher rate, and as one moves from the east of the study area towards the west, the disease rate and its sex ratio change dramatically. The rate rapidly decreases from east to west and the disease occurs in more males and in this direction shows a difference of 30 times in females and 10 times in males. Further toward the west, the incidence increases to a moderately high level (Mahboubi et al., 1973).

Unlike the narrow strip of northern Iran where the incidence rates are very well-documented, for the rest of the country, as mentioned, information is not based on population figures, but only on cases seen in different institutions. These results are given in Table 2 which points out that these data are not comparable, even in reports covering the same area.

TABLE 2   Esophageal Cancer--Incidence or Percentage of Relative Frequencies by Sex From Different Areas

Locality	Incidence 10^5 pop.		Relative Frequency		Investigator
	Male	Female	Male	Female	
Caspian Littoral					
Gonbad	93	110	46	49	Mahboubi et al. 1973[1]
Fowman	10.4	2.7	6	1.5	
Teheran Institutions	–	–[3]	3.36	2.68	Habibi, 1965
Excluding Skin	–	–	4.6	3.2	
Teheran, Fars, Isfahan and Caspian Combined	–	–	8.65	6.20	Habibi, 1975
Southern Iran	16.8	9.7	–	–	Sadeghi et al. 1977[2]
Southern Iran	–	–	1.7	3.1	Haghighi et al. 1971
Excluding Skin	–	–	2	3.5	
Iran	–	–	4.6	3.2	Dunham & Bailar, 1968

[1] Estimated from available data.

[2] Crude incidence rate.

[3] Figures not given.

RELATIVE FREQUENCIES

As shown in Table 2, Habibi was the first to report the relatively high frequency of esophageal cancer in Teheran (cases from different social classes and from different parts of the country). Habibi included skin cancer, which was reported in 21.6 percent of all cases and esophageal cancer at a 3.06 percent rate (3.36% for males and 2.68 for females) (Habibi, 1965). If one excludes skin cancer in Habibi's study, then this percentage would increase from 3.36 to 4.6% and 2.68 to 3.18%, respectively. A 1968 study by Dunham and Bailar from the National Cancer Institute used 16 world maps to show cancer distribution by site. In the esophageal cancer map, this group considered the Iranian distribution as moderately high and their figures for the relative frequency are 4.6 and 3.2 percent for males and females, respectively, based on information obtained from different institutions by communicating through correspondence (Dunham and Bailar, 1968).

Habibi's report was followed by several from other investigators with similar
results (Haghighi et al., 1971; Sadeghi et al., 1977). In 1975 Habibi presented
another report to the International Round Table on Geocancerology and studied
171,500 histological specimens from Iran of which 40,690 or 24% were malignant.
For every 5 male victims there were 4 females for all cancer sites. There were
3,082 cases of esophageal cancer or a 7.57% relative frequency (1,980 or 8.65%
for men and 1,102 or 6.20% for women). All these different, unrelated independent
reports suggest that esophageal cancer is prevalent all over the Iranian plateau
and even in the well-known low incidence area of Gilan (an island with a low incidence of esophageal cancer within the esophageal cancer belt of Asia) where the
incidence is not actually low compared to that of western countries.

An interesting feature of esophageal cancer epidemiology in Iran, as in a few
other areas in Africa and France is found in the Caspian Littoral, where the incidence changes sharply (more than 30 times in females) within a distance of a few
hundred kilometers and accordingly offers a unique situation for comprehensive
and multidisciplinary epidemiological studies.*

AGE

The onset of the disease is in persons at least 10 years younger than in western
countries, not only in the high incidence area of northeastern Iran, but almost
all over the country. Most victims are from 45-55 years of age instead of 60-70.
Cases of esophageal carcinoma have also been diagnosed in 14-year-olds in
southern, central and northeastern Iran.

LOCATION OF TUMORS WITHIN ESOPHAGUS

In nearly every report from Iran, the proportion of tumors located in the esophagus being unknown varies and may be as great as 56.5%, as suggested in a report
from the Caspian (Mahboubi et al., 1973).

Depending on the area, the proportion of tumors diagnosed in the upper, middle
or lower third of the esophagus vary greatly (Table 3). In the Caspian Littoral,
the information for subsite distribution within the esophagus applies predominantly to the lower two-thirds of the organ, as in most parts of the world, and is
in the lower one-third in more than 54% of the cases. Only 13% of the cases have
tumors in the upper one-third of the esophagus. Reports from the south indicate
that at least 32% of the younger victims (under 40 years of age) have tumors in
the upper one-third of the esophagus while in those 50 years or older, the
location is similar to that in victims from other parts of the world (Sadeghi
et al., 1977). The reports, for example, from all other countries combined were
as follows: upper third, 22%, and for middle and lower thirds, 44 and 34%,
respectively (see Table 3).

---

*These studies are still underway, and were supported jointly by the School of
Public Health and the Institute of Public Health Research, University of Teheran
and the WHO International Agency for Research on Cancer, Lyon, France.

TABLE 3   Percentage of Tumor Location in Esophagus

Study Area	Upper	Middle	Lower	Source
Caspian Littoral	13	32	55	Mahboubi et al., 1973
Southern Iran	32	middle & lower	68	Sadeghi et al., 1977
Central Iran	22	44	34	Habibi et al., 1975
World	10% cervical	40% upper half	50% lower half	Moertel, 1973

HISTOPATHOLOGIC TYPES

In one study from southern Iran (Sadeghi et al., 1977), 93% of the tumors were squamous cell carcinomas and the remaining 7% were adenocarcinomas. Another study from the same area (Haghighi et al., 1971) indicated that 99% were squamous cell carcinomas and 1% adenocarcinomas. In numerous reports from the Caspian area, there was no mention of histological types, but unpublished data from the Caspian area (annual reports) indicated that all specimens biopsied and examined were mostly well-differentiated squamous cell carcinomas. No adenocarcinomas were observed (Salmasizadeh, 1978).

ETIOLOGICAL CONSIDERATIONS

In much of the world, esophageal cancer is generally a disease of men, while in parts of Africa and Western countries it is etiologically associated with excessive consumption of strong alcoholic beverages and tobacco smoking. However, these factors do not explain the high incidence areas in some parts of Asia, especially Iran, where a negligible role of alcohol and tobacco was shown (Mahboubi et al., 1977). The other environmental factors suggested as possible etiological causes are food and drink consumption at high temperature, chewing tobacco in the form of nass, opium smoking, ingestion of lye and heavily spiced food, mechanical trauma, nutritional deficiency, and presence of known chemical carcinogens, such as nitrosamines, polycyclic aromatic hydrocarbons and aflatoxins. There have also been some suggestions about soil deficient in molybdenum, copper and zinc used for raising crops and the importance of zinc in tissue repair (Rose, 1967; Oleske et al., 1978). The result of an epidemiological study in the high and low incidence areas of Iran for determination of exogenous factors showed no significant differences between areas and revealed that in the high incidence area there was a low intake of vitamins A and C, riboflavin, animal protein and fresh vegetables and fruit. Analysis of food and water from high and low incidence areas did not show any significant differences (Iran/IARC), 1977). Another suggested factor is that of mouldy cereals which are contaminated by certain metabolites of Fusaria and used to make fermented foods or alcoholic drinks (fusarium extracts are suspected of carcinogenic activity).

Other suggested factors such as stress, psychic depression and genetic background need more detailed study. The result of a genetic marker study in the Caspian Littoral indicated that no systematic relationship between genetic distance and the language affiliation was observed (the language in Gilan and Mazandaran is Persian with Gilaki and Mazandarani dialects and in Gonbad is Turkoman Turkik). However, there were significant differences in G6PD deficiency in different geographical areas (Kirk et al., 1977). The one factor common to all study

populations was that esophageal cancer patients were from the lower socioeconomic
classes of their community and it was further indicated that nutritional deficiencies of vitamins, minerals and especially of zinc might play a very important
role in predisposition of organ sites or promotion in esophageal epithelium for
tumor development or generally in the overall alteration of the immune system
of the body. It has been suggested that zinc plays an important role in the
function of T-cells in cellular immunity (Oleske et al., 1978) and it is shown
that immune disorders increase tumor susceptibility.

SUMMARY AND CONCLUSION

Iran has 35 million inhabitants, out of which only 4 million who live in the
narrow strip of the Caspian Littoral, are covered by a cancer registry. For the
rest of the country, information on cancer incidence is based on data of relative
frequencies from pathology reports. Therefore there is no way to show the exact
incidence of any cancer types including esophageal cancer, except for the
one-tenth of the population for which there are reliable and population-based
data available. For the rest of Iran, it is apparently from available information
that the occurrence of esophageal cancer in Iran (and perhaps in the neighboring
countries of Iraq and Turkey) is at least twice that normally expected in western
countries, even in the low incidence areas of Gilan. On the other hand the situation is very striking in the high incidence area, because esophageal cancer
constitutes more than 40% of all registered cancer cases. (It is likely that part
of this high proportion might be due to underdiagnosed and consequent under-
reporting of findings for other cancer sites.) In western countries esophageal
cancer accounts for less than 2% of all malignant neoplasms (Table 4). It has

TABLE 4   Comparison of Selected Sites of Cancer in the United States and Caspian
Littoral of Iran (CLI)

| | Relative incidence frequency | | | |
| | U.S. | | C.L.I. | |
	Male (%)	Female (%)	Male (%)	Female (%)
Esophagus	1.6	.6	44	42
Stomach	4	2.6	15	09
Lung	22	7	04	02
Colorectal	14	15	03	02
Pancreas	3.4	2.8	01	0.3

also been shown that the sharp variations in esophageal cancer incidence (30 times
in females and 10 times in males) takes place within areas not more than 500 kilometers apart. This unique situation has provided a good natural laboratory for
epidemiological studies. Thus far, the intensified search for the etiology of
esophageal cancer has failed to pinpoint any particular factor(s), such as alcohol
and tobacco, N-nitroso compounds, nitrites, nitrates, polycyclic aromatic hydrocarbons, and food and water samples from high and low incidence areas. However,
nutritional and vitamin deficiencies, consumption of hot tea, opium residue and
genetic susceptibility deserve more detailed study in this area. One should note
that a universal factor that includes almost all esophageal cancer patients is
that they belong to the lower socioeconomic classes of their community.

REFERENCES

Armin, K. (1967). Some statistical data on cancer mortality in Iran. Internat.
    Path., 8, 27–29.
Cook, P.J., and D.P. Burkitt (1971). Cancer in Africa. Brit. Med. Bull., 27, 14.
Doll, R. (1967). Prevention of cancer, pointers from epidemiology. The Nuffield
    Provincial Hospitals Trust, p. 42.
Doll, R., C. Muir, and J. Waterhouse (1970). Cancer incidence in five continents,
    Vol. II, Union Internationale Contre Cancer.
Dunham, L.J., and J.C. Bailar (1968). World maps of cancer mortality rates and
    frequency ratios. J. Natl. Cancer Inst., 41, 155–203.
Habibi, A. (1965). Cancer in Iran. A survey of the most common cases. J. Natl.
    Cancer Inst., 34, 553–569.
Habibi, A. (1976). Apercu general sur le cancer en Iran. International Bimonthly
    Magazine, 31, 26–42.
Haghighi, P., I. Nabizadeh, S. Asvadi, and E. Mohallatee (1971). Cancer in
    Southern Iran. Cancer, 27, 965–977.
Haghighi, P., and K. Nasr (1971). Gastrointestinal cancer in Iran. J. Chron. Dis.,
    24, 625–633.
Joint Iran IARC Study Group (1977). Esophageal cancer studies in the Caspian
    Littoral of Iran: Results of population studies–A prodrome. J. Natl. Cancer
    Inst., 59, 1127–1128.
Kirk, R.L., B. Keats, N.M. Blake, E.M. McDermid, F. Ala, M. Karimi, B. Nickbin,
    H. Shahbazi, and J. Kmet (1977). Genes and people in the Caspian Littoral:
    A population genetic study in Northern Iran. Am. J. Phys. Anthrop., 46,
    377–390.
Kmet, J., and E. Mahboubi (1972). Esophageal cancer in the Caspian Littoral of
    Iran: Initial studies. Science, 175, 846–853.
Kmet, J. (1974). Epidemiology of the esophagus. Excerpta Med. Internat. Congress,
    3, 258–261.
Mahboubi, E., J. Kmet, P.J. Cook, N.E. Day, P. Ghadirian, and S. Salmasizadeh
    (1973). Oesophageal cancer studies in the Caspian Littoral of Iran: The Caspi
    an cancer registry. Brit. J. Cancer, 28, 197–214.
Mahboubi, E., J. Kmet, and S. Salmasizadeh (1974). The search for an environmental
    carcinogen in the etiology of esophageal cancer in the Caspian Littoral of
    Iran. Excerp. Med., 3, 253–257.
Mahboubi, E., N.D. Day, P. Ghadirian, and S. Salmasizadeh (1977). Negligible role
    of alcohol and tobacco in the etiology of esophageal cancer in Iran–A case
    control study. Cancer Det. Prevent., 2, 1149–1159.
Moertel, C.G. (1973). The esophagus. In J. Holland and E. Frei (Eds.), Phila-
    delphia, Cancer Medicine. Lea & Febiger, pp. 1519–1526.
Oleske, J., M. Westphal, S. Starr, S. Shore, D. Gorden, J. Bodgen, D. Caplan,
    and A. Nahmias (1978). Zinc therapy for acrodermatitis enteropathica. In:
    Infectious diseases.
Rose, E.F. (1967). A study of esophageal cancer in the Transkei. National Cancer
    Institute Monogr., 25, 83–96.
Sadeghi, A., S. Behmard, H. Shafiepoor, and E. Zeighmani (1977). Cancer of the
    esophagus in Southern Iran. Cancer, 40, 841–845.
Sarkissian, S. (1960). A study of carcinoma of esophagus in Iran. Acta Medica
    Iranica, 4, 10–13.
Segi, M., and M. Kurihara (1972). In: Cancer Mortality for Selected Sites in 24
    Countries, Vol. 6, p. 96.
Tuyns, A.J., and L.M.F. Masse (1973). Mortality from cancer of the esophagus in
    Brittany. Int. J. Epid., 2, 242–245.
Waterhouse, J., C. Muir, P. Correa, and J. Powell (1976). Cancer incidence in
    five continents, Vol. III. Lyon, IARC Scientific Publication No. 15.

Cancer of Oesophagus in Iran—Etiological Consideration

A. Modjtabai

Tadj Pahlavi Cancer Institute, Teheran University, Teheran, Iran

INTRODUCTION

Iran has a population of 35 million people and is one of the largest countries in the Middle East. Its official religion is Islam but from the ethnological standpoint the Iranians belong to an Indoeuropean race with some strains of Arab and Mongolian blood in certain parts of the country.

From the available information on the incidence of oesophageal cancer in Iran, it appears that this disease is common in most parts of the country, particularly in the northeast of the Caspian Littoral.

The population of the Caspian Littoral are not homogenous, neither from the geographical zones they occupy nor in their ethnic affiliations. Our study shows that they are also genetically heterogenesus.

The statistical studies carried out in the northeastern part of Iran by the International Agency for Research on Cancer (IARC) in the recent years have shown that the incidence of this disease varies among men and women and that the farther we move from northeast to northwest the incidence of this disease tends to decrease.

On the basis of studies undertaken by the Radiotherapy Department of Taj Pahlavi Cancer Institute on 1108 patients and also on the strength of studies carried out on 3985 cases of patients by the Department of Pathalogy of the above Institute, over a ten year period, indicate without doubt that the high incidence of this disease in the south and southeastern region of the Caspian Sea is more common than in other parts of the country, with a higher incidence among men than women in 55-65 year of age group.

The factors which may play a role in the etiology of this disease in Iran may be seemed as follows:

1. Tobacco:

In contrast to the published figures in other parts of the world that the use of alcohol and tobacco are the main factors for causing cancer of oesophagus the figures available in Iran fail to confirm the above conclusion. The people of that

part of Iran populated mostly by Turkamans hardly use more than ten to fifteen cig
arettes a day and yet it is considered as a high risk area. Furthermore, in this
area the women smoke even less than men and yet this disease is more common among
them in some parts of this area than among men.

2. Nass:

Nass is a substance composed of tobacco, wood ash and vegetable oil. It is chewed
in this part of the country which is considered a high risk area for this type of
disease.

The biochemical research carried out in this substance has failed so far to establish the existance of a carcinogenic substance, especially nitrozamine. For this
reason, we now believe that this substance alone cannot be responsible for the pathogenesis of cancer of oesophagus.

3. Alcohol:

This factor seems unlikely to play a significant role in the etiology of this disease:

a) The Islamic religion forbides its members to consume Alcohol.

b) In high incidence areas the disease is more common among women than men even
   though it is a fact that women, in general, consume less or even no alcohol at
   all.

c) In those parts of the country where a large number of non-Moslems live and use
   a considerable amounts of alcohol than their Moslem compatriots, the incidence
   of this disease nevertheless is very low among them.

4. Opium:

Aside from opium the following derivations from opium are used to an appreciable
degree in the high risk areas:

a) Shireh.   This product with opium as its base is produced by boiling a mixture of
             row opium and "sukhte" or burnt residue of opium, in water for 5 to 10
             minutes. After filtering this concusion a gumy residue is obtained
             which is then smoked through a pipe in a special manner.

b) Sukhteh. It is the lumpy residue of opium formed in the interior part of the
            pipe. It is either smoked through a pipe or eaten in required quanti-
            ties by the addicts.

Although a substantial number of the population in this region use opium, yet biological and clinical evidences fail to show relationship between the use of opium
and the use of opium and the existance of cancer of oesophagus.

The vast majority of those who use opium in this area use the so-called "sukhte".
For some time it was thought that since the burnt opium underwent chemical changes
in body, very probably in the process of such metabolic changes a carcinogenic substance came into existance. But the researches on this subject have failed so far
to establish the validity of this assumption.

On the other hand mutagenecity of burnt opium (sukhteh) or at least procaryotic
cells has been shown recently.

Sukhteh, the tar of opium smoke is mutagenic for at least salmonella strains of Ames. At the concentration of 25 micograms per dish the numbers of histidine revertant colonies of TA 100 and TA 1538 increase over 2-4 times compared with controls.

So there is not doubt that sukhteh is mutagenic on at least salmonella strains of Ames. Mutagenecity of sukhteh on other procayotes as well as eucaryotic cells has not been studied so far. We are taking steps to determine the mutagenecity of sukhteh on mammalian cells using mammalian cell culture system.

In this context two questions should be resolved:

1. Is the mutagenecity of sukhteh due to a presisting compound or is it due to the presence of a compound not already existing in the opium but synthezied during smoking processes?

2. In any situation is this mutagenic agent really carcinogenic or not?

5. Tea:

Drinking a large quantity of tea while hot by the vast majority of people of this area was considered as another probable etiological factor. But statistical figures obtained on 956 cases of cancer of oesophagus and 427 cases of larynx indicated that most people suffering from these two diseases actually consume a lesser amount of tea than the population as a whole.

6. Nutritional Study:

The nutritional pilot study by the Institute of Public Health, Tehran University, and IARC shows, very little sign of protein or caloric malnutrition.

a) Iron deficiency anaemia appeared to be common in women.

b) Riboflavin deficiency, especially in children were seen and varied from 9 to 22% and from 5 to 24% in the adults of different villages, and was uncommon in children under age 1. High frequency of riboflavin deficiency is consistant with the hypothesis of a dietary induced increase in susceptibility of oesophageal cancer.

c) Aflatoxin. The chemical analysis of food stuffs from the Turkaman area has eliminated the possibility that aflatoxin from these sources are responsible for the very high incidence.

d) As the food of the population of this area is limited mostly to a whole wheat, bread, and the manner it is prepared attention was focused on the question whether N-Nitrozamine, polycyclic aromatic hydrocarbones and aflatoxine existed in the bread used by them. The result showed that they did not exist to the extent to be a factor in the etiology of this disease.

7. As plants of poppy which belongs to fumaria species grow in the east of the Caspian Littoral where cancer of oesophagus has high incidence it was assumed that there might be a close relationship between the toxic substance in the poppy and cancer of oesophagus. At the present we are not able to verify this aaumption.

8. Histocampatibility:

Lymphocytes of 58 patients from different ethnic groups who had definite traces of oesophageal cancer and 121 normal individual from the corresponding population were typed by the Institute of Public Health Research, Tehran University. Based on a relatively small number of cases the frequency of HLA B40 seems noticeably to be high among the cancer patients in comparison with the normal controls. The increase frequency of B40 in oesophageal cancer patients from different ethnic group is suggestive of an association between this HLA antigen and greater risk of the disease, but on the basis of figures we have at our disposable it must be said that HLA B40 is common among the population of this area and therefore this factor cannot be said to play a significant role in the pathogenesis of this disease in this area.

EBV Virus:

Since these two diseases, namely Burkitt Lymphoma and NPC have been proved to be related, etiologically speaking, to EBV and in view of the fact that these two diseases from the standpoint of geographical pathology are observed in specific areas, it has been assumed that the cancer of oesophagus which is observed in specific regions of the world might be related, etiologically, to EBV. On the other hand, sera of 144 patients and their controls were assayed for the presence of anti EBV-VCA. Of all the patients 26% had titres higher than 1:160 in comparison with only 13% of control. In sera for anti CMV no significant differance between patients and their controls was observed, and it goes to show that no relationship whatsoever between EBV and oesophageal cancer exist. The result though not satisfactory, but seems to be encouraging.

Conclusion:

The cancer of oesophagus is a disease which is very prevalent in the north and northeastern regions of Iran.

Different factors have been supposed to be contributive to this type of cancer but none of them have been conclusive. Among the various factors mentioned above the exposure to a carcinogenic agent derived either from opium tars or wheat seem to play a significant role in the etiology of this disease. A genetic component also cannot be excluded, because the highest incidence occurs in a population who are mostly of Turkaman-Mongolian origin.

Inspite of the above statements more researchs must be carried out to determine the specific factors involved in the high incidence of cancer of oesophagus in the region. In this connection extensive researches are being carried out by IARC and Iranian research groups the results of which I hope to be available in a not long distant future.

Epidemiology of Oesophageal Cancer in Southern Africa

E. F. Rose

National Research Institute for Nutritional Diseases (East London Branch)
P.O. Box 192, East London, 5200, South Africa

ABSTRACT

Rates for oesophageal cancer in certain areas of Southern Africa are amongst the highest in the world. In others it remains low. Clues to etiology can be found in the variation in incidence between the sexes in specific geographical areas, different races and cultures and in the changing time pattern. An indepth study of a high incidence area, Transkei, over 23 years shows strong associations with geophysical environmental parameters which collectively would be expected to limit food production and induce trace element deficiencies. Results from 3 separate comparative studies undertaken in areas of high and low incidence implicate pipe smoking on the one hand and a lowered intake of vitamin rich foods on the other. The rising incidence evident in certain areas appears to be related to changing eating habits more than customs, suggesting increased susceptibility, through lack of protective foods, to carcinogens already present in the environment.

Keywords: oesophagus, cancer, geophysical, trace elements, smoking, vitamins, susceptibility, carcinogens.

INTRODUCTION

No disease has been more taunting to treat nor elusive to cause finding than cancer of the oesophagus since it was first described by GALEN in the second century A.D. Multiple contradictory theories have been proposed as etiological factors, none of which have been proved. Yet in the very nature of the disease lie the clues to it's causation, viz.: the high pockets of incidence amongst some peasant farmers living on a mono-cereal staple diet; the low socio-economic status of those most at risk in cities and the decrease in incidence in those countries whose standard of living has risen.

DEMOGRAPHY

The most characteristic feature of oesophageal cancer in Southern Africa is its changing pattern. This is reflected in time, in geographical area, amongst the races and between the sexes.

Spatial Distribution

A nation wide survey of hospital attendances (Oettle, 1963) shows an uneven distribution of the disease, where the highest attendance rate, apart from Bulawayo, Rhodesia (Skinner, 1965) was found in the south-eastern parts, particularly in Transkei (Fig. 1). Other areas of high incidence were where the greatest concentration of Transkeians worked.

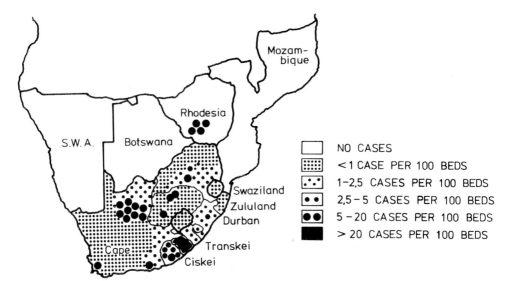

Fig. 1. Incidence of oesophageal cancer among Blacks, calculated per 100 hospital beds per annum.

Corroborative evidence is reflected in an 8 year survey of mine-workers (Harington and Bradshaw, 1977) where the highest number of oesophageal cancer cases came from the southern districts of Transkei. Hospital surveys indicate the relative frequency of a disease rather than the actual prevalence. This was well demonstrated in an indepth demographic survey in Transkei (Rose, 1973) where 5095 cases were identified at their home sites over 15 years, only 3281 of whom were recorded in hospitals draining the area. The pattern of frequency between the two groups, however, was the same (Rose and McGlashan, 1975). In Transkei where 50% of all tumors are oesophageal, there is a marked variation between districts being highest in the southern districts and central plains (Fig. 2).

Variation in Time

A characteristic of this disease in many parts of the world is the changing pattern with time (Segi, 1966). This is most dramatically demonstrated in the Black races in Southern Africa. Cancer surveys in Zululand, Natal and Transvaal undertaken before 1920 make no mention of the disease. In 3851 post-mortems performed in Johannesburg (Strachan, 1934) 24 oesophageal cancers were found in White men, 2 in White women and only 3 in Black men. Yet by 1954 (Higginson and Oettlé, 1960) it was the most commonly encountered tumor in Bantu males, viz.: 10.3% of all cancers admitted; by 1964 it had risen to 27.5%. The rise in the same period in females was 0.8% to 4.7%. The disease is increasing in the areas of lowest incidence in Transkei as well as in the Zulus of Durban (E. Bradshaw, personal communication). Keen (1978) has also commented on the increase in Northern Transvaal where, in some hospitals, the prevalence of liver cancer appears to be decreasing and oesophageal cancer increasing. Recent reports from Lesotho (Martin, personal communication) indicate that the disease is now being seen for the first time in some areas. In South West Africa, Botswana and Mozambique the incidence of oeso-

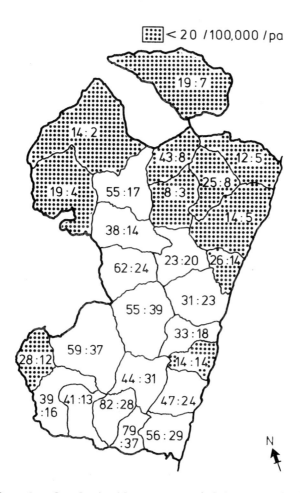

Fig. 2. Male : female incidence rates (African standard) of
oesophageal cancer in Transkei for 1965-1969.
Shaded districts average below 20 per 100 000 p.a.

phagus cancer remains low. Hospitals in the Ciskei and Transkei dating back to
1913 show a slowly increasing incidence in the Transkei since 1930, with an explo-
sive rise after 1940, the time of the first appearance of the disease in the Ciskei
(Fig. 3). Records from Baragwanath Hospital, Johannesburg, show a rising incidence
since its inception after 1945. This rise is paralleled in all hospitals of Transkei, whether in low or high incidence areas (Rose, 1977).

Racial Distribution

The population of Southern Africa which is multi-racial as well as multi-cultural,
provides an unique opportunity for studying the inter-relationship between disease
patterns, race and cultural habits. The largest group of people are Black Africans,
comprising many and diverse tribes. Next in order are the 2 White groups, followed
by Coloureds of mixed origin and Indians from Asia. Mortality data for the last 3
groups from 1949 to 1969 showed no change in oesophageal cancer mortality in Asian
and White males, nor in Coloured and White females (Bradshaw and Harington, 1975).

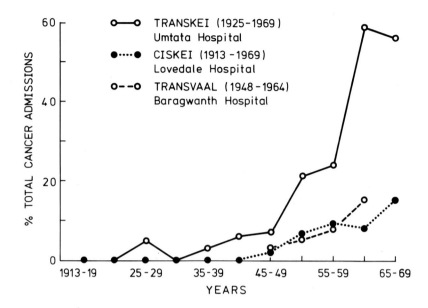

Fig. 3. Increase of oesophagus cancer admissions over time
in 3 widely dispersed hospitals.

Figure 4 demonstrates a slowly rising mortality since that time in both White and
Asian males. Coloured males on the other hand show a remarkable rise since 1954,
similar to that seen in Black people a decade earlier. The steady, but not so dramatic rise in Indian women is noteworthy, as is the recent rise in Coloured females. It appears that only White women have remained unaffected over the last
27 years. Histological records from the Frere Hospital, East London, reflect the
typical variation of incidence between Whites, Coloureds and Blacks (Table 1).
Here 1.7% of all cancers in White males and 0.3% in White females were oesophageal.
In Black and Coloured males it was 26% and 30% and 9% and 4% for their females.
There was a 15-fold difference between White and Black males, and a 30-fold difference between White and Black females.

TABLE 1 Histologically-proven Cancers in 3 Racial Groups
(1966-1967) seen at Frere Pathology Laboratory

Race	Total Cancers seen		Oesophageal Cancer		
	M	F	Males	Females	M:F Ratio
Whites	291	330	5	1	5.7 : 1
Coloureds	26	24	7	1	6.6 : 1
Bantu	326	450	86	40	2.9 : 1

A similar pattern between the races was described by Muir Grieve (1967) in the
Western Cape where the majority of Black people were migrant labourers from the
Transkei.

Sex Distribution

The sex distribution is as inconsistent as every other parameter related to this

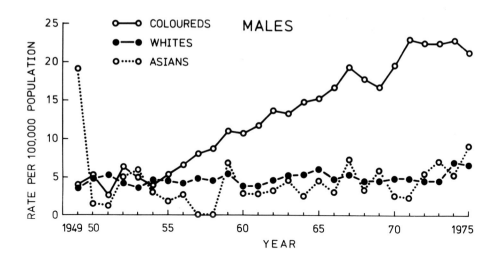

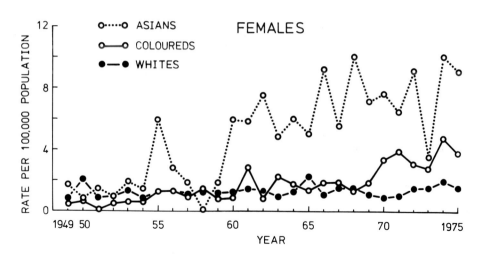

Fig. 4. Mortality rates for oesophageal cancer in three racial groups over 27 years in males and females.
(Age adjusted and standardized to UICC World Population).

disease and neither sex appears to be immune. Generally speaking, where the incidence of the disease is low the males appear to be more prone, but as the incidence
rises, so the sex ratio approaches unity, but this is not consistent. In 1954 in
Johannesburg the ratio of males to females was 26 : 1 (Higginson and Oettlé, 1960)
now it is 7 : 1. In the low incidence areas of Transkei the male to female ratio
is increasing. In the areas of high incidence the rise is in females. White females continue to have a low incidence and Indian females have a higher incidence
than Indian males. The rise in incidence in Coloured males preceded the rise in
their female counterparts by 10 years.

ASSOCIATION BETWEEN PHYSICAL ENVIRONMENT AND THE DISEASE

Consistent differehces of incidence rate in defined areas like the situation in Transkei encouraged the search for associated environmental variables which may be linked to the etiology.   The first clear finding associated with the disease was that a significantly greater number of persons with the disease lived and farmed on Beaufort sedimentary soils than on those soils derived from the more fertile volcanic dolerite (Marais & Drewes, 1962).   This finding initiated an investigation of the trace element profiles in the plants grown in gardens of cancer sufferers and areas where no oesophageal cancer was reported.   Deficiencies were found chiefly of Mo, Zn, Cu, Fe and Mg (Burrell, Roach and Shadwell, 1966).   On the presumption that lack of these elements might favour the formation of nitrosamines in plants, Roach set up an agricultural experiment, the results of which are not all available to date, but seem to indicate a relationship between lack of these elements and the presence of low levels of nitrosamines.   Certainly rats fed on food grown in gardens of cancer patients exhibited degenerative changes in basal cell nuclei of the oesophagus with some basal cell hyperplasia, mild dysplasia and cellular infiltration of the lamina propria (Van Rensburg and co-workers, 1974).

Arising from the findings of Marais and Drewes (1962) geophysical parameters in relation to clustering of cases were analysed (Rose, 1978).   The greatest clustering was found at an altitude of 1000-3000 feet where the soil was alkaline, on Beaufort sediments, thorn veld and in the lowest rainfall areas.   The correlation with rainfall demonstrated an inverse trend of cancer rate from areas of highest to lowest rainfall.   There were also significantly more cases than expected where the population was densest (Table 2).

TABLE 2 The Association of Environmental Factors with
Oesophageal Cancer Incidence in Transkei

Environmental Factor	Range	Characteristic Associated[*]
Population Density	56 - 150/sq. mile	Highest
Vegetation	10 Types	E.P. Thornveld[**]
Rainfall	600 - 1400 mm p.a.	600 - 800
Geology	7 Types	Beaufort Sediment[**]
Soil Type	6 Types	E.P. Semi-coastal belt[**]
Topography	0 - 8000 ft.	1000 - 3000

[*] P<0,01

[**] Inferior Types

A combination of these factors together with poor farming practices suggest a reduction of food production potential.   Many minerals are unavailable in alkaline soils and increasing populations would be competing for food grown under these conditions.

HABITS AND CUSTOMS

A marked difference was found in the habits and customs of people living in high and low incidence areas (Rose, in press).   Although these differences could be

related to tribal variations rather than causally to the differing cancer incidence, a number of factors were identical to those found in a case control study
which bridged tribal and geographical barriers.   The differences common to both
studies could be divided into two categories.

Firstly, in areas of high incidence and amongst cancer patients there was a
greater and different use of tobacco, potentially harmful medicinal plants (Roach,
Du Plessis and Nunn, 1969) and edible weeds (Mirvish, Rose and Sutherland, 1978).
Roasting food on the coals and the use of dung as fuel are also more common.   On
the other hand, more foods in the form of protein, vegetables and fruit were consumed by the people of the low incidence area.   Bradshaw and Schonland (1974)
showed an association between smoking, especially of pipes and oesophageal cancer
but were not able to show a significant correlation with alcohol or cigarette
smoking in two studies undertaken in the cities of Johannesburg and Durban.   Data
from the Transkei confirm these findings.   More tobacco is grown and smoked in
pipes in the high risk areas particularly by women who also suck the pipe residue
which is highly mutagenic (Hewer and associates, 1978).   Men of both areas smoke,
but in areas of low incidence they also use more commercial tobacco and cigarettes.

Although pipe smoking appears to be associated with the disease, 16 - 20% of cancer cases in Johannesburg (Hunt, 1977) and Transkei never smoked, and 20% of
Johannesburg controls and 58% of those in the Transkei claimed to be heavy pipe
smokers, starting before the age of 20.   Another fact to be considered is that
women who cling to their traditions smoke the most and are least at risk for
oesophageal cancer.

Therefore although potential carcinogens are more evident in the environment of
cancer sufferers, the association with lowered intake of protective foods should
not be ignored.

WESTERNIZATION AND URBANIZATION

Pockets of highest incidence of oesophageal cancer are found amongst peasant
farmers.   The disease is however not confined to rural areas.   In Denmark
Clemmenson (1965) found that urban males, but not females, had a higher incidence
than their rural counterparts.   True urbanization is difficult to assess in the
Black African.   In Hunt's series (1977) 58% had spent the major portion of their
life in towns but only 14% were born there.   Urbanization is not necessarily
synonymous with Westernization (Meyer, 1961).   The more educated Black people
usually assume a Western culture.   In Transkei there is a group of conservative
people, however, the "Qaba", who are antagonistic to Western ways, and wherever
they live they retain their traditional culture.   Intermediate are the "Qoboka",
people in transition not wholly commited to either group.   These are the people
most at risk for cancer of the oesophagus, more so in the men than the women,
with the "Qaba" females least at risk (Table 3).

TABLE 3 The Relationship between Oesophageal Cancer and
Acculturization in an High Incidence Area of Transkei[*]

| Acculturization | Observed cases over 15 year period | Crude rates per 10^5 p.a. | |
		Males	Females
"Qaba" (traditional)	124	45[**]	35[**]
"Qoboka" (semi-westernized)	137	88	58

[*]Kentani district - excluding sub-districts with a mixed population.
[**]Less (P < 0,01) than expected.

GENETIC SUSCEPTIBILITY AND CLUSTERING

Although this disease appears in all racial groups in varying degrees, the rates
are high wherever there is a predominance of Xhosa speaking people who originate
from Transkei.   However, in Johannesburg the Tswana people show the highest rate
relative to their population size, and the rates are rising in the other Black
races of Johannesburg.

Hammond and co-workers (1977) conducted HLA studies in South African Negroes and
found that HLA-BW-45 was significantly increased in oesophageal cancer cases.

In Transkei cases of oesophageal cancer tend to aggregate.   Although there are
many families in which there are a high proportion of first degree relatives with
the disease, we also have a high proportion of husband and wife and close neigh-
bours dying within a few years of each other.

The study on familial clustering is not yet completed and may show a significant
bias towards blood relations but at present a common environment seems more important than consanguinity.

DISCUSSION

In the very nature and inconsistency of this disease lie the clues to its
etiology.   All evidence points to a multi-factorial situation, the clarification
of which requires detailed knowledge regarding the interplay of factors culminat-
ing in the final fatal outcome.

In cities the disease appears to be strongly associated with a low socio-economic
status, alcohol and tobacco usage, but pockets of extreme incidence are invariably
found amongst peasant farmers who live chiefly on a monostaple grain diet which
suggests an imbalance between factors carcinogenic and those which protect.

Generally speaking South African Whites regularly consume more spirits and smoke
more commercial cigarettes than South African Blacks but on the whole have a
balanced diet.   Most South African Coloureds have a low standard of living and
are notorious for their drinking habits, particularly of wine.   This is not new
but their rising rate of oesophageal cancer is.   Indians are not particularly
heavy drinkers or smokers and have a varied diet.   However, the women whose rate
of cancer for the mouth, throat, oesophagus and stomach is greater than that for
males, chew more betel nuts than their menfolk.   Tobacco is rarely added to the
quid which consists of nut, leaf and small quantities of lime (Schonland and
Bradshaw, 1969).

The traditional diet of the Black races of Southern Africa has been wild game,
soured milk, sorghum, pumpkin, pulses and maize.   In 1938 Fox warned that with
such a simple but adequate diet there was a danger that small changes were capable of initiating serious deficiencies which would be less likely to occur with
a diet resting on a broader foundation.   With the opening up of the country and
increased population wild game has become scarce, and milk less readily obtainable.
Sorghum has been replaced by maize, both in the towns and country.   Westernization has promoted the use of refined maize meal and white flour which (denatured
as they are Fox, 1966) are more readily available and less trouble to prepare.
Consequently there has been an increase in carbohydrate consumption and a relative
decrease in protein with the emergence of nutritional deficiencies.   The drinking
of beer is traditional in South African Black people and smoking is an old custom
but eating habits have changed.   It appears that carcinogens can be found in any
environment to a greater or lesser extent but their action is minimal as long as
there is an equilibrium between them and those factors which protect.   When this
equilibrium is disturbed either by increase of carcinogens or co-carcinogens on

the one hand, or the decrease of protective factors on the other, that problems arise. All evidence regarding the genesis of the disease points to an imbalance between those factors which protect and those which cause insult to the epithelium of the oesophagus.

REFERENCES

Bradshaw, E. and J.S. Harington (1975). Changing pattern of cancer mortality in South Africa. S.A. Med. J., 49, 919-925.

Bradshaw, E. and M. Schonland (1974). Smoking, drinking and oesophageal cancer in African males of Johannesburg, South Africa. Br. J. Cancer, 30, 157.

Burrell, R.J.W., W.A. Roach and W. Shadwell (1966). Oesophageal cancer in the Bantu of the Transkei associated with mineral deficiencies in garden plants. J. Nat. Canc. Inst., 36, 201-214.

Clemmenson, J. (1965). Statistical studies in the aetiology of malignant neo-plasms. Acta. Path. 8 Microbiol. Scandin., suppl. 174, 112.

Fox, F.W. (1938) Some nutritional problems amongst the Bantu in South Africa. Premero Congresso Médico de Lourenco Marques, 3, 93-114.

Fox, F.W. (1966). Studies on chemical composition of foods commonly used in Southern Africa. S.A. Institute for Medical Research, Johannesburg.

Hammond, M.G., B. Appadoo and P. Brain (1977). HLA and cancer in South African Negroes. Tissue Antigens, 9, 1-7.

Harington, J.S. and E. Bradshaw (1977). Cancer of the oesophagus with special reference to gold miners from the Transkei and to Colored males. In W. Silber (Ed.), Carcinoma of the Oesophagus, Balkema, Cape Town.

Hewer, T, E. Rose, P. Chadirian, M. Castegnaro, C. Malareille, H. Bartsch and N. Day (1978). Ingested mutagens from opium and tobacco pyrolysis products and cancer of the oesophagus. Lancet (in press).

Higginson, J. and G. Oettlé (1960). Cancer incidence in the Bantu and Cape Colored races of South Africa. J. Nat. Canc. Inst., 24, 589-671.

Hunt, J.A. (1978). Squamous cancer of the oesophagus in urban South African Blacks. In W. Silber (Ed.), Cancer of the Oesophagus, Balkema, Cape Town.

Keen, P. (1977). The epidemiology of oesophageal cancer in South Africa. In W. Silber (Ed.), Carcinoma of the Oesophagus, Balkema, Cape Town.

Marais, J.A.H. and E.F.R. Drewes (1962). The relationship between solid geology and oesophageal cancer distribution in the Transkei. Ann. Geol. Surv., 1, 105-116.

Mayer, P. (1961). Townsmen and Tribesmen. Oxford University Press, Cape Town.

Mirvish, S., E.F. Rose and M. Sutherland (1978). Studies on oesophagus II enhance-ment of (3H) thymidine incorporation in rat oesophagus by Bidens pilosa, a South African edible plant, and by croton oil. "Cancer letters".

Muir Grieve, J. (1967). Cancer in the Cape division, South Africa. Oxford Uni-versity Press, London, New York, Toronto.

Oettlé, A.G. (1963). Regional variations in frequency of Bantu oesophageal cancer cases admitted to hospitals in South Africa. S.A. Med. J., 32, 434-439.

Roach, W.A., L.S. du Plessis and J.R. Nunn (1969). Carcinogen in a Transkeian Bantu food additive. Nature, 222, 1198-1199.

Rose, E.F. (1973). Oesophageal cancer in the Transkei 1955-69. Nat. Canc. Inst., 51, 7-16.

Rose, E.F. and N.D. McGlashan (1975). The spatial distribution of oesophageal carcinoma in the Transkei, South Africa. Br. J. Cancer, 31, 197-206.

Rose, E.F. (1977). Patterns of occurrence of oesophageal cancer with particular reference to the Transkei. In W. Silber (Ed.), Carcinoma of the Oesophagus, Balkema, Cape Town.

Rose, E.F. (1978). Demographic risk factors in causation of oesophageal cancer in the Transkei. In H.E. Nieburgs (Ed.), Cancer Detection and Prevention, Part II, Vol. 3, Marcel Dekker Inc. New York and Basle.

Schonland, M. and E. Bradshaw (1969). Upper alimentary tract cancer in Natal
    Indians with special reference to Betel chewing habit. Br. Journal Cancer,
    23, 670.
Segi, M. and M. Kurihara (1966). Cancer mortality for selected sites in 24
    countries. Tohoku University School of Medicine, Sendai, Japan, 4, 270.
Skinner, M.E.G. (1965). Malignant diseases of the gastro-intestinal tract in
    Rhodesian Africans with special reference to the urban population of Bulawayo.
    A preliminary report. Nat. Canc. Inst., Monograph 25, 57-71.
Strachan, A.S. (1934). Observations on the incidence of malignant disease in
    South African Natives. Journal of Pathology, 39, 209-211.
Van Rensburg, S.J., I.F.H. Purchase, E.F. Rose and W.A. Roach (1974). Structural
    alterations in the rat oesophagus epithelium after ingestion of the Transkei
    diet. S.A. Med. J., 48, 2361-2362.

Investigation of Etiologic Factors in Esophageal Cancer in Western France: Chemical Studies and Mutagenic Effect of Alcoholic Beverages

E. Walker*, J. J. Castegnaro*, E. Loquet** and J. Y. Le Talaer**

*Service des Cancérogènes, CIRC, Lyon, France
**Centre François Baclesse, Caen, France

INTRODUCTION

We have learnt from the investigations reported by Dunham and Bailer (1968) on countries with esophageal cancer mortality rates that France and Switzerland are the only 2 countries in Western Europe where the mortality rate exceeds 10 p. 100.000 in males.

Epidemiologic investigations conducted by the CIRC and published by Dr Tuyns (1973) have shown that France has 2 regions with exceptionally high mortality, Normandy and Brittany. The mortality rates in certain countries in these Western provinces are 6 to 8 times higher than those for the country as a whole, while overall mortality from esophageal cancer in France is already 2 to 3 times higher than that for the whole of Western Europe (Barrellier, 1974).

These same two provinces also have the highest mortality rates from alcoholism and cirrhosis of the liver. Further epidemiologic studies (Tuyns, 1973) conducted in the department of Ille and Vilaine (Brittany) have demonstrated the important role played by alcohol and tobacco in esophageal cancers. Findings show that for each of these substances there is a correlation between cancer risk and average daily intake, and that these risks combined have a multiplicative effect.

These observations prompted us to investigate the possible role played by some of the preferred alcoholic beverages in these regions, particularly apple cider and its distillates.

A series of investigations were conducted in an attempt to find answers to the following questions :

Do these beverages contain a particular substance that could be implicated in the etiology of cancer of the esophagus ?

With regard to this, do the beverages show a difference in composition according to geographic origin or mode of production (home-produced or industrially produced) ?

Three kinds of investigations were carried out : analytic, biologic and experimental.

In the first, the beverages were analyzed for the presence of certain know carcinogens, particularly Nitrosamines, which have been found to be organotropic to the esophagus in animals (Druckrey, 1961), certain aromatic polycyclic hydrocarbons and certain mycotoxins. ˙

Secondly, biological studies were conducted and the beverages and their fractions (Loquet, 1977) were examined for possible mutagenic effect using Ames' method (1973) of bacterial strains.

Finally, animal experiments were prepared. These are currently underway.

We would like to report on some of the results obtained in the first two sections of our investigations.

CHEMICAL INVESTIGATIONS

TABLE 1.   Breakdown of 268 samples

Home-produced apple brandy	94
Industrially produced apple brandy	39
Other spirits (whisky, cognac, rum	46
Apple cider	21
Beer	35
Wine	33

This table shows the breakdown of the different alcoholic beverages analysed, according to production method and type :

Home-Produced Apple Brandy

This apple cider distillate has an alcohol content that varies from 50° to 70°. It is produced directly at the farm, where it is consumed, undiluted, often in a cup of hot coffee. This is the beverage most commonly consumed by esophageal cancer patients.

Industrially Produced Apple Brandy

A cider distillate that is commercialized after dilution to 40°.

Other Spirits

Distillates of different beverages with an alcoholic content of about 40° (whisky, cognac, rum, etc...) were used for controls.

Two hundred sixty eight samples of alcoholic beverages were analyzed. They comprised : 154 apple beverages (133 apple brandies and 21 apple ciders, most of which were produced locally) and 114 other alcoholic drinks that are commonly used in the rest of the country.

The analyses compared the N-nitroso-compound content of those beverages possibly linked with cancer morbidity in Brittany and Normandy, with that of other beverages which are widely used in the whole of the country and are thus not considered to be particularly implicated in these regions.

VOLATILE NITROSAMINS CONTENT IN ALCOHOLIC BEVERAGES

Arithmetic Results of Analyses

Nitrosamine content was determined by gas chromatography and confirmed by mass spectography. We used a detector with selectivity for N-nitroso-compounds able to detect quantitites of 0.05 ug/l or more.

Table 2 and Table 3 give   results obtained for N-nitroso-dimethylamines, N-nitroso-diethylamines and N-nitroso-dipropylamines.

The beverage were divided into two groups : those with an alcohol content of 40° or more, and those with an alcohol content of 15° or under.

The tables give the number of positive samples, the maximum amounts and the arithmetic averages. Samples where these substances were not observed were retained in the calculation of the average amounts.

TABLE 2. Beverages with high alcoholic content

Beverage with alcohol content ⩾ 40 %	No of samples tested	N-nitroso-dimethylamines			N-nitroso diethylamines			N-nitroso dipropylamines		
		value max. µg/l	% of positive samples	average µg/l	value max. µg/l	% of positive samples	average µg/l	value max. µg/l	% of positive samples	average µg/l
Home-produced apple brandy	94	10	44	0,66	0,9	10	0,04	0,5	4	0,1
Industrially-produced apple brandy	39	3,6	51	0,38	2	36	0,15	2,6	23	0,13
Other fruit brandies	9	2,2	44	0,49	4,8	67	0,5	-	-	-
Whisky	8	0,7	75	0,26	0,4	38	0,1	0,4	25	0,09
Rhum	17	3	41	0,24	0,2	29	0,05	0,2	12	0,02
Cognac and Armagnac	12	1,6	66	0,33	0,9	42	0,15	0,3	8	-

The results show that almost all of the samples contained small amounts of the three nitrosamines NDMA, NDEA, NDPA; no evidence of other notrosamines was found.

These three compounds are found in the apple brandies as well as in the other beverages.

NDMA concentrations of 10 ug/l were found in some of the home-produced apple brandies, but amounts were mostly small and the averages was 0.6 ug/l.

The NDMA content of the industrially produced apple brandies was even lower; it was similar to that of the other beverages with high alcohol content.

TABLE 3. Beverages with low alcoholic content

Beverage with alcohol content ≤ 15 %	No of samples tested	N-nitroso-dimethylamines			N-nitroso diethylamines			N-nitroso dipropylamines		
		value max. μg/l	% of positive samples	average μg/l	value max. μg/l	% of positive samples	average μg/l	value max. μg/l	% of positive samples	average μg/l
Cider	21	1,8	29	0,22	2,2	10	0,19	1,1	5	-
Wine	33	0,6	15	0,05	0,3	3	-	-	-	-
Beer	35	8,6	97	1,8	0,8	9	0,06	-	-	-

More significant differences were found between the samples in this group. Small quantities of the three N-nitroso-compounds were found in the apple ciders. Whereas there was no evidence of NDPA in the wine and beer samples. The highest quantities of NDMA were found in the beer samples, with 34 positives samples out of a total of 35.

TABLE 4. Statistical evaluation of the results obtained for NDMA

	Home-produced apple brandy		Industrially produced apple brandy		Other spirits	
	log	arith	log	arith	log	arith
+ σ	2,90	795	2,68	479	2,62	417
average log x	2,12	132	2,04	110	2,06	115
- σ	1,34	22	1,40	25	1,50	31
	εf = 94		εf = 39		εf = 37	
	ND = 53		ND = 19		ND = 16	

	Wine		Cider		Beer	
	log	arith	log	arith	log	arith
+ σ	1,98	96	2,52	331	3,52	3320
average log x	1,62	42	1,84	69	3,00	1000
- σ	1,26	18	1,16	14	2,48	302
	εf = 33		εf = 21		εf = 35	
	ND = 28		ND = 15		ND = 1	

(The ND were given the value of 30 ppt = 30×10^{-9} g/l)
εf = total no. of samples
ND = no. of samples where NDMA was not detected

This table summarizes the distribution of NDMA positive samples. It can be seen that beer contains the greatest amounts of this substance, but most of the beverages showed low content, and the overall results ofr the whole group of samples were low.

MUTAGENICITY TESTING OF APPLE BRANDIES

In this part of our investigation, we attempted to detect the presence of chemical molecules that, because of their mutagenic action, may be potentially or directly carcinogenic.

We used bacterial strains of Salmonella Typhimurium mutants according to the method described by Ames.

This method obtains an overall effect, either directly, or after metabolization by an activated liver tissue extract.

Three types of apple brandy samples were examined : home-produced; industrially produced; experimentally produced.

Samples of these beverages were either tested directly or after fractionation.

Results of Direct Testing

One hundred fourty five samples were examined : 58 home-produced apple brandies, 28 industrially produced and 31 experimentally produced apple brandies; 28 samples of other alcoholic beverages. No mutagenic action was found.

Results of Mutagenicity Testing of Apple-Brandies after Fractionation

Each sample was separated into 3 fractions after distillation, yielding : an alcoholic fraction (A); an aqueous fraction (L); a solid residue (S).

This resulted in a concentration of the fractions. Each fraction was tested for mutagenesis, either directly or after metabolization.

RESULTS

Home-Produced Apple Brandies

Thirty samples were fractionated, yielding 90 fractions for investigation. Fourteen fractions - corresponding to 37 % of the original samples - were positive.

Industrially-Produced Apple Brandies

Eighteen samples were fractionated. Of the 54 fractions obtained, 2 were found to be positive; 11 % of the original samples were positive.

Other Distilled Spirits

In the 28 samples, 5 of the 84 fractions obtained were found to be positive; these corresponded to 18 % of the original samples.

RESULTS OF MUTAGENICITY TESTING

TABLE 5. Mutagenic effect : quantitative results

	A		L		S	
	−	+	−	+	−	+
Home-produced apple brandy	10	7	23		3	3
Industrially produced apple brandy		11				
Other spirits		18				

(Results in %)

This table gives a quantitative summary of the results of the mutagenicity tests according to fractions and types of beverage. Positive responses were obtained more frequently with the home-produced apple brandies. These positive responses are obtained either directly or after metabolization by an hepatic tissue extract. Thus it seemed that many substances could be implicated.

TABLE 6. Mutagenic effect : qualitative results

	A	L	S
Home-produced apple brandy	3,3	3,5	2,5
Industrially produced apple brandy	0	2,5	0
Other spirits	2,7	0	0

(Results in reversion rate)

This table gives a qualitative comparison of the results. The results are compared to those obtained for controls (spontaneous reversion rates), and were considered significant when the rates were more than double those obtained by the controls (2 T). Mutagenic effect seemed to be greater for the home-produced apple brandies. So, for the most part, mutagenic effect seems to be very low.

CONCLUSION

The small amounts of volatile N-nitrosamines found in the apple brandies correspond to the average content of these substances of other beverages or certain foods, and thus do not provide confirmation of the hypothesis that these substances could be linked to endemic esophageal cancer in Normandy and Brittany.

Furthermore, the mutagenic effects observed after fractionation and concentration of the same apple brandies are also slight, although they are higher and more frequent in the home-produced cider distillates. It is unlikely that the small amounts of N-nitrosamines found were responsible for these findings, but they could have been produced by some other, as yet unidentified, substances.

However, nitrosamines are known to induce esophageal tumors in animals. If they have an effect on humans, this would be co-carcinogenic either in association with the alcohol itself or with other unidentified substances. The series of experiments on laboratory animals currently being conducted may help to shed new light on the matter.

REFERENCES

Ames, B. N. and co-workers (1973). Carcinogens are mutagens : a simple test system combining liver homigenates for activation and bacteria for detection. Proc. Nat. Acad. Sci (USA), 70, 2281-2285.

Barrellier, M. T. (1974). Le cancer de l'oesophage en Basse-Normandie. Thesis, Caen.

Druckrey, H. and co-workers (1961). Carcinogene Wirkung von N-Methyl-N-Nitrosoanilin. Naturwissenchaften, 48, 722.

Dunham, L. J. and J. C. Bailar (1968). World maps of cancer mortality rates and frequency ratio. J. Nat. Cancer Inst., 41, 155-203.

Loquet, C. (1977). Contribution à l'étude et à la recherche des facteurs étiologiques dans le cancer de l'oesophage en Basse-Normandie. Sc. Thesis (Biology), Caen.

Tuyns, A. J. and L. M. Massé (1973). Mortality from cancer of the oesophagus in Brittany. Int. J. Epidemiol., 2, 241-245.

Esophageal Cancer: Early Diagnosis - USA

Benjamin F. Byrd, Jr.

Department of Surgery, Vanderbilt University School of Medicine,
Nashville, Tennessee
Surgical Service, St. Thomas Hospital, Nashville, Tennessee

In the United States cancer of the esophagus is fourth in relative frequency of the sites of cancer in the gastrointestinal tract[.] It ranks well behind cancer of the stomach, colon/rectum, and pancreas. Its relative incidence has not changed appreciably in the last 40 years in the overall population studies. However, evaluation of the death rates from cancer of the esophagus between 1930 and 1975 shows an essentially constant incidence of cancer deaths in white males at the 3.4 to 4.0 per 100,000 population. In white women the level runs at the 1.0 per 100,000 level and has been constant for the past 45 years. But when one looks at the non-white segment of the population in the United States, it is evident that there has been a dramatic increase in the incidence of esophageal cancer from 0.3 per 100,000 in non-white women in 1935, to 2.7 per 100,000 in 1975.[ ] In black males a similar dramatic increase has been seen from a level of 1.0 in 1930 to 9.8 in 1975.[ ] Even with these dramatic alterations of the incidence of cancer of the esophagus in non-white population, there are still many unanswered questions about the character of the change and its basic nature. Carcinoma of the esophagus has remained essentially a disease of advanced age groups and it is very rarely encountered prior to age 50 ranging in males from an incidence of 14.8 per 100,000 at age 50 – 59, to 33.0 at age 85 and up. In women it is about one third of this figure. A reflection of proportionate sex incidence followed without relation to age.

One would immediately surmise that there was some major difference in dietary habits or in personal habits such as the use of tobacco or alcohol which would account for this differentiation. Careful study has shown that there is some relation between heavy cigarette smoking as well as with the chewing of tobacco, which is accompanied by change in the epithelial lining of the esophagus. The facts, while impressive, seem to be secondary to the heavy ingestion of alcoholic beverages in addition to the use of tobacco. A study by Wynder and Bross[ ] shows that "Tobacco is an important factor in the development of cancer of the esophagus. This applies to all forms of tobacco smoke and to a lesser extent, tobacco chewing. The risk is somewhat greater for pipe and cigar smokers than it is for cigarette smokers." These observers went on to state that there is little evidence that alcohol acts as an independent carcinogen and seems to merely promote the effects of tobacco. In this same study it is evident that Plummer Vinson disease with associated iron deficiency and deficiency of vitamins B and C. may have some effect on the incidence of esophageal cancer.

It is difficult to identify a group which is at special risk for cancer of the

esophagus. The only dramatic relationship is the relation which cancer of the
esophagus occupies as a second focus of tumor. This association is especially mark
with cancer of the nasopharynx.[8] There is no other similar association with
gastrointestinal cancers below the esophagogastric juncture. Extensive
studies over the past 30 years of the records of patients[2] who present themselves
with carcinoma of the esophagus have shown no great improvement of the stage of
the disease when treatment is undertaken. There has been little characteristic
improvement in the survival rate for carcinoma of the esophagus with five year
survival rates averaging 2 to 4% regardless of treatment modality. The majority
of deaths occurred within 24 months of diagnosis without regard to the level of
the tumor or to the therapy protocol which is adopted.[2]

There are characteristic population groups which have been described in epidemiologic studies in China particularly[3] and in various other areas in the Mid East.
There are many interesting speculations generated from these geographically identified areas of high incidence of carcinoma of the esophagus. This has made these
areas and their inhabitants special subjects for study. In the United States
the only single area in which there is a continuing high incidence of esophageal
carcinoma is in the black population in the area of Charleston, South Carolina.[4]
Dr. Edward F. Parker is one of the outstanding authorities in the United States on
the surgical management of carcinoma of the esophagus. He has recently reported
an experience in this group with treatment by both radiation and surgery. The
patients with esophageal cancer seem to have the universal characteristic of
some dietary deficiency, but these have not been identified as a causative role
in the development of carcinoma in this section of the black population.

Clinical discovery of carcinoma of the esophagus in situ is such a rarity in the
United States that it is indeed a reportable entity. Sautis[7] reported in this year
two instances of carcinoma of the esophagus in situ and both of these were diagnosed by symptoms related to an inflammatory reaction, but a biopsy through a
fiberoptic esophagoscope confirmed the presence of squamous carcinoma in situ.
The patients are reported as well at two and three year intervals respectively.
The diagnosis of carcinoma of the esophagus must rely on a tissue diagnosis.
With the increasing use of fiberoptic esophagoscopy and the availability of trained
endoscopists, the diagnostic techniques will become more generally available.

The use of cytology has been well established in mass screening studies in China,
but at this time it is not a technically feasible process in the United States.
The geographically disseminated character of the relatively few occurring cases of
carcinoma of the esophagus makes impractical the adoption of brush cytology or radiography. These represent the only adequate screening studies that are currently
available. We must rely for early diagnosis on the occurrence of symptoms and
there has been no essential improvement in the stage of the disease at which patients present when reliance is on dysphagia, indigestion, or bleeding into the
intestinal tract.

The recent use of Galactosyltransferase Isoenzyme (GT-II) indicates the possibility of an enzymatic study capable of identifying a small population group
with a high incidence of gastrointestinal cancer. Currently 4/9 patients with
squamous cell carcinoma of the esophagus and 12/16 patients with adenocarcinoma
of the stomach were identified by serum electrophoretic studies of GT-II.
If group selection for more conventioan screening techniques is made possible
by GT-II assays, then this may be a new door opening for early detection of
esophageal carcinoma.[5]

References

1. Axtell, L.M., A. J. Asire, and M. H. Myers, ed. (1976). Cancer patient survival, report number 5. DHEW Pub. no. (NIH) 77-992, 64-69.

2. Gunnlaugsson, G. H., A. R. Wychulis, C. Roland, and F. H. Ellis (1970). Analysis of the records of 1,657 patients with carcinoma of the esophagus and cardia of the stomach. Surg., Gyn and OB, 130, 997-1005.

3. MacFarquhar, E., B. Beedham, and N. Macrae (1977). China. The Economist, Dec. 31, 1977, 13-42.

4. Parker, E.F. (1978). The case for surgery. Am.J.Dig.Dis., 23, 730-734.

5. Podolsky, D.K., M. M. Weiser, K. J. Isselbacher, and A. M. Cohen (1978). A cancer associated galactosyltransferase isoenzyme. N.Engl.J.Med., 299, 703-705.

6. Seidman, H., E. Silverberg, and A.I. Holleb (1976). Cancer statistics, 1976 - a comparison of white and black populations. Cancer Statistics, 1976, ACS Professional Education Pub., 1-29

7. Sotus, P.C., B. Majmudar, and P. N. Symbas (1978). Carcinoma in situ of the esophagus. JAMA, 239, 335-336.

8. Wynder, E. L. and I. J. Bross (1961). A study of etiological factors in cancer of the esophagus. Cancer,14, 389-413.

Introduction: Stratification of Esophageal Cancer

J. S. Abbatucci

*Professor of Radiology, Caen University of Medicine, Chief,
Department of Radiotherapy, Director of Centre François Baclesse,
Route de Lion-sur-mer, 14021 Caen Cedex, France*

INTRODUCTION

Various epidemiologic studies (Barrellier, 1974; Tuyns, 1970, 1973) have revealed a particularly high incidence of cancer of the esophagus in France, especially in the western regions of Normandy and Brittany.

A considerable number of cases of esophageal cancer are consequently seen at the Centre François Baclesse, the Regional Cancer Center of Normandy, and more than 2.000 patients were treated for this disease at our Center between 1960 and 1977. An analysis of the annual average figures for new esophageal patients shows that the number of cases continues to increase yearly.

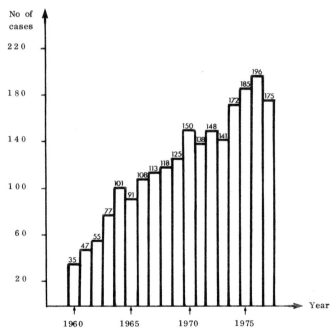

Fig. 1. Annual new patient figures for esophageal cancer.

The effective treatment of esophageal cancer understandably poses a major problem for our Center.

POPULATION ANALYSIS

All the cases of esophageal cancer seen at our Center (whether primarily medical, surgical or radiotherapeutic) are included in the population discussed here (Roussel, 1977). For the years 1968-1971, the represented close to 65 % of the total number of cases occuring in the whole of the department of Calvados (Barrellier 1974).

Ninety-five per cent of the cases were male; only 109 of the 2.175 recorded patient were women. The average age for the male population was 60 years, whereas for the women it was 70.

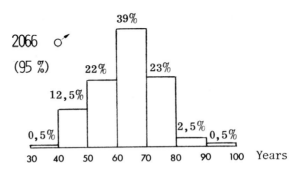

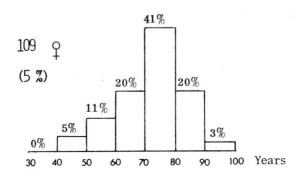

Fig. 2.   Cancer of esophagus : population
breakdown according to sex and age.

The primary tumor was most frequently located in the middle-third of the esophagus. Twenty per cent of the cases presented with upper-third lesions, and 20 % with lo-wer-third lesions.

TABLE 1   Tumor location

Middle third	58 %
Upper third	20 %
Lower third	22 %

The initial extension was reviewed in a group of 450 cases treated from 1972 to 1974. Limited forms corresponding to the U.I.C.C. definition T1 (under 5 cm in length, no circumferential involvement, no obstruction, no evidence of extra-eso-phageal spread) were found in less than 20 % of this group. Clinical or para-clini-cal extra-esophageal extension was present in 10 %, of whom 6 to 7 % had histologi-cally confirmed broncho-tracheal involvement. Extension to the regional lymph nodes occurred in the supra-clavicular chain (5 % of the cases showed clinical invasion), and more frequently in the sub-diaphragmatic areas, although these could be confir-med in laparotomized patients only, as was the case for invasion of the mediastinal nodes.

Metastatic spread was also frequent and was found in 12 % of the cases at the ini-tial examination, predominantly in the lungs and liver, and then in the bones.

Ten per cent of the cases presented with second cancerous lesions; half of these were previously treated lesions, the other half were simultaneous lesions. In the majority of the cases, the second tumor occurred in the head and neck area, predo-minantly in the hypopharynx. The etiology, evolution and prognosis for these le-sions are the same as those for esophageal carcinoma.

Recently, in our Center, Mandard, Rousselot and Tourneux (1978), carried out detai-led analyses of 35 specimens of esophagectomy for cancer to determine actual tumo-ral extension. They found extensive neoplastic parietal infiltration, with involve-ment of the peri-esophageal tissue in 22 cases (63 %). Carcinomatous lymphangitis was noted in 21 cases (60 %) and vascular involvement other than lymphatic in 13 (37,1 %). Lymph node metastases were present in 28 cases (80 %), with the following distribution :

TABLE 2.   Detailed analysis of 35 operative specimens

Oesophageal location	No of cases	N +	Site of nodal invasion		
			peri-eso-phageal	lesser curvature	other
Middle third	9	7 (77,7 %)	3	7	1
Middle and lower third)	8	4 (50 %)	2	4	2
Lower third	18	17 (94,4 %)	9	14	4
Total	35	28 (80 %)	14 (40 %)	25 (71,5 %)	7 (20 %)

A carcinoma in situ, distant to the primary tumor, was found in 6 cases (17,1 %).

A second invasive carcinoma was present in 5 cases : esophagus, 3 (8,6 %); stomach, 1; hypopharynx, 1.

It can be seen from this that lesion extension was extremely severe in this surgi-cal series.

STRATIFICATION OF ESOPAGEAL CANCER

In assessing cases for surgery, tumoral extension and second neoplastic lesions are considered in conjunction with other deficiencies (these were present in 22 % of the cases and were predominantly hepatic, but also cardio-vascular, pulmonary and renal) as well as the age of the patient (over 75 years of age in 10 %). The results was that more than two-thirds (69 %) of the patients were found to be inoperable at the initial examination and to warrant only palliative treatment. These figures are similar to the results published elsewhere (Parker, 1970; Seymour, 1965).

Of the 31 % found to be operable, a further 9 % did not receive surgery owing to the pre-operative discovery of distant metastases or of local extension rendering excision   useless or dangerous.

Consequently, a final figure corresponding to 22 % of the total population received surgery, in some cases combined with radiation therapy. Only some 10 % of these patients emerged with a potentially favorable prognosis, however, surgery having revealed infiltration of the neighboring organs or distant lymph-node or visceral invasion in the remaining 12 % (resection-anastomosis was performed for functional reasons in these cases).

Although these figures may appear to be somewhat pessimistic when compared to the majority of the surgical series in the literature, it is to be remembered that the latter usually concern highly selected populations due to the initial selection imposed by surgery. Consequently, although radical surgery does seem to offer the patient a better chance of long-term survival, proportionally few patients are really able to benefit from it.

The same stratification of our figures indicates that 23 to 45 % of the cases corresponding to the groups marked by an arrow in Fig. 3.- cases where extension remained local - would be potentially curable by radical radiation therapy in the event of further technical advances in this field. Similarly, chemotherapy may contribue to a favorable modification of these results.

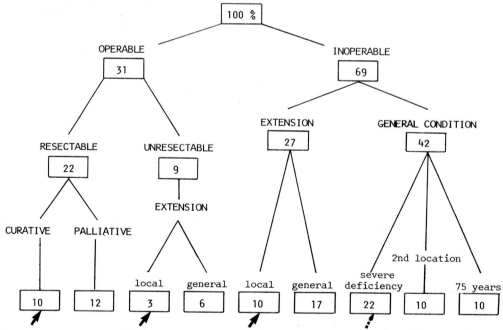

Fig. 3.   Cancer of esophagus : "Stratification" of population according to general health and disease extension.

CONCLUSION

Our experience at the Centre François Baclesse confirms the extreme severity of carcinoma of the esophagus, indicating that despite all the efforts made in that direction, therapeutic solutions to this disease are still far from satisfactory.

It would seem possible that some of the forms of this disease encountered elsewhere in the world are not really comparable to those occuring in France. Besides etiological dissimilarities, other marked variations, such as in sex ratios, may indicate different natural histories. It is, however, none the less evident that there is much need for progress in the search for therapeutic solutions. We sincerely hope that this international pluridisciplinary meeting will enable us to make definite steps in this direction.

REFERENCES

Barrellier, M. Th. (1974). Le cancer de l'oesophage en Basse-Normandie. Essai d'étude de Pathologie géographique. Thesis, Caen.

Parker, E. F., and co-workers (1970). Carcinoma of the esophagus. Ann. Surg., 171, 746-751.

Roussel, A., and co-workers (1977). Le cancer de l'oesophage dans l'ouest de la France. Analyse rétrospective d'une population de 1400 cas. Bull. Cancer, 64, 61-66.

Seymour, E. Q., and H. S. Pettit (1965). Pre-operative X Ray in therapy in cancer of the esophagus. Radiology, 85, 952-955.

Tourneux, J. (1978). Etude Anatomo-pathologique du cancer de l'oesophage. A propos de 36 pièces d'oesophagectomie. Thesis, Caen.

Tuyns, A. J. (1970). Cancer of the esophagus further evidence of the relation to drinking habits in France. Int. J. Cancer, 5, 152-156.

Tuyns, A. J., and L. M. F. Massé (1973). Mortality from cancer of the esophagus in Brittany. Int. J. Cancer, 2, 241-245.

The Surgical Treatment of Cancer of the Oesophagus

K. C. McKeown

Lately Senior Consultant Surgeon Memorial Hospital, Darlington, England

ABSTRACT

Surgical treatment for carcinoma of the oesophagus is based on an understanding of the modes of spread of the growth. Sub-mucous spread and satellite growths account for local recurrence, while regional lymphatic spread limits the scope for radical surgery in growths of the middle and upper oesophagus.

There are four operative problems; the mode of access, the extent of excision, the organ of replacement and the route of replacement. Surgical access is solved by the use of combined incisions, while the latter problems are still under discussion.

Based on a personal series of over 400 operations for oesophageal carcinoma a pattern of treatment has evolved appropriate for growths at various levels. The details of each mode of treatment is outlined, with special reference to the advantages of total three phase oesophagectomy.

Assessment of results on the basis of operative mortality, ability to swallow and survival time is presented.

INTRODUCTION

The surgical treatment of cancer of the oesophagus is based on a knowledge of the nature of the growth, the level at which it occurs and its modes of spread.

MODES OF SPREAD

Spread in the oesophagus takes place both circumferentially and longitudinally producing a stricture long in extent and often tortuous in shape.

Sub-mucous Spread

A characteristic feature is the tendency of the tumour to spread under the mucosa. This takes place directly by a process of burrowing, but may also occur by lymphatic permeation and embolism, giving rise to satellite growths at sites quite distant from the primary tumour (Fig. 1). It is therefore important to give a wide clearance well beyond the apparent margins of the tumour to allow for sub-mucous burrowing and prevent local recurrence at the anastomotic site. Total oesophagectomy will of course deal with the presence of satellite growths as well as the

345

rarer cases where multiple primary growths are present in the oesophagus.

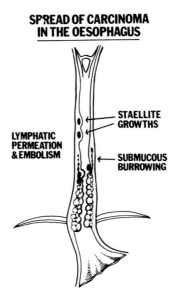

Fig. 1. Showing submucous and lymphatic spread

Mural Spread

The muscular wall of the oesophagus offers little resistance to the spread of the growth, and microscopic section often shows columns of cells spreading between the muscle fibres (Fig. 2).

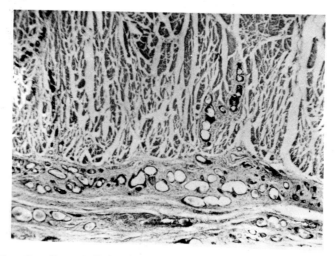

Fig. 2. Spread through the wall of the gullet. Columns of
malignant cells between muscle fibres.
(By kind permission of Annals of the Royal College
of Surgeons)

Extra-oesophageal structures such as the crura of the diaphragm, the bronchus and
the structures of the mediastinum are in consequence frequently involved. The
aorta, perhaps because of its constant movement, is less frequently involved.

Lymphatic Spread

The regional lymph nodes draining the various segments of the oesophagus are
illustrated in Fig. 3. Growths in the lower third drain to the para-cardial, the
splenic and coeliac lymph nodes, so that a planned radical 'en-bloc' excision of
the entire lymphatic drainage area is possible. In middle third growths, the
extensive hilar glands cannot completely be removed, while block dissection of
the cervical and superior mediastinal glands is a task even more daunting. Excision of carcinoma in the mid and upper segments of the oesophagus must therefore
be regarded as essentially a palliative procedure.

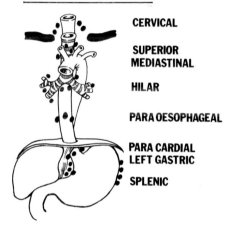

Fig. 3. Lymphatic drainage of the oesophagus

Distant Spread

With increasing survival after operation, the occurrence of metastatic spread to
bone and even to skin is now more frequently encountered. (McKeown 1972). As in
breast cancer, the possibility of distant spread having already taken place at the
time of operation must be considered a possibility, and may emphasise the importance of a systemic attack on the growths by chemotherapy.

SURGICAL TREATMENT

Four problems are presented in surgical treatment:

a) Surgical Approach
b) Extent of Oesophageal Resection
c) Organ of Replacement
d) Route of Replacement

Surgical Approach

The inaccessible situation of all segments of the oesophagus has presented difficulties of surgical access. Just as the problem of the approach to growths at
the pelvi-rectal junction has been solved by combined incisions, so too has the
problem of access to the oesophagus been solved in a similar manner.

Extent of Excision

Because of the mode of spread of cancer of the oesophagus a minimum clearance of
7cms must be given above and below the upper and lower margins of the growth.
The recent tendency towards total oesophagectomy not only attains this objective,
but also deals with the problems of satellite and multicentric growths. (Fig. 1).

Organ of Replacement

The essential criteria for the organ of replacement are that it must have the
requisite mechanical length, its blood supply must be adequate and amenable to
surgical manoeuvre, and that the mucosa must join readily with oesophageal mucosa.
The organs available are stomach, jejunum and colon and each organ appears to
meet these criteria in varying degrees.

Route of Replacement

Three routes for oesophageal replacement are available; pre-sternal, retro-sternal,
and posterior mediastinal. (Fig. 4).

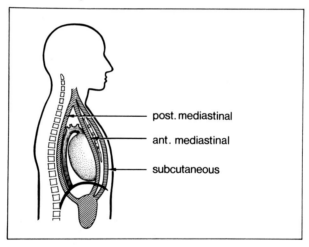

post. mediastinal

ant. mediastinal

subcutaneous

Fig. 4.   Routes for Oesophageal Replacement

Pre-sternal (sub-cutaneous)

The pre-sternal route is the least direct, but has the advantage that should stomal
leak occur this complication is not usually fatal.

Retro-sternal (anterior mediastinal)

The retro-sternal route occupies an intermediate position, in that it is more
direct than the pre-sternal route, but not so direct as the posterior mediastinal
route. At the same time, while not possessing the safety of the pre-sternal route,

leaks in the anterior mediastinum though serious do not have the fatality rate of those in the posterior mediastinum. It is, however, unsuitable for palliative resection because the tumour mass may obstruct the bypass. (Ong 1971).

Posterior mediastinal

The posterior mediastinal is the most direct and physiological and after re-construction swallowing is usually easy. It has however the danger that should stomal leak occur, this complication usually proves fatal.

DIVISIONS OF OESOPHAGUS

The exact surgical techniques to be used in the treatment of oesophageal cancer are largely determined by the site at which the growth occurs. The classical division of the oesophagus into three segments can, with advantage, be modified by further sub-divisions as shown in Fig. 5. This equates the site of the growth with the type of treatment.

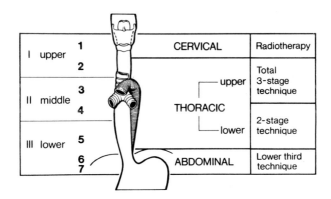

Fig. 5. Divisions of the oesophagus, showing relationship
between site of growth and type of treatment.
(By kind permission Proc. Royal Society of Medicine)

The upper third above the aortic arch can be considered as consisting of a cervical and a supra-aortic portion (Sites 1 and 2), the middle third to consist of an upper and lower segment (Sites 3 and 4), while growths in the lower third may be supra-diaphragmatic (Site 5) or infra-diaphragmatic (Sites 6 and 7).

MATERIAL AND DATA

Over the past 25 years, in the Darlington/Northallerton series, a pattern of surgical treatment has emerged appropriate for dealing with growths at various sites in the oesophagus. This work is based on 403 cases for which operation has been carried out. (Table I).

Of these, 237 were for growths at the lower third and 135 were for growths in the middle and upper segments. Two-stage oesophagectomy was performed in 66 cases and total three-stage oesophagectomy in 59 cases where the growths occurred in the upper thoracic oesophagus. (In the last few years more total three-stage operations have been carried out and the number has now reached almost 100). Anterior pre-sternal replacement was tried in 5 cases using the jejunum as organ of

replacement, but this technique was abandoned for various reasons (McKeown 1972).
If at all possible the growth, even though technically inoperable, was resected
and in only 6 cases was resection abandoned. In view of the poor medical condition and the extent of the growth 25 cases were intubed.

TABLE 1 Type of Operation (403 cases)

Operation	No of Cases	
Roux-en-Y	62	
Oesophago-anstrostomy	155	
Oesophago-duodenostomy	20	Total 237
2-phase	66	
Total 3-phase	59	
Anterior pre-sternal jejunal replacement	5	
Oesophago-pharyngo-laryngectomy	5	Total 135
Intubation	25	
Unresectable	6	Total 31
TOTAL		403

SITE OF GROWTH

As a result of experience gained in this series, the following details of treatment are outlined for growths at various sites, excluding cervical growths which
are best treated by radiotherapy or if this fails by oesophago-pharyngectomy
(Le Quesne and Ranger 1966).

Growths in the Lower Third Below the Diaphragm (Sites 6 and 7)

The surgical approach is by the classical left thoraco-abdominal incision as
shown in Fig. 6. (Ohsawa 1933, Adams and Phemister 1938).

With the patient in the left lateral position and the operating table split to
open out the operative field, excellent access is attained to growths at the lower
end of the oesophagus. This enables a radical 'en-bloc' excision of the growth,
together with locally invaded structures and the entire lymphatic drainage area.
(Allison and Borrie 1949).

For growths at the gastro-oesophageal junction (Site 7) total gastrectomy has
been the routine procedure and reconstruction by the Roux-en-Y anastomosis
(Fig. 7a). In cases where the growth is at Site 6 and where lymphatic glandular
involvement appears limited, the stomach may be sectioned obliquely at the level
of the gastric antrum and oesophago-antrostomy performed. (Fig. 7b).

Growths at the Lower Third Above the Diaphragm (Site 5)

While good access can be attained through the left thoraco-abdominal approach for
growths occurring in the lower third just above the diaphragm, certain problems
do arise because of the slightly higher level. In order to give adequate clearance above the growth, anastomosis has to be performed just below the aortic arch.
Aortic and cardiac movements, and the limited access for suturing make this
procedure difficult and dangerous. In these circumstances it is best to use the

two-phase technique described by Ivor Lewis (1946) and by Tanner (1947) and used
with such success by Franklin (1970, 1971).

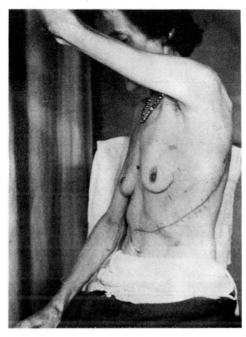

Fig. 6.   Left thoraco abdominal approach for growths in
          lower oesophagus

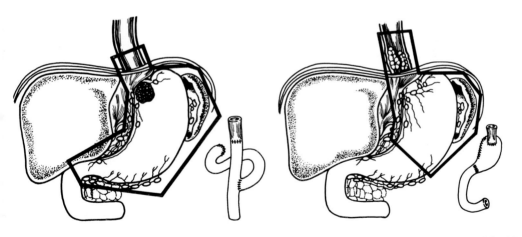

Fig. 7.   Extent of excision of carcinoma of the oesophagus

(a) At gastro-oesophageal   (b) Above hiatus (Site 5)
    junction (Site 7) with   with oesophago-gastrostomy
    Roux-en-Y

Phase 1: At laparotomy the stomach is mobilised with preservation of its blood
supply from the right gastric and the right gastro-epiploic vessels, and division
of the left gastric, left gastro-epiploic and the vasa brevia.

Phase 2: With the patient in the left lateral position the oesophagus is exposed
through right thoracotomy. After division of the vena azygus, the diaphragmatic hi
atus is freed and if necessary enlarged, so that the stomach can be pulled through
into the right pleural cavity. After resection of the tumour bearing segment
together with a ring of tissue round the cardia, the distal stomach is anastomosed
with the upper thoracic oesophagus.

Growths in the Middle Third (Sites 3 and 4 and sometimes 2)

Though the Ivor Lewis operation is very appropriate for growths in the lower thoracic oesophagus, problems arise in growths at a higher level where the anastomosis
has to be carried out above the aortic arch. In this situation working high up
under the dome of the pleura with long instruments and with poor illumination,
safe anastomosis is difficult to perform.

It is because of this that the addition of the third cervical phase greatly facilitates excision and makes anastomosis much safer. (McKeown 1969, 1972, 1973 and
1976). Figure 8 shows the surgical incisions for this three stage procedure.

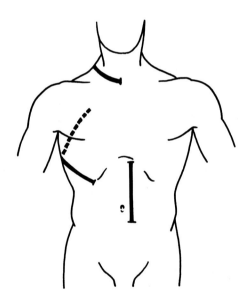

Fig. 8. Incisions for three phase oesophagectomy

The first stage is performed through an upper left paramedian incision. Mobilisation of the stomach and selective ligation of its blood vessels is carried out
in four stages so that an adequate blood supply is preserved (Fig. 9). The vasa
brevia are ligated individually and the left gastro-epiploic vessels tied and
divided close to their origin. Omental vessels from the right gastro-epiploic
artery are ligated separately to prevent bunching and shortening of the arcade.
The left gastric artery is tied close to its origin from the coeliac axis to
preserve the collateral anastomosis and particularly the oesophago-fundic branch
which supplies the dome of the fundus.

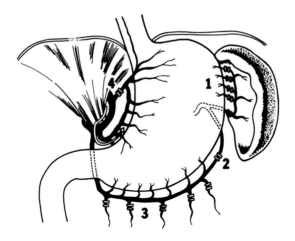

Fig. 9. Showing the four stages of ligation of the gastric
         vessels, vasa brevia, left gastro-epiploic, omental
         and left gastric vessels

Duodenal mobilisation is more extensive than in Kocker's manoeuvre in that the
entire head of the pancreas is mobilised so that 7cms of the inferior vena cava
are exposed, and the anterior wall of the aorta is demonstrated. In these circumstances, the entire head of the pancreas and the duodenum rotate to their
embryological position in the mid line. Pyloromyotomy as in the manner of
Ramsted's operation is performed if the sphincter is thick, while full pyloro-
plasty is performed in cases of stenosis due to former ulceration. If the pylorus
is wide no surgical intervention is required.

The second phase through a right thoracotomy mobilises the entire thoracic oesophagus with its tumour segment. Dissection is carried out high into the mediastinum and it is especially important to free the anterior wall of the oesophagus,
so that tracheal kinking does not occur when the stomach is pulled up in the
third cervical phase of the operation. Posterior dissection continues high up
into the retro-pharyngeal space.

The third cervical phase of the operation is performed in the right side of the
neck (Fig. 8). An oblique incision 7/9cms long is made in the supra-clavicular
region and dissection continued in front of the lower fibrous part of the right
sterno mastoid muscle, until the plane between the thyroid gland and the carotid
sheath is defined. Identification of the cervical oesophagus is facilitated by
the presence of the naso-gastric tube. After delivery of the entire thoracic
oesophagus and tumour into the neck, the gastro-oesophageal junction is closed
and the cervical oesophagus anastomosed to the dome of the fundus. A drainage
tube is inserted through a separate cervical stab wound down to the superior media
stinum.

ADVANTAGES OF TOTAL THREE PHASE OESOPHAGECTOMY

The advantages of this procedure are many. It provides wide excision, a single
anastomosis, less risk of infection, ease of anastomosis in the neck, it is well
tolerated, a full meal can be taken and there is absence of reflux even on bending.
Post operative radiotherapy is less hazardous.

Single Anastomosis

In colonic replacements three anastomoses are required in reconstruction, colo-
colic, colo-gastric and colo-oesophageal. Multiple suture lines increase the risk
of leakage, while the risks of infection occur early in the operation when the
bowel is first opened.

Less Infection

In the three phase technique the gut is not opened until the final cervical stage
of the operation. Dissection in the first two phases of the procedure are therefore carried out in an operative field that is not potentially contaminated as in
colonic or jejunal replacement. An additional feature is that the bacterial flora
of the stomach are less virulent than those of the colon. In view of these considerations this technique diminishes the risk of infection.

Ease of Anastomosis

One of the major causes of post operative mortality is stomal leak. Effecting an
anastomosis with long instruments and poor illumination deep in the confines of
the superior mediastinum is technically difficult and one misplaced suture is
enough to lead to fatal termination. In contrast the ease of anastomosis between
the stomach and cervical oesophagus in the superficial layers of the neck makes
accurate approximation of the mucosa a simple matter.

Well Tolerated

The addition of a third cervical phase does not increase operative mortality and
is surprisingly well tolerated even in patients of advanced age. The facility of
cervical anastomosis shortens rather than lengthens the operative time. Operative
time may be further shortened by the synchronous use of two operative teams.
(Royston, Dowling and Spencer 1975). There is also the additional advantage that
once the second phase is completed, spontaneous respiration may be restored so that
at the completion of this phase the patient may be in good cardio-pulmonary bal-
ance. (Franklin 1971).

Ability to Eat and Absence of Reflux

The outstanding feature of total gastric replacement is the patient's ability to
eat a full meal and the absence of reflux even in the head down position (Fig. 10).
The size of the gastric reservoir is not impaired and even a full meal does not
cause cardiac or pulmonary embarrassment. The absence of reflux is difficult to
explain, except to observe the pressure in the stomach appears to be negative and
to observe that a naso-gastric tube attached to an underwater drainage system
shows respiratory excursions comparable to that of intra-thoracic drainage.

Radiotherapy

The impairment of wound healing that occurs after radiotherapy has discouraged
many surgeons from using radiotherapy in any situation where intestinal anastomosis is likely to be adversely affected. In three phase oesophagectomy it has
been the usual procedure to makr any area of suspected infiltration in the hilum
by the insertion of Michels clips with a view to post operative radiotherapy. In
this operation the oesophago-gastric anastomosis and the site of the gastro-
oesophageal closure is well clear of the hilum so that the danger of breakdown
in the anastomosis following radiation therapy is obviated. The situation of the
gastro-oesophageal closure and the oesophago-gastric anastomosis in relation to
the marked glands is shown in Fig. 11.

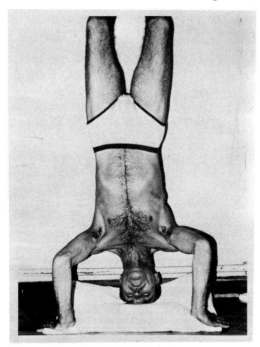

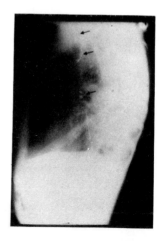

Fig. 11. Showing Michels clips
inserted at the hilum,
(lower arrow) and their
relationship to the
stapled oesophago-gastric
closure, and the oesoph-
Fig. 10. This patient experiences no reflux   ago-fundic anastomosis
even after a full hospital meal   (upper arrow)

ASSESSMENT OF RESULTS

Three factors of evaluation of the role of surgery must be considered:- operative
mortality, restoration of ability to swallow and length of survival.

Operative Mortality

The mortality rate after oesophagectomy depends on many factors. The condition
and age of the patient, the presence of concomitant disease, the level of growth,
the percentage of cases resected, and the complexity and type of the operative
procedure. In general terms age is not as important as the general and cardio-
pulmonary status of the individual. Mortality for resections of growths at the
lower end of the gullet is much lower than for those in the middle and upper
segments. The experience of individual surgeons is very important and the mortality rate is much higher in the earlier stages of the author's experience
(Collis 1971).

In presenting mortality figures only recorded series of considerable size have
been included. Table 2 shows the overall mortality for resections of growths
at all levels in series.

The different mortality rates for resection of growths at various levels of the
gullet is shown in Table 3.

Ability to Eat

Ability to eat depends largely on the type of anastomosis used for reconstruction
(Fig. 12). With Roux-en-Y anastomosis small frequent meals are required but
biliary reflux is rare. With oesophago-antrostomy and with oesophago-duodenostomy

used as a palliative procedure biliary reflux is often troublesome. In colonic
replacement swallowing is easier with iso-peristaltic anastomosis using right or
transverse colon, but reflux can be troublesome if a left colonic retro-peristal-
tic replacement is used. The reversed gastric tube gives adequate capacity for
eating, but reflux occurs if the tube is made too large (Gavriliu 1975). With
total three phase oesophagectomy a full meal can be taken and reflux is rare, even
in the head down position. (McKeown 1972, 1973, 1976).

TABLE 2 Overall Mortality Figures for Oesophagectomy for Carcinoma

Author	Date	No of Cases	Overall Mortality
Sweet	1956	327	17.4
Watson	1957	182	35.7
Nakayama	1959	975	5.8
Ellis	1960	138	16.0
Miller	1962	272	31.0
Logan	1963	342	25.0
Ong	1964	-	32.9
Lortat-Jacob	1970	1769	29.0
Leigh Collis	1971	350	14.3
Paris	1976	(57 surgeons)	16.0
Gavriliu	1976	352	14.4
McKeown	1976	392	9.6

TABLE 3 Mortality after Oesophagectomy for Growths at Various Levels

Author	Date	No of Cases	Mortality rate (%) site of growth			
			Oesophago-Gastric	Lower Third	Middle Third	Upper Third
Ellis	1955	579	14.8	18.4	16.7	-
Ellis	1965		10.1	13.0	13.7	-
Nakayama	1956	136	3.5	5.1	-	-
Miller	1962	272	20.0	25.0	32.0	
Lortat-Jacob	1970	1769	20.0	23.4	36.2	-
Leigh Collis	1971	400	11.0		13.0	
Gavriliu	1976	352	13.5	16.0	24.0	20.0
McKeown	1976	392	5.6		15.1	15.9

Survival Time

A characteristic feature of the survival time is the great wastage in the first
year after the operation. (Figs. 13a, 13b). This occurs both in growths in
the lower and upper segments of the oesophagus. If however the patient survives
the second year the outlook appears to improve. In considering the survival figures it must be remembered that the primary objective of treatment is to enable
the patient to swallow, and that many of the patients are in advanced years and
where the normal life expectation is so short. (McKeown 1973).

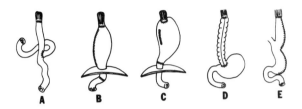

Fig. 12. Types of oesophageal replacement; A. Roux-en-Y,
         B. Oesophago-antrostomy, C. Total gastric
         replacement, D. Colonic replacement, E. Reversed
         gastric tube

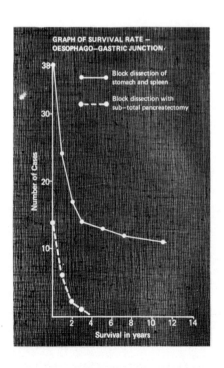

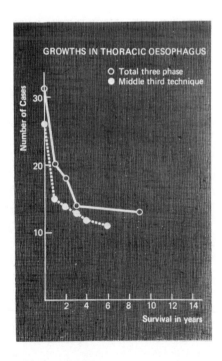

Fig. 13. Survival time after oesophagectomy
(a) Lower end   (b) Mid-third

CONCLUSION

A pattern of surgical treatment has evolved which has been outlined in this paper. Further improvement in the survival rates must be looked for by the use of chemotherapy, radiotherapy or a combination of both.

REFERENCES

Adams, W. E. and Phemister, D. B. (1938). Carcinoma of the lower thoracic oesophagus. (Report of a successful resection and oesophago-gastrostomy). Journal of Thoracic Surgery, 7, 621.

Allison, P. R. and Borrie, J. (1949). The treatment of malignant obstruction of the cardia. British Journal of Surgery, 37, 1.

Collis, J. L. (1971). Surgical treatment of carcinoma of the oesophagus and cardia. British Journal of Surgery, 58, 801.

Franklin, R. H. (1970). Personal communication.

Franklin, R. H. (1971). Grey Turner and the evaluation of oesophageal surgery. Annals of the Royal College of Surgeons of England, 49, 165.

Gavriliu, D. (1975). In M Ravitch (Ed.), Current Problems in Surgery. Year Book Medical Publications, Chicago.

Lewis, I. (1946). The surgical treatment of carcinoma of the oesophagus with special reference to a new operation for growths of the middle third. British Journal of Surgery, 34, 18.

Le Quesne, L. and Ranger, D. (1966). British Journal of Surgery, 53, 105.

McKeown, K. C. (1969). Total oesophagectomy. British Medical Association, Film No. 439.

McKeown, K. C. (1971). Surgical treatment for cancer of the oesophagus. In J. McFarland (Ed.) Postgraduate Surgical Lectures, 1 Butterworths, London. pp. 34-55.

McKeown, K. C. (1972). Trends in oesophageal resection for carcinoma. Annals of the Royal College of Surgeons, 51, 213-238.

McKeown, K. C. (1976). Total three-stage oesophagectomy for cancer of the oesophagus. British Journal of Surgery, 63, 259.

Ohsawa, T. (1933). Surgery of the oesophagus. Archiv. Fur Japanische Chirurgie, 10, 605.

Ong, G. B. (1971). In M. Ravitch (Ed.), Current Problems in Surgery. Year Book Medical Publishers, Chicago.

Ong, G. B. (1978). Personal communication.

Royston, C. N. S., Dowling, B. L. and Spencer, J. British Journal of Surgery, 62, 605.

Tanner, N. C. (1947). The present position of carcinoma of the oesophagus. Postgraduate Medical Journal, 23, 109.

Tratamiento Quirurgico del Cancer de Esofago. Experiencia de 1012 Casos

E. Lira

Cátedra y Servicio de Cirugía, Hospital Salvador. Santiago, Chile

ABSTRACT

1012 cases of Oesophageal Cancer are presented and were seen by the author during 25 years. Only the epidermoid cases of the body of the Oesophagus are considered, not the adenocarcinoma of the cardia.
On the tumors located in the inferior third, radical and palliative resective surgery was done. The latter is justified as there is a low mortality and morbidity with one to three years survival. In the upper location we have done only radical surgery. Palliative exeresis is not indicated because of high morbidity (19%), and short survival particularly associated with bronchial involvement.
Based on this criterion, in the upper localization we select the cases for radical surgery. Bronchoscopy is mandatory and was done by the author routinely over the last seventeen years. In 63% of this group we found bronchial compromise and surgery was not done. Scalene node biopsy indicated that in 50% of the cases palpable nodes were benign. However, biopsy should always be done in spite of palpable nodes before considering the patient inoperable because of this finding. If the scalene nodes are not palpable biopsy is not justified because of its low positivity.
336 resections and 487 explorations or palliative procedures are analysed. The few cured cases (4% in all the group and 12% of those resected) and the different palliative resources applied, justified the surgery employed and specialization in the management of patients with such a serious disease.

CONSIDERACIONES GENERALES

El cáncer del cuerpo del esófago es un carcinoma epidermoides en prácticamente todos los casos. Por excepción se presentan adenocarcinomas, la mayoría del tercio inferior de esófago y especialmente de la unión esofagogástrica; también se han presentado en nuestra serie tres leiomiosarcomas, dos melanomas y dos linfosarcomas.
El pronóstico de todos los tumores malignos del esófago es extraordinariamente grave, aunque se utilice cualquier terapéutica, nosotros nos extenderemos en el tratamiento quirúrgico, que además de curar algunos casos, permite emplear una serie de procedimientos paliativos que alivian a estos enfermos, todos en situación tan desesperada debido al tumor obstructivo.
La gravedad del pronóstico de esta afección se debe a diagnósticos y tratamientos tardíos. Aunque no haremos consideraciones clínicas señalamos de que un diagnóstico precoz, basado en síntomas o complicaciones previas a la disfagia lógica, ha permitido la mayoría de nuestras curaciones.
Después de 25 años de experiencia en cirugía esofágica, debemos confesar que a pesar de haber llega-

do a nuestra máxima habilidad técnica, el pronóstico de la cirugía de exéresis del cáncer esofágico ha mejorado escasamente y creemos que los pasos a seguir, deben llevarnos más a diagnosticar lesiones pequeñas que a mejorar o ampliar las resecciones.

La exéresis es el único tratamiento curativo. La exéresis paliativa la justificamos en las localizaciones bajas, no así en las localizaciones medias y superiores, en que sus resultados son pobres con alta morbi-mortalidad. Ello nos obliga a destacar los factores de inoperabilidad o irresecabilidad, evitando toracotomías inútiles y honerosas para el paciente, debiendo usarse otros procedimientos paliativos.

Al revisar en esta presentación nuestros resultados, en que se considera desde el primer paciente operado, le damos mayor relevancia a las técnicas actuales de tratamiento en cada localización de la lesión.

CASUISTICA

La serie analizada corresponde a pacientes asistidos por el autor en calidad de cirujano o ayudante responsable del equipo quirúrgico. Fueron atendidos 1012 pacientes en un lapso de 25 años -Junio de 1952 a Septiembre de 1977- en los Servicios de Cirugía de los Hospitales José Joaquín Aguirre y Salvador, de Santiago de Chile.

Para localizar la lesión empleamos el esquema de Resano (1951), (Lois, 1953), nos parece una clasificación muy práctica, anátomo-quirúrgica, en que los reparos radiológicos destacados nos señalan las vías de abordaje de la lesión. En las numerosas veces en que el tumor ocupa dos o más segmentos, debe considerarse como de la localización superior, al explorarse quirúrgicamente.

En la fig. 1, se señalan 1012 cánceres del cuerpo del esófago, y 485 cánceres del cardias o gástricos propagados, estos son todos adenocarcinomas y no son analizados en este estudio; sin embargo conviene destacar que numerosas veces, por lo avanzado de la lesión, no se pudo precisar si su origen fue esofágico o gástrico.

La frecuencia por sexo es similar a series extranjeras, más o menos dos tercios masculinos (63%) y un tercio femenino (37%).

La edad media es de 61 años, los hombres 62 y las mujeres 61.

Para referirse al tratamiento quirúrgico es indispensable analizar previamente nuestro criterio de operabilidad y resecabilidad.

En las localizaciones bajas, vale decir desde el hilio pulmonar a cardias, las exéresis paliativas están plenamente justificadas, son de morbi-mortalidad baja y se obtienen sobrevidas confortables y aceptables en cuanto a duración.

En las localizaciones altas, desde hilio pulmonar hacia arriba, las resecciones paliativas no se justifican, tienen mayor mortalidad, morbilidad y corta sobrevida por propagación traqueobronquial; ello nos obliga en estas localizaciones, a buscar todos los signos de inoperabilidad y creemos que la traqueobroncoscopía debe practicarse de rutina (Lira, 1957). Es así como en una serie de 300 casos (Lira, 1978) en que se practicó este examen en forma sistemática, en un 63% el hallazgo positivo de algún grado de compromiso traqueobronquial, contraindicó la exploración quirúrgica. Actualmente sólo intentamos cirugía de exéresis en las localizaciones altas con criterio de curación, es decir cuando creemos poder realizar una exéresis radical.

Hemos estudiado el rendimiento de la biopsia preescalénica (Lira, 1955). En una serie de 100 casos en que se practicó en forma sistemática concluímos lo siguiente: frente a ganglios palpables debe practicarse siempre; en 24 casos, 14 fueron negativos para cáncer, siendo los ganglios tuberculosos, antracóticos, inflamatorios o debido a sarcoidosis. Esto es de fundamental importancia porque puede considerarse como generalizada una lesión perfectamente operable.

Sin ganglios palpables, tuvimos una positividad baja, pero que puede recomendar este examen en lesiones de nivel hiliar hacia arriba (14% de positividad).

Cirugía de Exéresis y Resultados

Analizamos separadamente las técnicas empleadas y resultados obtenidos en cada localización.

Esófago cervical. En la Tabla 1 se analizan los procedimientos empleados. Las resecciones localizadas a esófago cervical han sido abandonadas. Actualmente empleamos un procedimiento original (Lira, 1962), en que la operación se efectúa en un tiempo y en decúbito dorsal. Primero se hace la exploración cervical que nos dice si el caso es extirpable y con o sin laringectomía. Resecado el tumor, digitalmente y en forma ciega se diseca desde el cuello el esofago sano hasta el arco aórtico, y desde el abdomen el infraaórtico; en el mismo tiempo operatorio se esqueletiza el estómago y se asciende por el mediastino anterior.

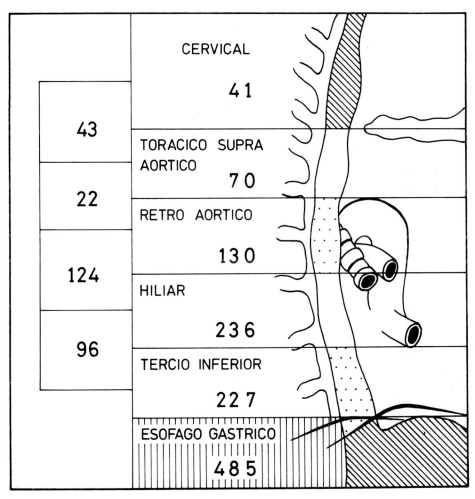

Generalizado a tres localizaciones   20
Doble localización: Retro Aortico y Gastroesofágico   1
                    Hiliar y Gastroesofágico   2

Fig. 1. Localización del cáncer de esófago. 1012 casos. Esquema de Resano

Tabla-1   RESECCIONES Y PLASTIAS EN CANCER
ESOFAGICO CERVICAL 18 EN 84 CASOS.

TIPO de RESECCION	TIPO de PLASTIA	Nº de CASOS	FALLECIDOS
ESOFAGECTOMIA CERVICAL	Cutánea.	3	1
ESOFAGEC. LARINGECTOMIA	Cutánea.	1	
ESOFAGECTOMIA TOTAL ■■	Faringogastrostomía por Mediastino poster.	2	
ESOFAGECTOMIA TOTAL ■■	Faringogastrostomía por Mediastino anter.	5	
ESOFAGEC. LARINGECTOMIA■■	Faringogastrostomía por Mediastino anter.	7	3
TOTALES		18	4 (22%)

■ EN 43 HABIA PENETRACION A ESOFAGO-TORACICO
■■ LA RESECCION Y PLASTIA SE EFECTUARON EN UN TIEMPO

Los pacientes operados con esta técnica han sido casi todos mayores de 70 años, con lesiones avanzadas, en que las resecciones han resultado paliativas. De 12 operados con o sin laringectomía hay 3 fallecidos en el post-operatorio inmediato dando una mortalidad de 25% (1 por trombosis mesentérica, uno por necrósis de la plastía en un cirrótico y uno por atelectasis obstructiva por mal manejo del traqueostoma). Hay una sobrevida de 5 años (Tabla 3).

Tabla-2   RESECCIONES Y PLASTIAS EN CANCER
ESOFAGICO TORACICO 318 EN 928 CASOS

TIPO DE RESECCION	TIPO DE PLASTIA	Nº de CASOS	FALLECIDOS
TORACOTOMIA DERECHA			
Resección parcial	Tubos Plásticos (Berman).	4	2
Resección parcial	Anastomosis Esofágica	3	1
Esofagectomía subtotal	Esofagogastrostomía derecha (Lewis)	4	1
Esofagectomía Thorex	Esofagostoma y Gastrostoma ■ ■	22	9 }20%)
Esofagectomía Thorex	Esofagogastrostomía por Mediastino anterior (II tiempo)	71	10
TORACOTOMIA IZQUIERDA			
Esofagectomía subtotal ■	Esofagogastrostomía supra Aortica (Garlock)	105	17 (16%)
Esofagectomía subtotal ■	Esofagogastrostomía Cervical (Sweet)	2	—
Esofagectomía subtotal ■	Esofagogastrostomía subcutánea.	1	1
Esofagectomía parcial ■	Esofagogastrostomía infra Aortica.	106	10 (9%)
TOTALES		318	51 (16%)

■ CON O SIN GASTRECTOMIA PARCIAL
■ ■ NO SE PRACTICO EL II TIEMPO

Esófago retro-aórtico. En la Tabla 2 se aprecian los diversos procedimientos empleados, todos han sido operados por toracotomía derecha, que permite una amplia disección del mediastino posterior. Desde hace 16 años practicamos la operación en dos tiempos, primero la exéresis con esofagostoma cervical y gastrostoma, en un segundo tiempo la plastía con estómago ascendido por el mediastino anterior.
En 22 pacientes de esta serie sólo se efectuó el primer tiempo, 9 fallecieron en el post-operatorio y 13 fueron rechazados para una plastía por diversas causas, fundamentalmente por malas condiciones

generales. En 71 se efectuó el segundo tiempo con 10 fallecidos en el post-operatorio. La mortalidad operatoria de esta técnica fue de 20%. De los 61 pacientes que sobreviven a la plastía hay 11 con sobrevidas mayores de cinco años (de 12 a 5 años). Tabla (3).

Tabla-3   SOBREVIDA A CINCO AÑOS DESPUES
          DE RESECCION EN CARCINOMA DE ESOFAGO

LESION	UICC	ATENDIDOS	RESECADOS	SOBREVIDA	PORCENTAJE
CERVICAL		84	18	1	
Resección Curativa					
Ganglios (-)	$T_2 N -$		4	1	10%
Ganglios (+)	$T_2 N +$		6		
Resección Paliativa			8		
RETRO Y SUPRA AORTICO		367	104	11	
Resección Curativa					
Ganglios (-)	$T_2 N -$		29	9	20%
Ganglios (+)	$T_2 N +$		24	2	
Resección Paliativa			51		
HILIAR		334	108	16	
Resección Curativa					
Ganglios (-)	$T_2 N -$		37	11	24%
Ganglios (+)	$T_2 N +$		30	5	
Resección Paliativa			41		
TERCIO INFERIOR		227	106	12	
Resección Curativa					
Ganglios (-)	$T_2 N -$		21	7	26%
Ganglios (+)	$T_2 N +$		25	5	
Resección Paliativa			60		
TOTALES		1012	336	40 del Total	12% 4%

Esófago hiliar. Empleamos el procedimiento de Garlock (Tabla 2) por vía izquierda en un tiempo con anastomosis supra-aórtica. De 105 pacientes fallecen 17 en el post-operatorio inmediato (16%) el 50% por dehiscencia de sutura de la anastomosis. De los 88 pacientes que sobreviven hay 16 sobrevidas a 5 años (de 25 a 5 años) (Tabla 3).

Esófago tercio inferior. Tabla 2. Se operan por toracotomía izquierda, generalmente con anastomosis infra-aórtica, en especial las exéresis que de partida se catalogan como paliativas. Habitualmente se asocia una gastrectomía proximal con disección de tronco celíaco.
La mortalidad operatoria es menor, 9% y la gran causa es la dehiscencia de sutura especialmente en pacientes con lesiones avanzadas. Hay 12 sobrevidas mayores de 5 años (Tabla 3) la gran mayoría de los pacientes aún con exéresis paliativas sobreviven de 1 a 3 años, ello justifica esta conducta ya que los no operados sobreviven promedio tres meses.

Desde hace 10 años, cada vez que nos ha sido posible practicamos en el pre-operatorio inmediato cobalto terapia masiva de 2000 r de acuerdo con el procedimiento de Nakayama (1961). Sin haber aumentado la morbi-mortalidad operatoria, aunque no hemos tabulado los resultados, creemos nos ofrece mayores curaciones en lesiones localizadas.
Como principio general, en cualquier tipo de resección, cada vez que ha sido posible hemos practicado una piloroplastía extra mucosa simple o doble.

En el post-operatorio, desde que iniciamos la cirugía del esófago, hemos sido partidarios de la
alimentación tardía al cuarto o quinto día. La sonda nasogástrica se emplea según tolerancia del
enfermo y los antibióticos de amplio espectro en todos los casos.
La gran causa de muerte ha sido la dehiscencia de sutura de la anastomósis; no reoperamos los enfermos, sino que esperamos el cierre tardío, previo asegurarnos un buen drenaje pleural o cervical. Si no ha habido un desprendimiento total o rotación de los segmentos afrontados y consegui-
mos una buena expansión pulmonar, curan un gran porcentaje de casos con o sin estenosis tardía.
En lo que se refiere a anatomía patológica, de acuerdo con la clasificación de la Unión Internacional contra el Cáncer (UICC) todos los casos con sobrevida a 5 años han correspondido a T2 y a
NX o NX + en que la positividad de los ganglios corresponde a periesofágicos y excepcionalmente a
celíacos.

Cirugía Paliativa sin Exéresis

La Tabla IV señala todos los procedimientos empleados. Gran valor le damos al recurso de practicar en casos inextirpables y sometidos a una toracotomía, la colocación de un tubo de Souttar
grueso por esofagotomía simple y dilatación tumoral. La esofagotomía la hacemos doble, según procedimiento original (Lira, 1967), para casos de localización muy alta dentro del tórax, en que la
dilatación debe efectuarse por la esofagotomía inferior (Figura 2). No hubo mayor mortalidad o
morbilidad que en la toracotomía exploradora (dos fallecidos en 51 casos). Preferimos el tubo de
acero inoxidable tipo Souttar grueso; el de plástico hasta ahora diseñado, fácilmente se desliza
según nuestra experiencia.

Tabla - 4   EXPLORACIONES Y PROCEDIMIENTOS PALIATIVOS
EN 1.012 PACIENTES CON CÁNCER ESOFÁGICO

EXPLORACIONES Y PROCEDIMIENTOS	Nº DE CASOS
LAPAROTOMÍAS EXPLORADORAS	2 0
GASTROSTOMÍAS	1 8 2
YEYUNOSTOMÍAS	7
TORACOTOMÍAS EXPLORADORAS	7 6
TORACOTOMÍAS EXPLORADORAS CON GASTROSTOMÍAS	9 4
ANASTOMOSIS SUPRATUMORALES	
CON ESTÓMAGO (INTRA-TORÁCICA)	3
CON YEYUNO (INTRA-TORÁCICA)	3
CON COLON (CERVICAL)	1
PROCEDIMIENTOS DE INTUBACIÓN	
ENDOSCÓPICAS.......................................	6
QUIRÚRGICAS (EN TORACOTOMÍAS).....................	5 1
MIXTAS (CON GASTROSTOMÍA).........................	4
DILATACIONES DIRECTAS	3 6
FARINGOTOMÍA Y ESOFAGOSTOMÍA CERVICAL	4
T O T A L E S	4 8 7

Desde 1961 en casos no resecables, en que se ha efectuado una toracotomía izquierda, realizamos
una gastrostomía transdiafragmática (Lira, 1978); para ello se incinde el diafragma, se efectúa
la gastrostomía alta, exteriorizándola por contra-abertura transrectal izquierda. La técnica es

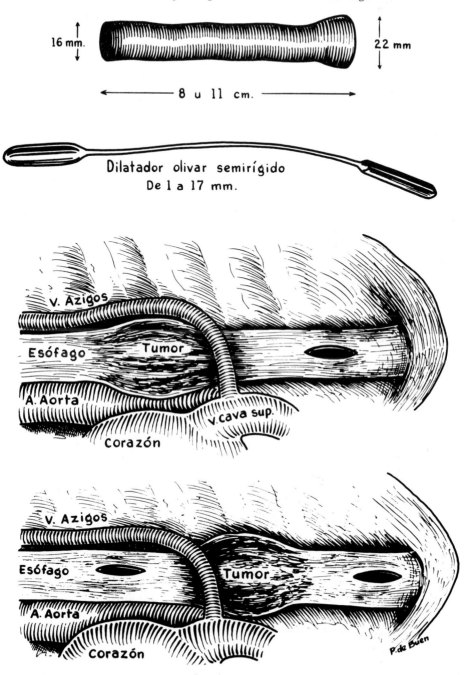

Fig. 2. Tubo de Souttar operatorio. En las lesiones muy altas la dilatación se hace de abajo hacia arriba, para ello debe practicarse una esofagotomía doble.

simple, empleando 5 minutos y por consiguiente acortando la anestesia al no usar el sistema clási-
co, en que una vez cerrado el torax se coloca el paciente en decúbito dorsal y prepara nuevamente
el campo operatorio y el equipo quirúrgico. El procedimiento lo hemos efectuado en 42 casos sin
mayor morbilidad o mortalidad atribuible a el.
En los casos en que la toracotomía no está indicada, practicamos dilataciones directas periódicas
y últimamente faringostomías o esofagostomías cervicales tratando de evitar la gastrostomía.

DISCUSION DE LOS RESULTADOS

Para los efectos del tratamiento, en el Servicio agotamos los procedimientos clínicos y de exploración en las localizaciones altas en busca de una generalización del proceso; ello debido a que
no justificamos la exéresis paliativas en lesiones por encima del hilio pulmonar. La traqueobroncoscopía ha tenido gran rendimiento y en la actualidad la consideramos imprescindible en localizaciones altas. Nos extraña las pocas publicaciones al respecto en la literatura mundial.
Sobre biopsia pre-escalénica no podemos ser tan categóricos, sólo señalamos que frente a ganglios
palpables y sin otro signo de generalización debe practicarse siempre, dado que en más de un 50%
los ganglios son benignos. Cuando no hay ganglios palpables su rendimiento es bajo y parece no
justificar su realización sistemática como en el cáncer bronquial. Faltan mayores series y nos
extraña a su vez que en la literatura los casos analizados sean de series muy reducidas que no per-
miten sacar conclusiones.
Sobre tratamiento, deseamos discutir sólo nuestro criterio actual frente a las diversas localizaciones.
El cáncer de esófago cervical es el único que puede curar con radioterapia; en nuestra experiencia
hay dos casos curados, pero con obliteración de esófago y que ha obligado en uno a una plastía con
colon y en otro a una gastrostomía definitiva ya que el paciente ha rechazado la plastía. Preferimos la esofagectomía total con o sin laringectomía, según el procedimiento preconizado por nosotros, que es bien tolerado ya que se hace sin abrir la cavidad toráxica.
En las localizaciones retro y supra aórtica el abordaje lo hacemos por la derecha efectuando un
Thorex. En un segundo tiempo efectuamos la plastía con estómago por mediastino anterior; nuestra
mortalidad operatoria de un 20%, cifra muy inferior a las series publicadas con plastías intra-
toráxicas o cervicales por mediastino posterior. El procedimiento se puede efectuar en un tiempo
en pacientes más jóvenes y en buenas condiciones generales.
En las localizaciones hiliares usamos la técnica de Garlock, exéresis y esófago gastrostomía intra
toráxica supra aórtica por vía izquierda, con la ventaja de su realización en un tiempo.
En las localizaciones de tercio inferior de esófago, usamos la esófago-gastrostomía supra o infra-
aórtica generalmente con resección del estómago proximal, en un tiempo por vía izquierda.
La piloroplastía la practicamos cada vez que hay campo operatorio, con la idea de evitar la dilatación gástrica por vagectomía de necesidad; el no realizarla y la alimentación precoz las creemos las principales responsables de las dehiscencias de sutura de las anastomósis.
Para reconstruir el esófago, siempre hemos usado el estómago, creemos que es el procedimiento más
simple, breve y de menor morbilidad.
Los resultados post-operatorios ya fueron analizados al revisar la casuística; somos categóricos
en señalar que los casos curados corresponden a tumores pequeños, o en todo caso en que la lesión
está limitada a la pared del órgano; cuando ya hay ganglios para esofágicos o de la segunda barre-
ra las curaciones son de excepción.
Del total de nuestra serie sobreviven 5 años 40 pacientes que corresponde al 4%. Considerando sólo las exéresis corresponden al 12% y considerando las resecciones curativas aplicables a 176 casos al 22% (grados T2 NX- y T2 NX + de la clasificación de la UICC).
Concluimos señalando, que dominada la técnica quirúrgica, nuestros esfuerzos deben orientarse a un
diagnóstico de tipo precoz. Estamos convencidos que si se diagnostica la lesión en una etapa aná-
tomo patológica en que no haya invasión de la capa muscular del órgano el tratamiento de exéresis
va seguido de curación en casi todos los casos.

RESUMEN

Se presentan 1012 pacientes con carcinoma del cuerpo del esófago atendidos en 25 años por el autor.

Se hacen consideraciones desde el punto de vista de seleccionar los casos que justifiquen una exé-resis paliativa o radical. Papel principal lo juega la endoscopía traqueobronquial, efectuada desde hace 17 años sistemáticamente por el autor en las localizaciones superiores y medias. En el 63% de los casos en que se practicó el examen hubo algún compromiso traqueobronquial. La biopsia pre-escalénica permite concluir que frente a ganglios palpables, más del 50% son de etiología be-nigna, lo que obliga a practicar siempre la biopsia, antes de considerar generalizado el proceso por ese simple hallazgo; cuando no hay ganglios palpables su rendimiento es bajo y parece no jus-tificar su realización sistemática como en el cáncer bronquial.

En lo que se refiere a tratamiento, las localizaciones bajas justifican las exéresis paliativas; son de baja mortalidad 9% y se obtiene una sobrevida de 1 a 3 años. En las localizaciones altas no se justifica, por su mayor morbilidad, mortalidad (19%), y corta sobrevida por propagación traqueobronquial.

Se analizan 336 exéresis practicadas en las diversas localizaciones y 487 procedimientos explora-torios o tratamientos paliativos sin exéresis. Los pocos casos curados y los diversos recursos paliativos aplicados en la mayoría de los enfermos, justifican plenamente la cirugía empleada y una cierta especialización en la atención de pacientes con tan grave afección.

Las 40 sobrevidas a 5 años (1 cervical, 11 retro-aórticas, 16 hiliares y 12 tercio inferior) co-rresponden a 176 resecciones catalogadas como curativas, grados T2 NX- o T2 NX + de la clasifica-ción de la UICC, es decir al 22%. Considerando todas las resecciones al 12% y todos los casos a-tendidos al 4%.

BIBLIOGRAFIA

Lira, E., D. Podestá, y A. Alcazar. (1957). Aporte de la Traqueobroncoscopía en Cáncer al Esófa-go. IV Congreso Latinoamericano de Cáncer. Buenos Aires, Argentina.

Lira, E., (1962). Cáncer del Esófago Cervical. Nuevo procedimiento de exéresis y de reconstruc-ción. Archiv. Soc. Cirujanos de Chile, 14:387

Lira, E., E. Valenzuela, G. Duran, y J. Safian. (1963). Biopsias pre-escalénicas en cáncer de esófago y cardias. Estudio de 100 casos. II Congreso internacional de cáncer del Pacífico Sur y IV Congreso chileno de cáncer. Santiago, Chile. Actualidades en cancerología, pág. 416,

Lira, E., y J. Huenchullan. (1967). Tubo de Souttar operatorio como tratamiento paliativo del cáncer esofágico. IV Congreso latinoamericano de cáncer. Buenos Aires, Argentina.

Lira, E., (1978). Gastrostomía transdiafragmática, un nuevo recurso quirúrgico. Rev. chilena de Cirugía (en prensa).

Lira, E., E. Rivas, and A. Aguayo. (1978). Tracheo-Bronchoscopy in esophageal cancer. Follow up study on 330 cases. XII International cancer congress. Buenos Aires, Argentina. Workshops Vol 2, pag. 218.

Lois, J. (1953) Clasificación de J.H. Resano para el cáncer del esófago toráxico. Arch. Soc. Cirujanos de Chile. 5: 511.

Nakayama, K. (1961). Carcinoma esofágico y del cardias. Experiencia de 3.000 casos. J. Intern. Coll. Surg. 35:143.

Resano, J. H. (1951). Traitement Chirurgical du cancer du segmunt juxta - hilaire de l'oesophage Presse med. 59:1200.

Radiotherapy in the Treatment of Carcinoma of the Esophagus

A. Bosch and Z. Frias

*Division of Radiation Oncology of the Department of Human Oncology,
Univ. of Wisconsin Center for Health Sciences, 1300 University Avenue,
Madison, Wisconsin 53706, U.S.A.*

ABSTRACT

Carcinoma of the esophagus constitutes 1% of the 700,000 new cancer cases seen
yearly in the United States; less than 5% survive to five years. Despite the marked improvement of surgical techniques, the results of this treatment modality remain poor. Most centers still consider radiotherapy for carcinoma of the esophagus a palliative modality of treatment and only the very advanced, incurable cases
are referred for irradiation, frequently after exploratory surgery has been performed and the tumor found unresectable due to metastatic disease or to invasion of
surrounding organs.

Further improvement in treatment results should come from a better understanding of
the etiological and environmental factors, prevention and early diagnosis. Better
preoperative evaluation and selection of cases for radical surgery will reduce the
operative morbidity and mortality. Preoperative irradiation of all cases, or at
least of borderline operable cases, may improve surgical results by preventing local recurrence and dissemination at the time of surgery. Radiotherapy results will
improve with treatment of patients in earlier stages, better tumor localization,
and use of megavoltage irradiation that will allow a better distribution of the
dose in the tumor. Hyperthermia, radiosensitizers and high LET particulate radiations should be considered as adjuvant to current radiation modalities.

KEYWORDS

Esophagus, Cancer of esophagus, Radiotherapy, Treatment cancer esophagus.

INTRODUCTION

Carcinoma of the esophagus is not frequent in the United States. Around 7000 new
cases are seen annually and they represent 1% of the 700,000 cancer cases diagnosed
annually. The problem of cancer of the esophagus is thus of a lesser magnitude
than in countries such as Africa, China, India, Puerto Rico, Brazil, Japan (Waterhouse and co-workers, 1976), Iran, France, and others.

Cancer of the esophagus is generally diagnosed in advanced stages of the disease,
and treatment results still remain poor, in spite of advances in surgical techniques
and of the use of megavoltage units in radiotherapy. The results obtained in various cancer centers where a large number of cases of esophageal cancer are treated is

369

shown in Table 1. In the majority of institutions, more than half of the patients receive no treatment or only palliative treatment for relief of symptoms; the 5-year survival for these patients is zero. Selected cases are treated radically and with curative intent with either surgery, radiotherapy, or a combination of both modalities, but the results obtained are poor. Usually less than 5% survive to 5 years, the overall 5-year survival considering all cases seen in one institution being under 3%.

TABLE 1   Total Experience with Cancer of the Esophagus

Author	Time Period	Entire Series	Treatment Modality			
			None or Palliative	Surgery	Radiation	Combined Rad & Surg
Cliffton (1968)	1926-65	1786 (1.4)	403 (0)	345 (3.0)	912 (1.0)	126 (6.0)
Pearson (1966)	1931-64	1640 (5.4)	882 (0.4)	443 (9.9)	315 (12.7)	-
Petrov (1967)	1945-65	1344 -	-	249 (2.8)	-	-
Nakayama (1967)	1946-65	4816 -	-	1900 (6.3)	-	64 (37.5)
PRESENT SERIES	1950-74	331 (4.2)	189 (0)	81 (12.3)	61 (6.6)	-
Leborgne (1963)	1950-59	361 (2.5)	67 (0)	0 -	294 (3.1)	-
Desai (1969)	1965-66	1120 (2.2)	884 (0)	31 (*)	205 (9.2)	-

( ) Parentheses indicate percent 5-year survival.
(*) Survival of 19% at 3 years.

Treatment modalities employed in the management of cancer in general and of esophageal cancer, in particular, are modified according to the results obtained at the various institutions. Such an evaluation of treatment modalities is only possible in cancer centers where a large number of cases are treated, and where surgeons and radiotherapists are conscious of the problem and collaborate in trying to improve the results. This evolution has not yet occurred in the majority of treatment centers. Esophageal cancer cases are usually referred to the department of surgery where the operable cases are selected and those considered inoperable because of advanced age, poor general condition, medical contraindications to surgery, cases with local or metastatic spread of the disease, plus those who are found to be unresectable at exploration are then referred for radiotherapy.

RADIOTHERAPY TECHNIQUES

The different treatment techniques used in radiotherapy are shown in Table 2. Radon seeds were used in the past, and the seeds were implanted into the tumor transthoracically at the time of exploration when an unresectable tumor was found. Seeds also were implanted endoscopically, and perforation of the esophagus during this procedure was a common complication. Bougies containing radium sources also were employed in the treatment of this type of tumor but the short distance of the radioactive source from the tumor does not permit a good distribution of the dose.

External irradiation is the treatment modality most commonly employed. Opposed fields are only used when the tumor dose is to be less than 5000 rad. A three-field distribution is the recommended technique and the one usually employed in the treatment of esophageal cancer. Multiple fields (six to eight) were used with orthovoltage units, but are less employed with megavoltage. Rotation is another technique used to deliver a homogeneous dose to the tumor while partially protecting adjacent structures.

TABLE 2   Radiotherapy in Carcinoma of the Esophagus

1.   Insertion of radon seeds
     a)   transthoracic exploration
     b)   endoscopy
2.   Bougie containing radium tubes
3.   External irradiation
     a)   opposed fields
     b)   three fields
     c)   multiple fields
     d)   rotation

Table 3 shows the results obtained with these irradiation techniques.   The 1-year
survival ranges from 11 to 44 percent in the different series and the 5-year survival is less than 10 percent, usually 3% except for Pearson's series where the
5-year survival was 22 percent.

TABLE 3   Results of Radical Radiotherapy

Author	Time Period	Radiation Source	No. Cases Treated	1-Year Surv. No. %		3-Year Surv. No. %		5-Year Surv. No. %	
Guisez (1925)	1909-24	Ra Bougie	270	30	(11)	7	(3)	3	(1)
Cliffton (1963)	1926-69	KV, MeV	912	-		-		7	(1)
Pearson (I) (1966)	1931-47	Ra Bougie, KV	154	30	(19)	-		3	(2)
Lederman (1945)	1936-40	Ra Bougie	33	1	(3)	0	(0)	-	
Ebenius (1964)	1943-49	KV Rotation	119	-		13	(11)	-	
Leborgne (1963)	1950-57	KV Rotation	294	-		-		9	(3)
PRESENT SERIES	1950-74	1-4 MeV	61	24	(39)	7	(11)	4	(7)
Wara (1976)	1950-73	60 Co, 1-4 MeV	103	23	(22)	-		1	(1)
Pierquin (1976)	1953-60	22 MeV	115	-		-		3	(3)
Frazier (1970)	1953-60	22 MeV	90	13	(11)	-		1	(1)
Lederman (1966)	1955-62	60 Co	196	37	(19)	6	(3)	-	
Pearson (II) (1966)	1956-64	4 MeV	144	63	(44)	-		32	(22)
Desai (1969)	1965-66	60 Co	205	67	(33)	-		19	(9)

The range of tumor dosage with curative intent is from 5000 rad in four weeks to
6000 or 6500 in six or six and a half weeks, the patients treated daily (Marcial
and co-workers, 1966).   Doses above 6500 rad have shown to control the local tumor
in a large number of cases, but the morbidity and mortality due to the treatment
is also considerably higher (Doggett and co-workers, 1970).   Split-course techniques also are favored by some radiotherapists (Holsti, 1969; Levitt and others,
1970), but results are similar to the other techniques.

The volume to be irradiated should be carefully determined by means of endoscopy
and esophagogram.   Tumor infiltration of the submucosa for a considerable distance
beyond its gross demonstrable margins is common, but to irradiate a large volume
in order to include 5 cm or more of the demonstrable tumor may necessitate a substantial reduction in the total tumor dose.   Pierquin and co-workers in 1966 irradiated the entire esophagus with a 22 MeV betatron; the results were disappointing.

PREOPERATIVE IRRADIATION

Preoperative irradiation is used with the purpose of preventing metastases and local recurrences as a result of its inhibiting effect on the reproductive capacity

of the cell, of controlling metastatic spread in lymph nodes, and of facilitating surgical resection by inducing tumor shrinkage and, therefore, rendering resectable cases initially considered nonresectable. Surgical resection of the primary tumoral region will reduce the incidence of local failure with irradiation alone.

Preoperative irradiation is currently used in selected cases who initially are considered as surgical candidates. The irradiation techniques are similar to the ones used for radiotherapy alone, and they generally differ in the total dose and number of fractions which are usually smaller. The preoperative treatment modalities may consist of a short course of 2000 to 3000 rad in 3 to 10 fractions delivered in 3 to 14 days, or of a longer course with doses of 5000 to 6000 rad in 20 to 30 fractions in 4 to 6 weeks. In the first case, surgery is performed within a few days after completion of the radiation course; when a more prolonged course is used, surgery is performed 4 to 6 weeks after completion of radiotherapy. The results obtained with preoperative irradiation are shown in Table 4.

TABLE 4   Preoperative Irradiation

Author	Time Period	Preop. No.	Resected No. %	1 Yr. Surv. No. %	3 Yr. Surv. No. %	5 Yr. Surv. No. %
Fraser (1978)	1950-73	18	7 (39)	-	4/7 (57)	4/7 (57)
Cliffton (1968)	1956-63	81	42 (52)	18/42 (43)	14/42 (33)	2/42 (5)
Akakura (1965)	1956-64	42	37 (88)	24/37 (65)	17/37 (46)	-
Nakayama (1967)	1957-64	191	-	38/64 (59)	20/57 (35)	3/8 (38)
Marks (1976)	1960-73	332	101 (30)	-	23/101 (23)	14/101 (14)
Parker (1976)	1962-67	138	47 (34)	-	11/47 (23)	9/47 (19)
Groves (1973)	1964-71	38	24 (63)	6/24 (25)	-	2/20 (10)

Thirty to fifty percent of the cases are found not resectable after preoperative irradiation, and of those resected, only 40 to 50% are alive at the end of one year; the 5-year survival in all of the series is based on a small and very selected number of cases and lacks statistical significance.

FAILURE OF THE VARIOUS TREATMENT MODALITIES

When dealing with carcinoma of the esophagus, rather than evaluate the results of treatment which are always poor, we should evaluate the reasons for failure of this disease. With the purpose of evaluating treatment failures we reviewed our experience at the University of Wisconsin Hospitals for a period of 25 years; we consider our experience to be similar to that of most university hospitals and large general hospitals in the United States.

During the period 1950 to 1974, three hundred thirty-one cases with the diagnosis of carcinoma of the esophagus were seen in our institution. Eighty-two percent (270 cases) were male and 18% (61 cases) were female. The median age was 65 years, the youngest patient being 36 years old, and the oldest 91. The location of the tumor was distributed as follows: 18% (61 cases) in the upper third of the esophagus, 57% (188 cases) in the middle third, and 25% (82 cases) in the lower third. Thirty-five percent of the patients had lesions measuring 5 cm or less, and the remaining 65% had lesions over 5 cm. In 95% (313 cases) the pathologic diagnosis was squamous cell carcinoma, in 4% (14 cases) adenocarcinoma, and 1% other types.

Only 30% (99 of the 331 cases) had tumor localized to the esophagus. Infiltration of the surrounding structures and/or metastases were found at the time of diagnosis in 28% (93 cases) and in 32% (108 cases) extension of the tumor to surrounding structures or metastasis to lymph nodes or organs was found at the time of surgical exploration. Spread of the tumor was determined on follow-up in 5% (15 cases), and at autopsy in 5% (16 cases).

Of the 99 cases with localized disease, 26 received palliative treatment in view of the locally advanced stage of the disease or poor general condition. Seventy-three patients were treated with curative intent, 46 of them with irradiation and 27 with surgery. The 26 patients treated with palliative intent died with evidence of persistent or recurrent disease. Forty-two of the 46 cases treated with irradiation also died with persistent or recurrent tumor and only 4 were alive at the end of 5 years. Of the 27 cases treated with surgery, 13 died within 30 days post operation, 7 died with recurrent disease, and 7 were alive 5 or more years after treatment. Three out of the 108 cases in which extension of the tumor or metastasis was found at exploration survived 5 years or more; one of the patients had a squamous cell carcinoma of the lower third infiltrating stomach, and the other two had metastases to the periesophageal lymph nodes.

Figure 1 shows the distribution of the extent of the disease and results of the 331 cases of esophageal carcinoma in our series.

LOCALIZED 99 cases (30%)			SPREAD 232 cases (70%)					
RADICAL TREATMENT 73 cases (22%)		PALLI-ATION	SPREAD AT DIAGNOSIS 93 cases (28%)		SPREAD AT EXPLORATION 108 cases (32%)		AFTER TREAT-MENT	AT AUTO-PSY
RADIOTHERAPY 46 cases	RESECTION 27 cases	26 cases (8%)	EXTENSION 41 cases (12%)	METASTASES 52 cases (16%)	EXTENSION 28 cases (8%)	METASTASES 80 cases (24%)	15 cases (5%)	16 cases (5%)
DWD 42 cases	//// DWD ////	DWD			1 case alive 5 yrs	2 cases alive 5 yrs		

5-yr Survivors:
7 Resection
4 Radiotherapy

Postoperative Deaths:
13 cases

DWD = Died With Disease

Fig. 1.   Extent of disease and results in 331 cases of esophageal carcinoma.

Surgery as well as radiotherapy are local treatment modalities and neither is effective in controlling disease in these patients who usually present with generalized disease at the time of diagnosis.

PALLIATIVE RADIOTHERAPY

Since the majority of patients with cancer of the esophagus are diagnosed at an advanced stage of the disease, and since treatment results are indeed poor, palliative treatment thus becomes important, and patients may be offered alleviation of

their symptoms, mainly dysphagia, and improvement of their general condition for
the remaining months of life.

In our series, the patients who received palliative radiotherapy with doses of 5000
rad or more had a better survival than those who received palliation with lower doses, or who had other palliative measures, or who received no treatment. Figure 2
shows the survival according to treatment modality. Figure 3 shows the survival of
the patients in our series with the different palliative treatment procedures. Patients who received palliative radiotherapy had a longer survival than those who
underwent other procedures to improve their dysphagia and nutritional intake or who
received no treatment.

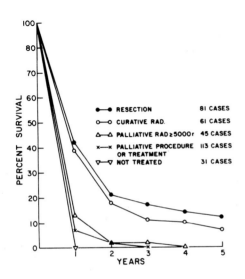

Fig. 2. Survival according to
treatment.

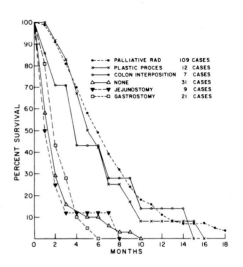

Fig. 3. Survival with palliative
treatment or no treatment.

IMPROVEMENT OF TREATMENT RESULTS

To improve the results of treatment in carcinoma of the esophagus there are some
areas which need to be further developed and are listed in Table 5.

TABLE 5 Possibilities for Improvement of Treatment Results
in Carcinoma of the Esophagus

1. Prevention
    a) Reduction in Alcohol Intake
    b) Reduction in Tobacco Consumption
    c) Better Nutrition
2. Early Diagnosis
    a) Exfoliative Cytology of Populations at Risk
    b) Radioesophagogram of Populations at Risk
3. Improvement of Treatment Modalities
    a) Surgery
        Better Selection of Cases
        Reduction of Operative Mortality
        Adjuvant Preoperative Irradiation

TABLE 5   Continued:

　　　　　　　　b)　Radiotherapy
　　　　　　　　　　Better Selection of Cases
　　　　　　　　　　High Energy Irradiation
　　　　　　　　　　High LET Particulate Radiations
　　　　　　　　　　Better Tumor Localization (CAT)
　　　　　　　　　　Preoperative Irradiation
　　　　　　　　　　Adjuvant Radiosensitizers
　　　　　　　　　　Adjuvant Hyperthermia
　　　　　　　　　　Adjuvant Systemic Treatment
　　　　　　　　　　　(if available someday)

Areas which require special attention are epidemiology, prevention, early detection and treatment modalities.

Epidemiologic studies should be undertaken in areas of high incidence such as Africa, China, India, Puerto Rico, Brazil, Japan, Iran, Northwest France and others. Prevention of carcinoma of the esophagus may be enhanced by reduction in alcohol intake and tobacco consumption, and also by improving the nutrition of populations at risk.

Early diagnosis by means of exfoliative cytology (Chinease Academy of Medical Sciences and Honan Province, 1973; Villardell, 1974) or radioesophagogram (Bosch and co-workers, 1977) may be of value in high risk populations. Also of importance is to reduce the patient and physician delay in diagnosis and treatment.

The surgical results may be improved by better selection of cases amenable to surgery, experience of the surgeons in the management of patients with carcinoma of the esophagus, reduction in the morbidity and operative mortality which is related to the experience and expertise of the surgeon and selection of the cases and possibly adjuvant preoperative radiotherapy.

The radiation results may be improved by better selection of cases for curative treatment. Use of high energy treatment units, ^{60}Co or other equipment should be utilized, and high LET particulate radiations should be investigated. Better tumor localization by means of computerized transverse tomography should be pursued as well as evaluation of optimal doses and treatment volume for preoperative irradiation and adjuvant modalities such as hyperthermia, radiosensitizers, and systemic cytotoxic therapy.

REFERENCES

Akakura, I., Y. Nakamura, T. Kakegawa, Y. Hoshino, T. Tsuzuki, H. Yamashita, S. Ikari and M. Yamada (1965). The combined treatment for carcinoma of the esophagus with radical resection and the preoperative irradiation. Keio J. Med., 14, 145-157.
Bosch, A., R. Dietrich, A. E. Lanaro and Z. Frias (1977). Modified scintigraphic technique for the dynamic study of the esophagus. Int. J. Nuclear Med. Biol., 4, 195-199.
Chinese Academy of Medical Sciences and Honan Province (1973). Early detection of carcinoma of the esophagus. Chinese Med. J., 1, 95-98.
Cliffton, E. E. and J. T. Goodner (1968). Integrated treatment of carcinoma of the esophagus. In B. E. Rush and R. H. Greenlaw (Eds.), Cancer Therapy by Integrated Radiation and Operation, Charles C. Thomas, Springfield, Illinois, pp.60-66.
Desai, P. B., E. J. Borges, V. G. Vohra and J. C. Paymaster (1969). Carcinoma of the esophagus in India. Cancer, 23, 979-989.
Doggett, R. L. S., J. M. Guernsey and M. A. Bagshaw (1970). Combined radiation and

surgical treatment of carcinoma of the thoracic esophagus. Front. Radiation
    Ther. Onc., 5, 147-154.
Ebenius, B., L. Edling, and I. Gynning (1964). Rotation roentgen therapy of eso-
    phageal cancer. In G. T. Pack and I. M. Ariel (Eds.), Treatment of Cancer and
    Allied Diseases, Vol. 4, Harper and Row, New York, pp. 600-610.
Fraser, R. W., W. M. Wara, A. N. Thomas, P. M. Mauch, N. H. Fishman, M. Galante,
    T. L. Phillips and F. Buschke (1978). Combined treatment methods for carcino-
    ma of the esophagus. Radiology, 128, 461-465.
Frazier, A. B., S. H. Levitt and L. S. DeGiorgi (1970). Effectiveness of radiation
    therapy in the treatment of carcinoma of the esophagus. Am. J. Roentgenol.,
    108, 830-834.
Groves, L. K. and A. Rodriguez-Antunez (1973). Treatment of carcinoma of the eso-
    phagus and gastric cardia with concentrated preoperative irradiation therapy
    followed by early operation. A progress report. Ann. Thor. Surg., 15, 333-345
Guisez, J. (1925). Malignant tumors of the oesophagus. J. Laryngol. Otol., 40,
    213-232.
Holsti, L. R. (1969). Clinical experience with split-course radiotherapy. A ran-
    domized clinical trial. Radiology, 92, 591-596.
Leborgne, R., F. Leborgne and L. Barlocci (1963). Cancer of the esophagus. Results
    of radiotherapy. Brit. J. Radiol., 36, 806-811.
Lederman, M. and J. Clarkson (1945). Radium treatment of cancer of the oesophagus.
    Brit. J. Radiol., 18, 22-28.
Lederman, M. (1966). Carcinoma of the oesophagus, with special reference to the
    upper third. Part I. Clinical considerations. Brit. J. Radiol., 39, 193-204.
Levitt, S. H., A. B. Frazier and K. W. James (1970). Split-course radiotherapy in
    the treatment of carcinoma of the esophagus. Radiology, 94, 433-435.
Marcial, V. A., J. M. Tome, J. Ubiñas, A. Bosch and J. N. Correa (1966). The role
    of radiation therapy in esophageal cancer. Radiology, 87, 231-239.
Marks, R. D., H. J. Scruggs and K. M. Wallace (1976). Preoperative radiation the-
    rapy for carcinoma of the esophagus. Cancer, 38, 84-89.
Nakayama, K., H. Orihata and K. Yamaguchi (1967). Surgical treatment combined with
    preoperative concentrated irradiation for esophageal cancer. Cancer, 20, 778-
    788.
Parker, E. F. and H. B. Gregorie (1976). Carcinoma of the Esophagus. JAMA, 235,
    1018-1020.
Pearson, J. G. (1966). The radiotherapy of carcinoma of the oesophagus and post-
    cricoid region in South East Scotland. Clin. Radiol., 17, 242-257.
Petrov, B. A. (1967). Resection of the thoracic esophagus for cancer. Cancer, 20,
    789-792.
Pierquin, B., A. Wambersie and M. Tubiana (1966). Cancer of the thoracic oesopha-
    gus: Two series of patients treated by 22 MeV betatron. Brit. J. Radiol., 39,
    189-192.
Villardell, F. (1974). Exfoliative cytology of the esophagus. In Handbuch der
    inneren Medizin Dritter Band/Erster Teil, Funfte Auflage: Disease of the
    Esophagus, Springer-Verlag, Berlin, Heidelberg, New York, pp. 218-234.
Wara, W. M., P. M. Mauch, A. N. Thomas and T. L. Phillips (1976). Palliation for
    carcinoma of the esophagus. Radiology, 121, 717-720.
Waterhouse, J., C. Muir, P. Correa and J. Powell (Eds.) (1976). Cancer Incidence
    in Five Continents, Vol. 3. IARC, Lyon. 584 pp.

Cancer of the Esophagus: Combined Chemotherapy and Radiation Therapy

A. Roussel

Radiation Therapy Department, Centre François Baclesse,
Route de Lion-sur-mer, 14021 Caen Cedex, France

ABSTRACT

Methotrexate was administered prior to radiation therapy in the treatment of 254 cases of esophageal cancer at the Centre François Baclesse. A first series of 144 patients received intra-muscular doses of 10 mg/day for 8 days; in a second series of 110 cases, the drug was administered sub-cutaneously in 4 daily doses at a rate of 0.05 mg/kg for 4 days. All cases received irradiation doses of 60 grays. Muco-cutaneous and liver tolerance was less satisfactory in the second series, but survival was identical for both series (33.5 % and 35.5 % at 1 year and 9 % and 7 % at 3 years respectively). These results were more satisfactory than those obtained with radiation therapy alone (26 % at 1 year and 3 % at 3 years) and close to those obtained with combined radiation therapy and surgery (41 % at 1 year and 12 % at 3 years).

Unfortunately, these results cannot be used to make valid comparisons of the actual efficacy of the different therapeutic modalities as the criteria for patient selection for the different series varied too greatly. A true evaluation of the effectiveness of radiation therapy as compared with surgery, and more particularly, of the combined modality of radiation therapy + chemotherapy, can only be obtained with randomized studies.

Keywords : Cancer, Esophagus, Chemotherapy, Radiotherapy

INTRODUCTION

The various epidemiologic studies conducted internationally in recent years have made it possible to ascertain the incidence of esophageal cancer throughout the world (Audigier, 1973; Barrellier, 1974; Tuyns, 1970a). Several regions of high incidence have been identified, and it is now known that France has the highest mortality rate due to this disease in Europe : 14 per 100.000 for the male population. In the French provinces of Normandy (where our Center is located) and Brittany, which are the most affected regions if the country, this rate rises to 40 per 100.000 (Tuyns, 1973).

Etiological studies have revealed an indiscutable link between esophageal carcinoma and alcohol and tobacco usage in France (Tuyns, 1970b, 1977); the afflicted population in Iran, on the other hand is free of alcohol consumption. Chinese studies

377

have suggested links with dietary factors in that country. Moreover, sex ratios
vary widely from country to country : in France there is a male predominance of
19/1, whereas in England the ratio is 1/1. This information leads us to believe
that we are in fact dealing with several different diseases rather than one distinct
type. Although the esophageal lesions all share a uniformly poor prognosis, we feel
that we should proceed with caution when comparing the therapeutic modalities and
results in the different countries.

The majority of the patients present with very advanced lesions - whether invasion
is local, regional or metastatic - and are already beyond a stage where local radiation therapy or surgery is sufficient to obtain cure. For this reason, various
attempts have been made over the past 15 years to combine chemotherapy with surgery
or irradiation in the hope of obtaining better results. Three chemotherapeutic
agents have been used for this purpose at the Centre François Baclesse.

Methyl-hydrazine was administered orally or intra-venously to 39 patients in increasing doses to reach 250 mg/day; improved tumoral regression with radiation therapy seemed to be obtained, but severe digestive intolerance caused us to terminate
utilization (Couedic, 1967; Robillard, 1967).

Bleomycin, widely used by Japanese authors, was administered prior to irradiation
in 3 cases only; total doses of 150-300 mg were given in injections of 15 mg every
second day. Radiation therapy was then delivered to a maximum dose of 60 grays.
One case developed pulmonary complications with cutaneous fibrosis, and the remaining 2, tumoral necrosis with fistula. Use of this treatment was immediately discontinued.

However, several cases were given post-irradiation intra-muscular injections of a
combination of 15 mg Bleomycin + 10 mg Methotrexate weekly for 10 to 12 weeks. This
treatment is easily administratered and well tolerated; however, its introduction
is still very recent and it is at present too early to evaluate the results.

Methotrexate prior to irradiation therapy. This treatment is discussed more fully
below.

MATERIAL AND RESULTS

From 1960 to 1977, 2.175 patients were treated for esophageal carcinoma at the
Centre François Baclesse. Ninety-five per cent were men. The average age of the
total population was 62,5 years, and for the male population it was 10 years less
than for the female population.

Thirty-two per cent of these patients received purely palliative treatment, if any,
due to the advanced stage of their disease or the extremely poor general state of
their health at initial examination (Roussel, 1977); more than half of them succumbed ot their disease within 3 months, none survived over 1 year.

The treatment given to the remaining 68 % varied according to the year, but three
main therapeutic modalities were used :

1.   Radiation therapy alone

2.   Combined irradiation and surgery

3.   Combined chemotherapy and radiation therapy

Overall survival rates of 32,5 % at 1 year and 5,6 % at 5 years were obtained.

A combined treatment of Methotrexate and irradiation was attempted for the first time in 1967-1968. One hundred forty four patients were treated with the following protocol :

A) Methotrexate : 10 mg intra-muscularly for 8 days

B) Free interval : 4 to 8 days

C) Telecobalt irradiation in a volume limited to the lesion, using arctherapy to a maximum dose of 55 to 70 grays.

This treatment was very well tolerated and there were no cases of major complications. Isolated leukopenia temporarily developed in 20 % of the cases, and tempo- rary pancytopenia was noted in 6 %. Mucosal reactions occurred in one-third of the cases but were well tolerated when the chronology of the protocol was followed; in a few cases, radiation and methotrexate were given simultaneously, and treatment had to be interrupted temporarily as severe esophagitis developed and aggravated the initial dysphagia.

The results obtained were encouraging (Robillard, 1970; Roussel, 1974, 1975) : sur- vival was 33,5 % at 1 year, 9 % at 3 years and 5 % at 5 years, showing a definite improvement on the results obtained in 1965-1966 for a series of 116 patients trea- ted with radiation therapy alone using the same technical and dosimetric modalities.

TABLE 1   Survival accoding to the treatment (1965 - 1968)

	No cases	1 year	2 years	3 years	5 years
1965-1966 Radiotherapy alone	116	23 %	7 %	4 %	2,5 %
1967-1968 +Methotrexate +Radiotherapy	144	33,5 %	12,5 %	9 %	5 %

The combined treatment Methotrexate and irradiation was resumed in 1972 as soon as the results of the first series became available. At this time, the drug was being administered subcutaneously in other protocols for the treatment of solid tumors, and this method was thus adopted for our second series, which included 110 patients. The treatment protocol comprised :

1. Subcutaneous injections of Methotrexate; 0,5 mg/10 kg (body weight) every 6 hours for 4 days; total : 16 injections.

2. Free interval : 8 to 12 days.

3. Radiation therapy, using two methods :

A) One-half of the cases received irradiation to the mediastinum and the supra- clavicular and celiac nodes, to a dose of 40 grays using anterior and posterior fields. A supplementary dose of 20 grays using arctherapy or four ablique fields was then given to the lesion only, which thus received a total of 60 grays.

B) The second sub-group was given a dose of 60 grays to the lesion only.

Reactions to this treatment were more marked than in the previous series : Lethal toxicity 2 %; Leucopenia 30 %; Pancytopenia 10 %; Skin and mucosae 25 % (moderate 15 %; severe 10 %). Mucocutaneous and hematologic reactions were more frequent, and there were 2 deaths due to aplasia. The most severe complications developed in patients who weighed 70 kg or more. This was due to the fact that dosage was calculated according to body weight, with the result that the heavier patients received overdoses; this would not have happened if dosage calculations had been based on body surface.

The maximum total dose was consequently limited to 52 mg, and with the aid of liver and renal check-ups we were able to avoid new cases of major complications.

The survival rates were exactly the same as those for the first series : 35,5 % at 1 year, 7 % at 3 years.

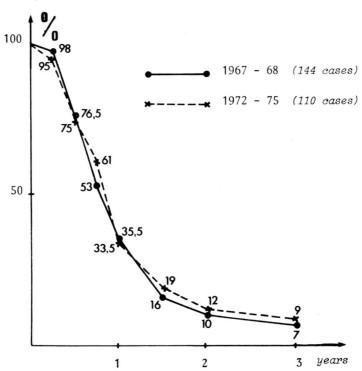

Fig. 1. Association Methotrexate radiation survival curves according to two periods.

Once again, they were more satisfactory than those obtained in the series treated with radiation therapy alone (26 % at 1 year and 3 % at 3 year) and came close to those obtained by combined radiation therapy and surgery (41 % at 1 year and 12 % at 3 years).

TABLE 2   Results according to the treatment (1972 - 1975)

	1 year	2 years	3 years
Methotrexate + Radiotherapy	35,5 %	10 %	7 %
Radiotherapy alone	26 %	7,5 %	3 %
Radiotherapy + Surgery	41 %	15,5 %	12 %

As has been stated, two different radiation therapy plans were used in this second series, one including the mediastinum and the supra-clavicular and celiac nodes, and the other limiting irradiation to the esophageal lesion. The results showed no significant difference between the two sub-groups and wide field irradiation to include all the nodal areas was discontinued. Our current protocol irradiates the uppper mediastinal and supra-clavicular nodes for high lesions and the lower mediastinal and celiac nodes for the lower lesions.

DISCUSSION

A comparison of the survival curves for the patients treated from 1972 to 1975 with Methotrexate and radiation therapy on the one hand, and combined radiation therapy and surgery on the other, shows better long-term results for the surgical series. However, the Methotrexate group has a better short-term prognosis owing, of course, to post-operative mortality.

The two curves cross exactly as the point of median survival, which in both cases falls between 9 and 10 months. The accumulated delay of the surgical cases as illustrated in the first part of the curve (area contained between the two curves) is only compensated after the second year. Thus, for the whole series, the beneficial results obtained by surgery only appear after a certain time. Moreover, this analysis does not take into account the initial patient selection for each group which is usually more advantageous for the surgical series.

The radiation therapy series, on the other hand, often included the most advanced cases. The results obtained in the series where radiation therapy alone was used are poor, but could not, in fact, have been otherwise; the selection requirements for the other two protocols makes it impossible to give a true assessment of radiation therapy efficacy, as the series that are being compared differ too greatly in composition. This is, in fact, a major drawback in many studies.

An analysis of the prognostic factors within each group is therefore significant.

TABLE 3   Prognostic factors importance according to the therapeutic protocols (%)

	(127 cases) + Radiotherapy Surgery	(110 cases) + Methotrexate Radiotherapy	(226 cases) Radiotherapy alone
Age > 70	4	25	29
Weight lost ⩾ 25 %	1	2	4
Undifferenciated carcinoma	9	16	12
Bronchus or tracheal involvement	0	5	10
Supraclavicular nodes	1	6	6
Metastasis	1	3	4
2nd carcinoma	7	14	13
Other visceral pathology	8	17	32

However, our data are incomplete, and local extension, for example, is not recorded as it can only be ascertained by open thoracic examinations, as is the case for celiac extension, and it is thus not possible to make valid comparisons between the groups.

Prognosis worsens for patients over age 70 : these patients represent 20 % of the total population, but only 4 % of the surgical series as compared to 25 % and 29 % in the other two series.

Weight loss is an extremely important factor when it exceeds one-fourth of the normal body weight, as chances of survival beyond 1 year become pratically nil.

Each prognostic factor is, of course, significant in itself, but its importance varies within each therapeutic category because of the initial patient selection.

The stricter the selection for a specific therapeutic modality, the better the results obtained by that treatment, but these are applicable to a proportionally limited number of patients. What is to be done for the remaining patients, that is to say, the majority ? One obvious answer is to increase the possibility of early diagnosis, thereby enabling physicians to initiate treatment at a less advanced stage of disease. However, given prevailing conditions, our present task must be to develop a treatment that would most immediately benefit the greatest number of patients

Esophageal lesions are known to spread early and extensively, and for this reason we feel chemotherapy to be a choice treatment modality, either in combination with surgery (although, as we have already stated, the latter has severe limits), or, preferably, in combination with radiation therapy.

In any case, a real assessment of these different modalities in the treatment of esophageal carcinomas cannot be made without randomized studies. Two studies are currently being conducted by the EORTC Digestive Tumors Cooperative Group : the first, comprising operable cases, is aimed at assessing the possible benefits of pre-operative radiation therapy; the second, comprising inoperable cases, is based on our experience in Caen and is aimed at evaluating the possible benefits of combining Methotrexate and radiation therapy.

We would like to suggest that, one the results of these two studies have been obtained, we should have the courage to initiate further trials to compare the best modality of each within a homogenous population, that is, within groups of patients that are, a priori, operable. It is our belief that this is perhaps the only way to resolve the dilemma posed by the choice of treatment modalities.

REFERENCES

Audigier, J. C. (1973). Mortalité par cancer du tube digestif en France dans 2 périodes 1961-63 et 1967-68. Thesis, Lyon.
Barrellier, M. Th. (1974). Le cancer de l'oesophage en Basse-Normandie. Essai d'étude de pathologie géographique. Thesis, Caen.
Couedic, Y. (1966). Association radio-chimiothérapique dans le cancer inopérable de l'oesophage. Thesis, Paris.
Robillard, J., and Y. Couedic (1967). Résultats comparés de 80 cas de cancers de l'oesophage traités soit par télécobalt, soit par association télécobalt-méthyl-hydrazine. J. Radiol. Electrol., 48, 867-871.
Robillard, J., and co-workers (1970). Le traitement radiothérapique des cancers de l'oesophage (à propos de 237 cas inopérables). J. Radiol. Electrol., 51, 785-789.
Roussel, A., and co-workers (1974). Résultats dans 600 cas de cancers de l'eosophage traités au Centre François Baclesse de 1964 à 1971. J. Radiol. Electrol., 55, 485-489.
Roussel, A. (1975). Bilan des cancers de l'oesophage traités au Centre François Baclesse depuis 1964. Ouest Méd., 28, 381-386.

Roussel, A. (1977). Le cancer de l'oesophage dans l'Ouest de la France : analyse rétrospective d'une population de 1400 cas. Bull. Cancer, 64, 61-66.

Tuyns, A. J.(1970a). Geographic study on esophageal cancer in Europe. IARC Internal Techn. Rep., 70/007.

Tuyns, A. J. (1970b). Cancer of the esophagus : further evidence of the relation to drinking habits in France. Int. J. Cancer, 5, 152-156.

Tuyns, A. J., and L. M. F. Massé (1973). Mortality from cancer of the esophagus in Brittany. Int. J. Epid., 2, 241-245.

Tuyns, A. J., G. Pequignot, and O. M. Jansen (1977). Le cancer de l'oesophage en Ille et Vilaine en fonction des niveaux de consommation d'alcool et de tabac. Des risques qui se multiplient. Bull. Cancer, 64, 45-60.

Le Traitment Radio-chirurgical du Cancer de l'Oesophage Thoracique — a propos de 153 Cas

J. Gary-Bobo, H. Pujol, C. Solassol and A. Gary-Bobo

Centre Régional de Lutte contre le Cancer de Montpellier, Montpellier, France

ABSTRACT

It would appear that pre-operative radiotherapy early in the treatment of oesophageal cancer has avoided in many cases (especially those in an advanced stage), the appearance of local recurrences, which cause death very rapidly during the first year in those patients having surgical treatment only. This treatment, however, which is only localized to the mediastinum, has not prevented the appearance of metastases at a later date.

It is obvious, therefore, that though we have improved local prognosis by localized and regional treatment, and the association of radiotherapy and surgery, we have not been able to act on the residual cancerous disease, and something else is needed. This "something else" must be chemotherapy, but at the present time we do not know which product, at which dose, and at which moment, this chemotherapy should be applied to be most effective.

INTRODUCTION

Le cancer de l'oesophage reste un des plus meurtriers de tous les cancers. Son pronostic est assombri, d'une part par les difficultés de diagnostic, et d'autre part par le peu d'efficacité des moyens actuels de traitement.

Nous rapportons ici une expérience pilote d'association radio-chirurgicale dans le traitement du cancer de l'oesophage thoracique effectuée au Centre de Montpellier de 1966 à 1974.

Jusqu'en 1965 le cancer de l'oesophage thoracique était un cancer à traitement chirurgical exclusif pour les cas opérables et la radiothérapie par télécobalt n'avait sa place que pour le traitement palliatif.

De 1956 à 1958, par exemple, 755 cas de cancers de l'oesophage thoracique ont été traités au Centre et dans le Service de Chirurgie thoracique du Professeur NEGRE : 131 cas seulement ont été opérés avec exérèse et reconstitution immédiate et 530 considérés comme des traitements palliatifs ont été irradiés par télécobalt. Le pourcentage de survie des malades opérés était de 15 % à 5 ans tandis que sur les malades déclarés au-delà de toute possibilité chirurgicale et irradiés la survie était de l'ordre de 4 à 5 %.

La présence d'un certain pourcentage de survie à 5 ans par radiothérapie seule nous a amené à envisager l'association radiochirurgicale pour le traitement loco-régional du cancer de l'oesophage thoracique et c'est le résultat de cette expérience que nous présentons aujourd' hui.

METHODE THERAPEUTIQUE

La méthode thérapeutique utilisée a été conçue pour raccourcir au maximum le temps du traitement et donner aux malades le maximum de confort le plus rapidement possible dans son foyer : l'ensemble thérapeutique radiothérapie et chirurgie ne dure pas plus d'un mois contrairement aux autres méthodes d'association qui s'échelonnent sur une année pratiquement. La technique utilisée a été la suivante :

1°) Irradiation par télécobalt en rotation complète de 360° pour les localisations du tiers moyen ou par 4 à 5 champs convergents fixes pour les tiers supérieurs et les tiers inférieurs. La dose administrée et contrôlée à l'axe de rotation par des pastilles de fluorure de lithium est de 40 gray tumeur en 8 séances et 9 jours (NSD 1600).

2°) Dans la semaine qui suit et plus fréquemment dans les 4 jours suivants l'irradiation : oesophagectomie par voie droite ou gauche selon la localisation avec reconstitution immédiate de la continuité.

3°) Si le temps chirurgical ne peut être complété du fait de l'extension des lésions ou de découverte de métastases, un complément d'irradiation de 20 gray tumeur en 8 jours est administré et pour certains cas, en plus, une chimiothérapie au long cours.

LES RESULTATS

La série que nous rapportons comporte 234 cas s'étendant de 1966 à 1974.
Un certain nombre de malades (81 cas) n'ont pu bénéficier du traitement complet. Le temps chirurgical a dû être réduit à une simple laparotomie ou à une thoracetomie exploratrice pour les raisons suivantes :

- Extension locale ou ganglionnaire   :   50 cas
- Métastase   :   24 cas
- Contre-indication d'ordre général   :   7 cas

La survie de ces malades est très brève puisque 3 seulement ont dépassé 2 ans, la majorité des malades décédant dans les 8 premiers mois malgré une tentative de traitement complémentaire. Il faut noter d'ailleurs que lorsqu'on associe à la radiothérapie une chimiothérapie la survie des malades, tout en restant assez courte, est nettement allongée.
En ce qui concerne les 153 malades ayant reçu un traitement complet (irradiation concentrée accélérée et chirurgie immédiate) il faut noter que l'audace de l'équipe chirurgicale, ayant augmenté avec les bons résultats obtenus, a fait augmenter automatiquement le pourcentage des décès post opératoires (19 % en moyenne : 30 cas) mais on peut affirmer qu'en aucun cas les causes de décès post opératoire n'ont pu être imputés particulièrement aux conséquences de l'irradiation et que tous relèvent de causes habituelles de décès post opératoires des cancers oesophagiens traités par chirurgie seule.
Tous les malades ayant eu au moins 5 ans de surveillance les résultats peuvent être étudiés en survie directe non corrigée selon deux localisations anatomiques pour l'oesophage thoracique (zone tiers su-

périeur, tiers moyen et jonction ; zone tiers inférieur et jonction
avec le tiers moyen) et selon la nomenclature T.N.M. : T2, T3.

Pour les cancers localisés au tiers moyen la survie directe non corrigée est :

	Pour les T2 :			
		a 1 an	:	70 %
		a 2 ans	:	34 %
		a 3 ans	:	28 %
		a 4 ans	:	20 %
		a 5 ans	:	10 %

	Pour les T3 :			
		a 1 an	:	36 %
		a 2 ans	:	28 %
		a 3 ans	:	28 %
		a 4 ans	:	14 %
		a 5 ans	:	7 %

Pour les cancers localisés au tiers inférieur la survie directe
non corrigée est :

	Pour les T2 :			
		a 1 an	:	49 %
		a 2 ans	:	33 %
		a 3 ans	:	27 %
		a 4 ans	:	20 %
		a 5 ans	:	16 %

	Pour les T3 :			
		a 1 an	:	56 %
		a 2 ans	:	33 %
		a 3 ans	:	33 %
		a 4 ans	:	22 %
		a 5 ans	:	22 %

DISCUSSION

L'examen de ces résultats permet de noter plusieurs points :

- les résultats obtenus avec les néoplasies du tiers inférieur bien
que moins nombreux sont, à partir de la 5ème année, meilleurs que
ceux des néoplasies du tiers moyen alors qu'à la 3ème année les résultats sont à peu près équivalents.

- l'extension locale de la tumeur reste un facteur important dans la
survie du malade, moins cependant pour le tiers inférieur de l'oesophage.

- un phénomène apparait très nettement c'est la disparition d'un
grand nombre de malades à partir de la 3ème année mais surtout entre
la 4ème et la 5ème année ramenant les résultats de survie à un taux
peu élevé. Nous avons voulu analyser les causes de ces échecs : il
apparait très clairement qu'un nombre important de métastases à distance (foie, cerveau, poumon) ou de reprise évolutive en dehors de
la zone irradiée sont la cause principale de décès des malades (28 %).

CONCLUSION

L'expérience d'association radio-chirurgicale du cancer de l'oesophage thoracique pratiquée au Centre de Montpellier avec une forte
dose d'irradiation concentrée pré-opératoire et une chirurgie im-

médiate a amené de grands espoirs au cours des premières années de
surveillance de malades traités, puisque le taux de survie était
autour de 30 %. Malheureusement entre la 3ème et la 5ème année une
grande partie des malades disparait.
Il semble donc que l'apport de la radiothérapie accélérée pré-opératoire a permis d'empêcher (surtout pour les stades avancés) un
bon nombre de récidives locales. Par contre ce traitement radio-
chirurgical exclusivement localisé au médiastin n'a pas empêché
l'apparition de métastases tardives à distance.
Il parait donc évident, d'après cette série, que le traitement loco-
régional par association radio-chirurgicale améliore le pronostic
local mais n'agit pas sur la maladie cancéreuse résiduelle. Il est
donc indispensable de faire quelque chose de plus qui doit être
vraisemblablement de la chimiothérapie mais, actuellement, nous ne
savons ni à quel moment, ni quel type de chimiothérapie doit être
pratiqué pour être le plus efficace.

Combination Treatment Methods in Esophageal Cancer

P. B. Desai

Tata Memorial Hospital, Bombay, India

ABSTRACT

Cancer of the esophagus is the 4th commonest malignancy encountered and about 850 patients are seen every year. Nearly 50%
have lesions which are beyond any definitive attempt at cure
(Desai, 1969).

Radiotherapy and surgery individually have failed to give satisfactory salvage beyond 10 to 15%; the author has, therefore, in
an attempt to increase patient salvage judiciously used a combination of pre-operative radiotherapy with one stage surgery and
used cytotoxic drugs as an adjunct with irradiation and surgery.

End results of over 100 patients (pre-operative radiotherapy +
one stage surgery) over a 15 year period and 50 patients (radiotherapy and chemotherapy) over a 5 year period, indicate that in
early lesions, the former combination achieves a significant salvage (36% at 5 years) and the latter has increased significant
palliation in advanced lesions at 3 years. The use of cytotoxic
drugs concomittantly or sequentially along with radiation and
surgery in selected cases is a potent source for further clinical
research. Early diagnosis and adequate treatment will give results comparable to any squamous cancer elsewhere in the body.

THE EMERGENCE OF COMBINED MODALITY.

Surgeons and Radiotherapists involved in the treatment of cancer
in general and that of the esophagus in particular were quick to
realise the poor over-all results obtained by either method. A
study of selected patients treated by cobalt 60 teletherapy and
surgery individually over the last two decades and published previously by the author (Desai, 1969) revealed very poor control
rates. Pinto (1975), reporting from the same Institution an unselected material treated by radiotherapy showed even poorer results. This experience is similar to that of other series reported in the literature (Flavell, 1963; Guinn, 1971; Gunnlaugsson,

1970; Huguier, 1970; Resano, 1963; Smithers, 1961). The main
causes of failure are the large tumour bulk, residual disease,
local recurrences in the esophagus, the mediastinum and distant
metastasis.

In an attempt to increase the cure rates the author, therefore,
combined radiotherapy as a pre-operative modality in certain selected cases of middle 1/3 esophageal cancers. There is little
doubt about the benefit that this combined modality confers on
the lesion. As shown (Fig. 1 - a.b.c.d.) cancers under the effect of radiotherapy shrinks, becomes,necrotic, becomes less vascular and facilitates the surgical procedure.

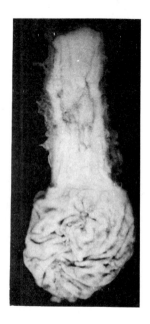

Fig. 1-a

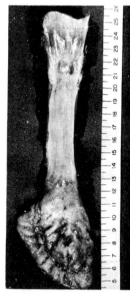

Fig. 1-b

Fig. 1-c

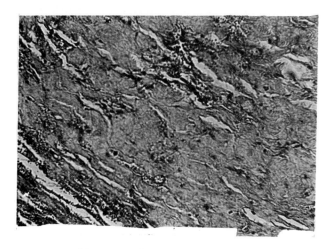

Fig. 1-d

Fig. 1-a.b.c.d. shows three operative specimens after pre-operative radiotherapy. The bulk of cancer tissue shrinks leaving behind shallow necrotic ulcerations. Histologically (d) the tumour
cells are barely viable and mostly necrotic. Surgery 3 weeks
after radiotherapy 3000 rads in 10 or 5 fractions.

This combination was utilised mainly for cancers of the middle
1/3 as the author believes that the low esophageal cancer is as
much a surgical problem as the high supra aortic esophageal cancer is a problem for the radiotherapist. Surgical attempts in
the latter region are apt to be prolonged and complicated involving total esophagectomy and a replacement procedure. The morbidity and mortality are usually unacceptable. There is hardly a
series published with gratifying results.

Patients with middle 1/3 esophageal cancers who underwent this
combination therapy between 1961 and 1973 were then analysed to
see the efficacy of this combination in comparison with those
treated by radiation and surgery alone.

It is necessary to stage the disease while computing the end result obtained by a particular method of treatment. It is quite
improper to judge the efficacy of pre-operative radiation in a
case where distant nodal metastasis are present away from the
field of radiation. Table I gives the end-results of various treat
ment modalities.

TABLE I   End Results of Treated Cases of Cancer
                of Mid Thoracic Esophagus.

Mode of Treatment	Number of cases	5-Year survival rate.
Radiotherapy alone	400	36 (9%)
Surgery alone	31	5 (16%)
Pre-operative Radiation and Surgery		
Node -ve	22	8 (36%)
Node +ve	47	3 (6%)

A few pertinent observations can be made from this study:

1.   In patients with lesions which were advanced and who had node metastasis at surgery, the combination conferred no benefit as the long term survivors were actually the lowest in this group.   It is obvious that nodal metastasis beyond the area of pre-operative radiation is a crucial factor and in all such patients, full radiotherapy and cytotoxic drug combination with nutritional support would be a better alternative.   The incidence of node metastasis is directly proportional to the size of the primary cancer and lesions more than 7 cms. are best treated with radiation and chemotherapy.

2.   Lesions which are small (T_1 or T_2) - less than 5 cms. - where lymph node involvement is unlikely are more suitable for combination (pre-operative radiotherapy + one stage surgery) therapy as shown by the results.   It is in this group of patients that the control rate is quite significant - as obtains for any squamous cancer elsewhere in the body.   The author continues to use this combination in selected patients who are younger (below 60) and have a resilient cardiovascular status; - selection of patients is imperative if one has to achieve satisfactory results.   It is more pertinent, despite criticism, to select patients especially in esophageal cancer where over-all treatment results are still very poor.

The Role of Cytotoxic drugs as an adjuvant with Radiotherapy and Surgery.

It is interesting to study the main causes of failure after radiotherapy or surgery based on actual analysis of case material.

An appropriate combination of Radiation, Surgery and Chemotherapy as indicated may increase patient salvage.

Radiotherapy Failures
(Total number treated 400)
——(Desai, 1974 (a))

Possible Increase in
Patient Salvage by
Combining

Extensive local disease
(68% of the treated group)

Chemotherapy

Local Recurrence in esophagus after
full irradiation
(22% of the treated group)

Pre-operative irradiation
and surgical excision.

Mediastinal, Supraclavicular and
coeliac axis node involvement
(50% of the treated group)

Extended field irradiation
and chemotherapy

Liver, Lungs and distant metastasis (28% of the treated group)

Chemotherapy

Surgical Failures
(Total Resections - 400)
  (Desai, 1974 (b))

Possible Increase in
Patient Salvage by
Combining

Residual Nodal Disease Mediastinum, Neck, Coeliac
(65% of the operated group)

Pre-operative irradiation
and post-operative chemo-
therapy.

Liver, Lungs and Distant metastasis (20% of the operated group)

Post-operative chemo-
therapy

Local Recurrences at the Stoma
or in the esophagus
(10% of the operated group)

Adequate surgery

It is quite obvious, therefore, that in order to increase patient salvage a judicious combination of Radiotherapy, Chemotherapy and Surgery have to be instituted.

Radiotherapy and Chemotherapy

In patients with involvement of more than 7.5 cms. of the upper
and mid esophagus a combination of radiotherapy and chemotherapy
as a definitive treatment has now been used in over 50 patients
over the last 5 years. Surgery has now been given up for such
lesions as there were few (8%) survivors for more than 18 months
as seen in the operated group. The drugs used have been Bleomycin, Methotrexate and Mitomycin - separately or in various
combinations. While chemotherapy has not yet made a significant
dent in the salvage of patients with solid-tumours - the effects in conjunction with radiotherapy appear to be significant.
Table II and Fig. 2 a.b.c.d. gives the data on patients so treated and the improvement on esophagograms.

TABLE II   Combined Radiotherapy and Chemotherapy
(Methotrexate, Mitomycin-C, Bleomycin)

for

High and Mid Esophageal Cancers > 7.5
cms. on Esophagogram

Adjunctive Drug used	Year	Total Number of Patients Treated	Survival in Years				
			1	2	3	4	5
Mitomycin-C	1973	18	12	4	2	2	2 (11%)
Mitomycin-C + Methotrexate	1974	12	5	3	1	1 (8%)	-
Mitomycin-C + Methotrexate	1975	23	9	5	4 (15%)	-	-
Bleomycin + Mitomycin-C	1976	30	14	11 (37%)	-	-	-

The number of patients treated is small and the follow up short.
Nevertheless in this group of patients, a combination of Radiotherapy and Chemotherapy ensures a better palliation and survival
rates than extensive surgery which involve replacement procedures.
Further time should elapse before a definitive statement can be
made. Unlike surgery, no patient loss due to treatment has
occurred.

There appears to be a significant advantage at 12, 18 and 36
month periods and one hopes that these results will hold for a
longer period. The over-all results have been poor due to the
advanced state of the disease to begin with. Further clinical
research with this combination in smaller lesions is, therefore,
warranted. This may further increase the salvage rates. It is
too early to report on this combination for early cases as the
number of patients treated are small and the follow up short.

It has been found difficult to adminster intensive single agent
chemotherapy or polychemotherapy in most patients with advanced
cancer of the esophagus due to the poor general and nutritional
status.

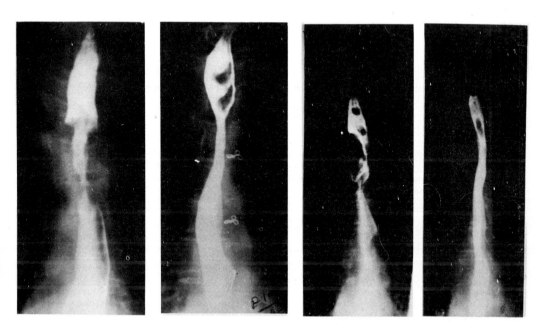

Fig.2-a   Fig.2-b   Fig.2-c   Fig.2-d

(a.b) Female age 52 with cancer mid esophagus (squamous ca.) and
bilateral supraclavicular nodes. Treated with Radiotherapy and
Mitomycin-C. Survival 8 years free of disease.

(c.d) Male age 57, supra aortic, excavating cancer treated with
cobalt 60 teletherapy and Mitomycin-C and Methotrexate. Survival 3 years alive with residual supraclavicular nodes. Extensive
surgery has little place in such cases where irradiation and
cytotoxic drugs afford good palliation.

The disadvantages and hazards of combination treatment should not
be underestimated. Chemotherapy has to be withheld in atleast
35% of patients due to marrow depression. Seventy percent of patients who complete the initial radiation and chemotherapy become
extremely weak, develop dysphagia for a while due to severe muco-
sitis and esophagitis and have to be fed parenterally for varying lengths of time. Thirty percent of patients who are in good
general health to begin with tolerate treatment well, though most
complain of weakness, retrosternal burning and loss of weight.
Sepsis, pulmonary infections, pharyngitis and esophagitis are the
usual complications particularly during the leucopenic phase and

careful supportive care with parenteral nutrition, antibiotics
and transfusions when necessary have to be instituted. No patient loss has occurred though one patient developed huge pulmonary abscess. Feeding Gastrostomy has been used in a few patients.

The usual dosage used is:

  Bleomycin, 15 mgm. I.V. twice weekly x 3 weeks   ) Along with
) Radiothe-
  Methotrexate 15 mgm. I.V. twice weekly x 3 weeks   ) rapy.
)
  Mitomycin-C 6 mgm. I.V. twice weekly x 3 weeks   )

Mitomycin-C has often been used alone upto a total dose of 60
mgms. Bleomycin and Mitomycin has been the usual combination.
Chemotherapy has been continued for a period of 12 months with
drug free intervals of 3 months in between four such cycles during the year.

Chemotherapy and Surgery

In patients where surgical excision has been satisfactory and no
node involvement has occurred, it is probably unwise to adminis-
ter chemotherapy. The presence of infiltrated nodes in the specimen and in a situation where disease has been left behind are
definite indications for post-operative chemotherapy. This is
usually commenced after 2 to 3 weeks when post surgical patients
begin to take normal diet. Twentyfour patients after esophageal
resections who fall in the latter group are undergoing chemotherapy and it is too early to make a definitive statement. seven of these have succumbed due to disease within 20 months.

CONCLUSION

A complementary attitude of different treatment disciplines is
imperative in cancer treatment and more so in a serious disease
like esophageal cancer where the survival and control rates are
poor. Just as combination of pre-operative radiotherapy and
surgery has significantly increased the survival rate in early
mid esophageal cancers, it is possible that a combination of radiotherapy and chemotherapy in advanced cases may ultimately improve patient salvage in cancers of the esophagus. Extended
field radiotherapy and chemotherapy and post surgical chemotherapy are important avenues of clinical research in late esophageal cancers and may increase over-all patient salvage.

REFERENCES

Desai, P.B., E.J. Borges, V.G. Vohra and J.C. Paymaster (1969).
       Cancer of the Esophagus in India. Cancer, vol. 23,
       No.4, pp. 979-989.

Desai, P.B.(a) (1974). A Critical Evaluation and Rationale of
       Pre-operative Radiation in the Treatment of Cancer of
       the Middle Thoracic Esophagus — An Experience based on
       100 Resections. Ind J. of Surg., vol. 36, No.8, pp.
       309-311.

Desai, P.B.(b) (1974). Lessons Learnt in Esophageal Surgery for
       Cancer — A Personal Experience of over 15 Years and 300
       Resections. Ind. J. of Surg., vol.36, No.8, pp.299-308.

Flavell, G.L. (1973). The Oesophagus. London-Butterworth, 1st
       Edition.

Guinn, G.A., H.P. Jordan and C.V. Stewart (1971). Appraisal of
       Therapy of Cancer of the Esophagus. Amer. J. of Surg.
       Vol. 122, pp. 703-705.

Gunnlaugsson, G.H., R.W. Adam, R.Charles and F. Henry Ellis Jr.
       (1970). Analysis of 1657 Patients with Carcinoma of
       Esophagus and Cardia. S.G.O., Vol.130, No.6. pp.997-
       1005.

Huguier, M., F. Gordin, J.N. Maillard and J.L. Lortat-Jacob
       (1970). Results of 117 Esophageal Replacements. S.G.O.
       vol. 130 . No.6. pp. 1054-1058.

Pinto, J.M., R.L. Bhalavat and P. Gangadharan (1975). Radiothe-
    = rapy in Cancer of the Esophagus. Ind. J. of Surg. vol.
       12. No.4.

Resano, D. (1957). in Bull. Soc. Int. Chir. quoted by Flavell
       (1963).

Smithers, D.W. (1961) in Tumours of the Esophagus. London, E & S
       Livingstone Ltd., 1st Edition.

Chairman's Summary—Panel on Oesophageal Cancer

D. J. Jussawalla

Panel discussions on oesophageal cancer were held in two sessions:

The etiology, epidemiology and early diagnosis were discussed in the first session; the therapeutic and prognostic factors were reviewed in the second session.

Dr. Calum Muir from the IARC in Lyon, discussed the time trends presented by the disease and reported that the mortality rates in Finland and Switzerland tended to show a decline with the passing years, whereas in France the mortality had shown an increasing trend of late. This changing pattern was first noticed around 1960. It was very interesting to note that in the French-speaking part of Switzerland the mortality rates appeared to show an increasing trend as opposed to the situation in other parts of the country. The M/F ratio in general was heavily tilted towards the males in most countries. The ratio, however, tended to even up in countries such as Finland and India (Bombay) where the incidence of the disease was higher, and in Iran (where a near endemic situation seemed to exist for generations) the M/F ratio was in fact reversed.

Dr. Mahboubi reported on findings from Iran. He was of the view that the disease was probably dependent in almost 90% of cases on environmental factors. Numerous and differing agents were suspect in different countries. One factor common to all communities, however, was the low socio-economic status of the victims.

Ms. Rose from South Africa reported that an unprecedented rise in oesophageal cancer incidence had been observed in a number of black races in Africa in the second half of this century. She stressed the fact that the causal relationship between carcinogens and the disease, however, yet remained equivocal. Betel-nut chewing, the use of tobacco and alcohol by urban males, pipe smoking and pipe residue contamination (having a high nitrosamine content) were found to be common habits in the high incidence areas of the Transkei region. Investigations were currently in progress to assess the interplay of carcinogens, protective factors and inherited susceptibilities in the etiology of the disease.

Dr. Lyon's paper (from Utah) presented data from the U.S. from the 2nd and 3rd National Cancer Surveys and from selected population-based registries. The one outstanding characteristic noted was the striking increase of this cancer in the black population with the male rates increasing eight-fold and the female rates five-fold between 1935 and 1974. The Mormon population of Utah, known for its abstinence from smoking and minimal usage of alcohol, did not demonstrate any rise in incidence in contrast with the rest of the State population, which presented a four-fold increase.

Dr. Hirayama from Japan presented data to show that smokers were at moderately high risk, but when this group also imbibed alcohol habitually the risk factor increased three-fold. He further reported that the risk from Braken Fern was also significant and that case control studies were currently under way to assess the part played by it in the etiology of the disease. Dr. Hirayama, however, suggested that a combination of carcinogen(s) and a localising agent was necessary for the occurrence of this disease.

Dr. Talaer's paper analysed the possible etiological factors prevalent in Western France. Studies conducted in Brittany were presented to demonstrate the role played by alcohol and tobacco in the etiology of this cancer. Each of these factors individually demonstrated a correlation between the cancer risk and the average daily exposure to the two habits. A combination of these factors apparently had a multiplicative effect. These observations led to an investigation of the role played by different alcoholic beverages in the etiology of oesophageal cancer, particularly apple cider and its distillates. The results, however, did not reveal any link between these suspect agents and the endemic high risk of oesophageal cancer in the populations of Normandy and Brittany.

Dr. Mojtabai from Iran presented a paper on the etiology of the disease and analysed the probable factors which could play a part in the extremely high incidence noted in the Caspian littoral. Tobacco, opium, tea, soil composition, iron and protein deficiency, alcohol, HLA and EBV involvement, were all examined to establish a causal relationship, but to no purpose.

Dr. Martinez from Puerto Rico presented the results of research studies undertaken during the past 20 years. He was of the view that a balanced diet was essential for maintaining a healthy oesophageal epithelium and normal physiology of the immune mechanism of the body. He correlated dietary deficiency with the low socio-economic status of the oesophageal cancer patient. The disease was, in his opinion, probably induced by a deficiency of a number of essential factors, caused by ingestion of alcohol and tobacco which depressed the immune competence of the body. The ingestio of alcohol could prevent the detoxification of carcinogens to innocuous chemicals, through damage to the liver cells. Subsequent to a change in cellular protoplasm, Dr. Martinez was of the view that the initating factors could well be:

1) thermal in nature, caused for example by drinking very hot tea, coffee and other beverages;
2) or mechanical, caused by swallowing coarse food due to mastication problems;
3) or due to action of caustics — accidental ingestion of lye, etc., in childhood;
4) or due to chemicals such as alcoholic beverages, tobacco, potent nitrosamines and micotoxins.

Any one or more of the above factors were probably responsible for the occurrence of oesophageal cancer. Different countries perhaps had different factors at work in their populations. He recommended closer collaboration between epidemiologists and other scientists, to identify all the causative factors.

Dr. Mandard's paper on early diagnosis presented the results of macroscopic studies undertaken in Caen (France) on in-situ cancer in 39 speciment removed surgically. Lugol's iodine test showed that normal oesophageal mucosa was iodine-positive whereas in-situ and invasive cancers were always iodine-negative. He recommended the use of this test for early endoscopic diagnosis of oesophageal cancer.

Dr, Byrd from the U.S. recommended that estimation of $G-T_2$ isoenzyme levels could be utilised to identify high-risk groups in a population.

Dr. Jussawalla presented his data from the Bombay Cancer Registry. He stressed the point that the carcinogenic process in oesophageal cancer still remained largely unknown and even knowledge of premalignant conditions was yet quite vague. Bombay

represented a mid-point in the world map of incidence of this cancer. In various
parts of the globe, the rates varied from 190 per 100,000 (in the south Caspian
region) to a low 1.1 per 100,000 in the New Zealand Maoris. Bombay presented age-
adjusted rates of 15 for males and 11 for females. Time-trend analyses over a
period of ten years showed that there was a slight increase of this cancer in the
male population of Bombay. He also stressed the fact that in a few high risk areas,
the M/F ratio tended to increase in favour of females and pointed out that perhaps
this was one area where epidemiological investigation could help to specifically
identify causal factors. In Bombay city the highest incidence was found in areas
where the poorer sections of the population lived.

In the second session, Dr. Abbatucci from Caen (France) stressed that the French
experience was not quite comparable with the situation reported from other countries,
because of differing etiological agents at work. Variations in the sex ratio
apparently indicated a different pattern of the disease. Because of the early
metastases only 10% of patients were able to benefit from curative surgery and
barely 20% were potentially curable, even by radiotherapy.

Dr. Lira from Chile stated that the vast majority of oesophageal cancers were epidermoid in character and stressed the fact that in this viscus cancer was found to
be curable only in the lower third. He then referred to an interesting finding from
his Institute, where bronchoscopy was routinely undertaken. This test revealed that
62% of patients had bronchial involvement, especially if the disease was present in
the upper two-thirds of the thoracic oesophagus. He pointed out, however, that only
14% of palpable cervical nodes were found to be involved by cancer, so that enlarged
nodes in this area whould not rule out surgery. He presented cases in whom adequate
surgical removal was indicated even if trans-sternal tracheostomy had to be performed.

Dr. McKeon from England gave an excellent exposition of the current status of surgical treatment of this cancer. He pointed out that submucosa spread occurred not
only by continuity but also through emboli, and that spread to different sites was
often seen. From the surgical point of view he felt that the following factors
should always be considered:

1)   accessibility of the cancer
2)   the organ of replacement to be employed following excision of the lesion, and
3)   the route utilised for bringing the replacement organ into position.

He suggested that the usual description of cancer in this area by sites (upper,
middle and lower third oesophagus) should be further sub-divided into cervical and
supra-aortic in the upper region, the upper and lower segments in the middle zone,
and supra and infra diaphragmatic areas in the lower segment. For all lesions
above the diaphragm, the right-sided Lewis-Tanner approach was ideal. He stressed
the fact that it was always possible in the vast majority of cases to bring the
stomach up even to the level of the pharynx for anastamosis, if adequate mobilisation is undertaken not only of the duodenum but also of the pancreas, from the
posterior abdominal wall. A good surgical technique should seek to satisfy three
criteria in order to ensure:

1)   a low mortality risk
2)   long survival
3)   good functional ability to swallow.

According to Dr. McKeon, surgery in this area had already reached its peak possibility and any improvement in the salvage rate could now only be brought about by
employing additional therapeutic modalities.

Radiotherapy techniques and results were presented by Dr. Bosch from the U.S.A. and
Dr. Leborgne from Uruguay. Both underlined the fact that the average life span of
these patients was barely 9/10 months and the 5-year survival rate was no more than

2.4%. This dismal situation still demanded an adequate solution everywhere
throughout the world.

Dr. Garry Bobo's paper (from France) on combination treatment employing surgery
and radiotherapy once again underlined the fact that end results of any form of
treatment currently available were far from satisfactory.

Dr. Roussel, also from France, presented the results of combination therapy employing methotrexate and radiotherapy in 254 patients. The immediate survival rate was
similar to that obtained with a combination of radiotherapy and surgery. He agreed,
however, that adequate comparison could not be made of the relative efficacy of the
two different combined modalities as the crtieria for selection varied in the two
groups.

Dr. Amiel from France commented on different chemotherapeutic combinations utilised
in the treatment of this cancer.

Dr. Desai from India presented the results of combination therapy and the surgical
technique employed at the Tata Memorial Centre in Bombay. The immediate results
were better when preoperative radiotherapy was employed.

Dr. Schieppati from Argentine analysed the various prognostic factors.

In summing up the Panel Discussions, Dr. Jussawalla commented that a number of
common themes seemed to be running through the papers presented in Session 1, which
stressed:

1)   That environmental causes were mainly responsible for the occurrence of this
     cancer but that they differed in different countries around the world;

2)   That the M/F ratio varied in areas having different risk factors — the females
     tending to be involved more frequently in the high risk areas;

3)   That a low socio-economic status was apparently responsible for an unbalanced
     diet which led to problems in maintaining a healthy epithelium. It was sugges-
     ted that perhaps this factor caused a deficiency in the riboflavin vitamin C
     and iron levels;

4)   That the etiology and pathogenesis of the disease were associated with carcin-
     ogens in the environment, in the presence of a co-carcinogen which acted as a
     selected localising agent. The incidence of the disease showed an increase
     whenever two or more carcinogens were implicated in the presence of a localising
     agent;

5)   The carcinogens implicated were:
     (a)   aflotoxins
     (b)   nitrosamines
     (c)   polycyclic hydrocarbons
     (d)   opium and its burnt residue.

It was also evident that HLA and other genetic factors apparently did not play an
important role in the etiology of this disease.

Index

The page numbers refer to the first page of the article in which the index term appears.